Guides to Clinical
Aspiration Biopsy

Infectious and Inflammatory Diseases and Other Nonneoplastic Disorders

Guides to Clinical Aspiration Biopsy

Series Editor: Tilde S. Kline, M.D.

Prostate
Tilde S. Kline, M.D.

Thyroid
Sudha R. Kini, M.D.

Retroperitoneum and Intestine
Kenneth C. Suen, M.B., B.S., F.R.C.P.(C)

Lung, Pleura and Mediastinum
Liang-Che Tao, M.D., F.C.A.P., F.R.C.P.(C)

Head and Neck
Ali H. Qizilbash, M.B., B.S., F.R.C.P.(C)
J. Edward M. Young, M.D., F.R.C.S. (C)

Liver and Pancreas
Denise Frias-Hidvegi, M.D., F.I.A.C.

Breast
Tilde S. Kline, M.D.
Irwin K. Kline, M.D.

Flow Cytometry
Philippe Vielh, M.D.

**Infectious and Inflammatory Diseases and
Other Nonneoplastic Disorders**
Jan F. Silverman, M.D.

Guides to Clinical Aspiration Biopsy

Infectious and Inflammatory Diseases and Other Nonneoplastic Disorders

Jan F. Silverman, M.D.

Professor and Director of Cytology
Department of Pathology and Laboratory Medicine
East Carolina University School of Medicine
Greenville, North Carolina

IGAKU-SHOIN   New York • Tokyo

Published and distributed by

IGAKU-SHOIN Medical Publishers, Inc.
One Madison Avenue, New York, N.Y. 10010

IGAKU-SHOIN Ltd.,
5-24-3 Hongo, Bunkyo-ku, Tokyo

Library of Congress Cataloging-in-Publication Data

Silverman, Jan F.
Fine-needle aspiration of infectious and inflammatory diseases and
  other nonneoplastic disorders / Jan F. Silverman.
    p. cm.—(Guides to clinical aspiration biopsy)
  Includes bibliographical references and index.
  1. Biopsy, Needle.   2. Communicable diseases—Cytodiagnosis.
3. Inflammation—Cytodiagnosis.   I. Title.   II. Series.
[DNLM: 1. Biopsy, Needle.   2. Communicable Diseases—diagnosis.
3. Cytodiagnosis.   4. Inflammation—diagnosis.   5. Virus Diseases—
diagnosis. WC 100 S586f]
RB43.S55 1991
616.07'58—dc20
DNLM/DLC
for Library of Congress   91-7022
                                                                          CIP

ISBN: 0-89640-207-X (New York)
ISBN: 4-260-14207-0 (Tokyo)

Printed and bound in the U.S.A.

10 9 8 7 6 5 4 3 2 1

Dedicated to: Mary, Mischell, Jeff, Laura and Dobo

Preface

While FNA biopsy has been used primarily for the diagnosis of neoplasia, it has become increasingly apparent that many nonneoplastic mass lesions are sampled. Until recently, the main emphasis in the literature and practice has been on the aspiration biopsy cytologic diagnosis of benign and malignant neoplasms. This is ironic since the technique of aspiration biopsy cytology was originally used to obtain samples for the diagnosis of infectious diseases. Recently, there has been a renewed interest in nonneoplastic aspiration biopsy because of the increasing need for rapid diagnosis of opportunistic infections in immunocompromised patients associated with the acquired immune deficiency syndrome (AIDS), organ transplantation and aggressive treatment of neoplastic diseases. It is evident that the cytopathologists and cytotechnologists not only need to be able to recognize specific infectious agents in aspirated material, but also to avoid potential false-positive diagnosis of malignancy in benign lesions and false-negative diagnosis of malignancy in those neoplasms having a prominent inflammatory component.

The majority of the cases illustrated and discussed in the different chapters were seen at Pitt County Memorial Hospital, East Carolina University School of Medicine. The chapter by Jamie Covell and Philip Feldman on identification of infectious agents consist of cases seen primarily at the University of Virginia Medical Center, while Dr. Kardos' chapter on FNA of the lymph node consists of cases seen at the Medical College of Virginia, Richmond, VA and Baptist Memorial Hospital, San Antonio, TX.

We employ both Papanicolaou and Diff-Quik stains for the smears from aspirated material. In addition, ancillary techniques, including cell block, culture, histochemistry, immunocytochemistry, and/or electron microscopy are used when indicated and sufficient material is available. We cannot overly emphasize the importance of these ancillary techniques. Close cooperation and dialogue with clinicians, radiologists, and the microbiology laboratory are imperative for making the most accurate diagnosis.

This book is an outgrowth of our personal experiences and workshops given by Drs. Feldman, Kardos and myself at the annual meetings of the American Society of Cytology and American Society of Clinical Pathologists. I was honored and delighted when Dr. Tilde Kline asked me to write a monograph on the topic following attending one of the workshops. I hope that pathologists and cytotechnologists find this work of benefit in their daily practice.

Jan F. Silverman, M.D.

Acknowledgments

First, I would like to thank the contributors of chapters to this monograph. Dr. Harry Adams gives the clinician's perspective on the value and utility of FNA biopsy of infectious disease. Drs. John Christie and Donald Callihan detail the microbiology laboratory workup of aspirated material, while Jamie Covell and Dr. Philip Feldman describe the cytomorphologic features of various types of microorganisms in FNA specimens. Dr. Thomas Kardos succinctly presents the major cytologic patterns of nonneoplastic aspiration and also discusses the cytomorphology of nonneoplastic lymph node aspiration biopsy. I also want to thank Drs. Saul Kay and Jack Frable, Medical College of Virginia, Richmond, VA for their contribution to my education. They both are lifelong mentors and role models. I very much appreciate the contribution my colleagues have made in the establishment and workings of the fine-needle aspiration biopsy service at East Carolina University School of Medicine. This monograph would not be possible without the support of Ernest Larkin, MD, Kim Park, MD, Jim Finley, MD, Keith Nance, MD, and Marsha Unverferth, M.Ed. SCT(ASCP), CMIAC, Lisa Berns, BS, CT(ASCP), Joan Brueckner, BA, CT(ASCP), Jan McCool, BS, SCT(ASCP), Angrid Emerson, BS, Regina McAnally and Dannette Christman. I appreciate Dr. Tim Benning's critical review of the manuscript and Elbert Kennard and John Artois for printing the black and white illustrations. A very special thanks to Trish Robbins for her excellent preparation of this manuscript. I also appreciate the support Dr. H. Thomas Norris, Professor and Chairman, Department of Pathology and Laboratory Medicine, East Carolina University School of Medicine, has given to the cytology division and this project. Last, and perhaps most of all, I want to thank Mary, my wife for her patience, cooperation, and understanding when I was away from home or on the third floor writing this book.

Foreword

Historically the needle aspiration biopsy has made important contributions to the diagnosis of infectious disease and benign nonneoplastic conditions. As far back as 1904 Greig and Gray described the diagnosis of sleeping sickness made from aspiration biopsy of lymph nodes. While the resurrection of aspiration biopsy in the seventies was directed principally toward diagnosing neoplasms, the importance of recognizing both specific infectious disease and reactive processes has not been lost.

Infectious disease may present with a mass lesion and is therefore frequently in the differential diagnosis of any aspirated "tumor." Human immunodeficiency virus (HIV) infection has resulted in a great increase in the numbers and types of infectious lesions. Aspiration biopsy can procure specimens not only to identify the infection in unusual sites, but also to determine the etiology by morphologic and microbiological methods. The immunocompromised patient being treated for cancer provides the same challenge for aspiration biopsy with a differential diagnosis that may include recurrent or metastatic tumor versus an opportunistic infection or iatrogenic complications.

In Guides to Clinical Aspiration Biopsy: Infectious and Inflammatory Diseases and Other Nonneoplastic Disorders, Dr. Silverman and his colleagues detail both the breadth and depth of aspiration biopsy as applied to these clinical problems. The importance of morphologic interpretation and the triage of the aspiration samples for additional microbiologic studies form the cornerstone of this monograph. It is a great pleasure to recognize friends and former faculty members whose contributions to the application of aspiration biopsy are so thoroughly and completely set forth in the pages of this monograph.

William J. Frable, M.D.
Director of Surgical and Cytopathology
Virginia Commonwealth University,
Medical College of Virginia
Richmond, Virginia

Contributors

Harry G. Adams, M.D.
Associate Professor and Section Head
  of Infectious Diseases
Department of Medicine
East Carolina University School of Medicine
Greenville, North Carolina

Donald R. Callihan, Ph.D., MT(ASCP)
Manager, Microbiology
Department of Pathology
Pitt County Memorial Hospital
Greenville, North Carolina

John D. Christie, M.D., Ph.D.
Associate Professor
Department of Pathology and Laboratory Medicine
East Carolina University School of Medicine
Greenville, North Carolina

Jamie L. Covell, B.S., CT(ASCP)
Assistant Professor of Pathology (Cytology)
University of Virginia Medical Center
Charlottesville, Virginia

Philip S. Feldman, M.D.
Professor and Director of Cytopathology
Department of Pathology
University of Virginia Medical Center
Charlottesville, Virginia

Thomas F. Kardos, M.D.
Clinical Assistant Professor
University of Texas Health Science Center
And
Director of Cytology
Department of Pathology
Baptist Memorial Hospital
San Antonio, Texas

Contents

7. Breast   139

8. Head and Neck Including Thyroid   169

9. Thoracic Lesions   201

Key to Abbreviations

ABC   Aspiration Biopsy Cytology
NAB   Needle Aspiration Biopsy
FNA   Fine Needle Aspiration

Guides to Clinical
Aspiration Biopsy

Infectious and Inflammatory Diseases and Other Nonneoplastic Disorders

1

History of Nonneoplastic Aspiration and Technique

HISTORICAL PERSPECTIVE

The earliest report of needle aspiration biopsy and description of the procedure was probably by Kun, a physiologist from Strasbourg,[1] while Greig and Gray were the first to describe aspiration biopsy for the diagnosis of infectious disease.[2] In 1904, Drs. Greig and Gray performed fine needle aspiration (FNA) biopsy of lymph nodes from 15 patients with sleeping sickness. The authors demonstrated actively motile trypanosomes in the aspirates and believed that "examination of fluid removed from lymphatic glands will prove to be a much more rapid and satisfactory method of diagnosing early cases of sleeping sickness than the examination of the blood."[2] Cohen and associates recently reviewed Greig and Gray's writings and commented that their cytologic methods and observations remain in use and are recommended in commonly used medical texts nearly 80 years after the authors first described their experience.[3] For the next 20 years lymph node aspiration was used as a valuable means of documenting the presence of filariasis, bubonic plague, and spirochetes in secondary syphilis.[4,5] In 1921 Guthrie reported FNA biopsy of lymph nodes using air-dried Romanowsky-stained smears.[5] In his series, cytologic findings of infectious and neoplastic diseases were described including cases of syphilis, tuberculosis, simple adenitis, and trypanosomiasis. The author reported using special stains for organisms including Ziehl-Neelsen stain for acid-fast bacilli along with dark field examination for spirochetes. Guthrie also reported the presence of streptococci and staphylococci in lymph node aspirates along with cytologic features of lymphoid hyperplasia including the "presence of large numbers of lymphoid cells in varying stages of maturity, plus the presence of polymorphonuclear neutrophilic leukocytes." Guthrie commented on the potential shortcomings of the procedure, including the possibility of spreading infection by needle puncture of infected glands, although this did not occur in his experience. Other early reports of FNA biopsy for diagnosis of infectious and inflammatory diseases include

Leyden's description of the first transthoracic aspiration biopsy for the diagnosis of pneumonia in 1883[4,6] and Proscher's use of lymph node aspirates for the diagnosis of spirochete infection in 1907.[4,6]

Starting in 1925, physicians from Memorial Hospital in New York began to use aspiration biopsy extensively. Classic reports by Martin and Ellis[7] and Stewart[8] describe the Memorial Hospital experience in over 2,500 aspirates. The procedure used at Memorial Hospital included using prior anesthesia and skin incisions followed by aspiration biopsy, predominantly with 18-gauge needles. Air-dried smears were prepared and stained with hematoxylin and eosin. Although the majority of their biopsies were for neoplastic conditions as would be expected at a major cancer center, benign conditions were also encountered including tuberculosis, syphilis, and actinomycosis of cervical lymph nodes.[7,8] Although a series of publications ensued from Memorial Hospital, the technique was not widely adopted in the United States at that time.[9,10] Beginning in the 1940s, a number of European physicians described their experience with aspiration biopsy. Noteworthy pioneers in the field were Paul Lopez-Cardozo, Nils Soderstrom, Sixten Franzen, Josef Zajicek, and Torsten Lowhagen among others.[11,12,13] These clinician-cytopathologists have described the cytologic features of innumerable benign and malignant entities. In the last 10 years, FNA biopsy has undergone a revival in the United States. Much of the heightened interest in aspiration cytology can be attributed to individuals such as Frable and Kline along with other investigators.[6,14] Although aspiration biopsy has been used primarily to diagnose neoplastic conditions, a number of reports have described its utilization for the diagnosis of infectious and inflammatory diseases. The renewed interest in nonneoplastic aspiration biopsy has coincided with increasing numbers of reports of usual and unusual infections in immunocompromised patients related to the AIDS epidemic, organ transplantation, and aggressive treatment of neoplastic diseases. In addition, with the wider application of FNA biopsy for the documentation of neoplastic processes, it is not surprising that more nonneoplastic lesions are encountered. The purpose of this book is to describe and summarize cytologic features of nonneoplastic aspirates and to detail the cytologic criteria used to avoid potential false-negative or false-positive diagnosis of malignancy. Rapid identification of specific infectious agents will also allow for appropriate prompt treatment and avoidance of unnecessary surgery.

PROCEDURE AND TECHNIQUE

In the FNA workup of inflammatory and infectious diseases, the following procedures and techniques are recommended. For superficial lesions, a 22-gauge, 1-inch or 1.5-inch needle is attached to a disposable 20-ml syringe fitted into a commercially available holder, allowing one-handed aspiration (Fig. 1.1). Deep masses are aspirated percutaneously with a 22-gauge biopsy needle under fluoroscopic, ultrasound, or computed tomographic (CT) guidance. The procedures employed in stereotactic biopsies of the brain are discussed in Chapter 12. For superficial lesions, at least two aspirations ("passes") are performed on almost all cases. The aspirated material is expressed onto slides and smeared with another slide, similarly to the preparation of a bone marrow aspirate. Approximately half the smears are immedi-

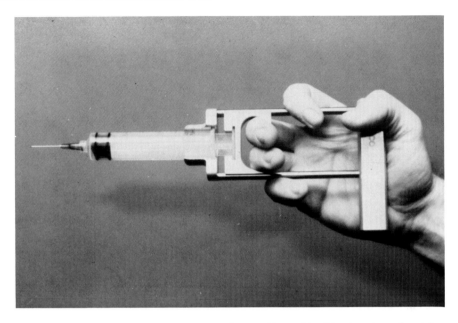

Fig. 1.1. 22-gauge, 1-inch needle is attached to a disposable 20-ml syringe fitted into a commercially available holder, allowing one-handed aspiration.

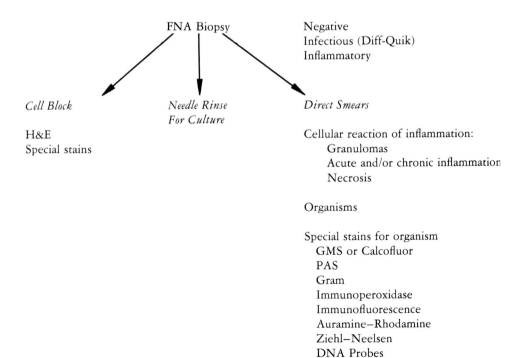

FNA Biopsy

Negative
Infectious (Diff-Quik)
Inflammatory

Cell Block

*Needle Rinse
For Culture*

Direct Smears

H&E
Special stains

Cellular reaction of inflammation:
  Granulomas
  Acute and/or chronic inflammation
  Necrosis

Organisms

Special stains for organism
  GMS or Calcofluor
  PAS
  Gram
  Immunoperoxidase
  Immunofluorescence
  Auramine–Rhodamine
  Ziehl–Neelsen
  DNA Probes

Fig. 1.2. Workup algorithm for FNA in inflammatory and infectious disease.

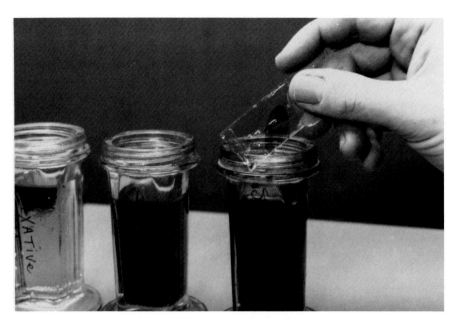

Fig. 1.3. Immediate Diff-Quik staining of selected smears from each pass can be performed within 30 seconds and thereby lends itself to a quick-read interpretation of the material. (From Silverman JF: Cytologic Diagnosis In Acquired Immunodeficiency Syndrome. In: *Pathology Of Aids And Other Manifestations Of HIV Infection,* Ed. Joshi: VV. New York, Igaku-Shoin, 1990.)

ately wet-fixed with sprayed 95% ethyl alcohol for Papanicolaou staining. The remaining smears are air-dried and stained by a modified rapid Wright stain (Diff-Quik stain, manufactured by Dade Diagnostics, Inc., Aquada, Puerto Rico; distributed by American Scientific Products). Usually two air-dried smears from each pass are chosen for rapid Diff-Quik staining. The staining can be performed within 30 seconds and thereby lends itself to a quick-read interpretation of the material[15] (Fig. 1.3). Specimens obtained by clinicians and radiologists are usually immediately brought to the laboratory, stained, and examined microscopically with a preliminary report given by telephone or by a quick trip to the radiology department where films and clinical details are reviewed. When the FNA biopsy is performed by the pathologist, immediate examination can be facilitated by having a cart containing the stains and a microscope taken to the site (Fig. 1.4).

Triage of FNA Specimens

The critical step in the workup of the FNA biopsy is the rapid examination of Diff-Quik stained smears (Fig. 1.2). The immediate interpretation can answer a number of questions:

Is the specimen adequate or representative?
Is the lesion inflammatory or neoplastic?
Is the lesion benign or malignant?
Is the malignant lesion primary to the site or metastatic?
Are additional ancillary studies needed (Table 1.1)?

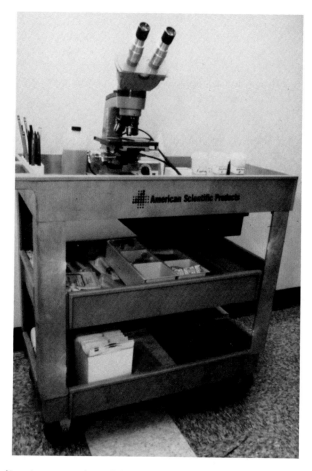

Fig. 1.4. Immediate interpretation of the aspirate is facilitated by having a cart that contains the stains and a microscope. (From Silverman JF: Cytologic Diagnosis In Acquired Immuno-deficiency Syndrome. In: *Pathology Of Aids And Other Manifestations Of HIV Infection,* Ed. Joshi: VV. New York, Igaku-Shoin, 1990.)

If the immediate evaluation of Diff-Quik stained smears is negative for malignant cells or shows cytologic findings consistent with an infectious or inflammatory condition, then needle rinses for culture are submitted (see Chapter 3). Previously prepared, sterile 2-ml tubes are used for the needle rinses. These tubes are available in the radiology department and on the cart used by the pathologist. The microbiology workup for pulmonary cases includes Gram stain, routine culture, fungus culture and smear, AFB culture and smear, and legionella culture and smear. For nonpulmonary cases, the workup includes Gram stain, anaerobic and aerobic culture, and smears and culture for fungi and AFB. If the clinical or cytologic findings suggest a viral process, then material is submitted to the virology laboratory. If specific organisms or a granulomatous process is identified in the Diff-Quik smear, then the workup can be tailored to confirm the cytologic impression. When a cell block is available, H&E and special stains for organisms are also performed on the histologic portion of the specimen. Examination of the direct smears is done to categorize the cellular reactions into those showing acute and chronic inflammation,

TABLE 1.1. Role of Immediate Interpretation

Determine adequacy of the aspirate and thereby decrease false–negative rate.
Preliminary diagnoses, similar to frozen section in surgical pathology.
Achieve a lower rate of pneumothorax in lung aspiration.
Identify cases needing additional aspirate(s) for microbiologic studies.
Identify cases needing additional aspirate(s) for electron microscopy, immunocytochemistry, flow cytometry, cytogenetics, or molecular biology studies.

granulomatous inflammation, or necrosis. A search for organisms is also performed which is facilitated by special stains. The algorithm for the workup of inflammatory and infectious diseases is presented in Figure 1.2, and a more complete discussion of the microbiology laboratory workup is presented in Chapter 3.

Use of Romanovsky Type Stains in the Immediate Interpretation of Fine-Needle Aspiration Biopsies and Their Value in Infectious and Inflammatory Cases

The fine-needle aspiration experts at the Karolinska Institute in Stockholm were the first to use Romanovsky stains on a large scale in aspiration cytology.[16] The May–Grunwald–Giemsa stain was the most popular stain used, providing good metachromasia to identify stromal fragments and parachromatin definition in benign and neoplastic cells, as well as defining the morphologic features of hematopoietic cells. Therefore, it readily lends itself to the workup of infectious and inflammatory diseases. In contrast to other stains such as metachrome B, the May–Grunwald stain does not fade after complete drying with xylene, Permount, and a coverglass. The main disadvantage of the stain is that it is inconvenient to use, since the Giemsa working solution has to be prepared fresh daily and the May–Grunwald working solution is prepared fresh once a week.

In the late 1970s a much more convenient Romanovsky type of stain called Diff-Quik became available from Harleco, a division of American Hospital Supply. Staining of air-dried smears is accomplished in three steps, taking about 20–30 seconds. The first step consists of fixation in methyl alcohol followed by staining with solution I, which utilizes L-xanthene, an eosin variant (step II). The third step is staining with solution II, a mixture of Azure A and methylene blue. The Diff-Quik stain has proved convenient and durable with retention of good staining quality of the smears.

Personal preference, habits, and historical considerations of various investigators and institutions seem for the most part to dictate which stains are used in FNA cytology. The Scandinavians, heavily influenced by their hematologic background, have in general preferred the May–Grunwald–Giemsa stain. In contrast, American cytopathologists, whose experience is mainly based on exfoliative cytology, have primarily used the Papanicolaou stain. We use the Diff-Quik stain for the immediate interpretation of FNA biopsies and both Diff-Quik and Papanicolaou stain for evaluation of the entire case. The advantages and limitations of Diff-Quik staining when compared to the Papanicolaou stain has been previously detailed[16-19] (Table 1.2). The Diff-Quik stain has some technical advantages. For example, immediate fixation is not required because staining can be performed on air-dried smears. In

TABLE 1.2. Diff-Quik Stain Versus Papanicolaou Stain

Diff-Quik	*Papanicolaou*
Air-dried smears	Immediate fixation with 95% alcohol
Less cell loss	Greater cell loss with alcohol fixation
Staining takes 20–30 sec	Rapid staining takes 5–10 min
Smears are usually examined wet without coverslipping	Smears are coverslipped
Cells are larger and architectural patterns better demonstrated	Cells are smaller owing to shrinkage secondary to alcohol fixation
Cytoplasmic granules and inclusions better seen	Granules present, but not as evident
Metachromatically stained mucin and colloid better seen in Diff-Quik stain	Mucin and colloid not visualized as well
Bacteria better demonstrated	Fungi and viruses better seen
Keratinization poorly demonstrated	Cytoplasmic keratinization is demonstrated
Nuclear and nucleolar detail not as well visualized	Nuclear features well demonstrated including features of small cell carcinoma and presence and absence of nucleoli
Hematologic disorders well demonstrated	Hematologic disorders not as well visualized, although nuclear cleavage characteristic of some lymphomas better seen with this stain

Modified from Silverman JF, Frable WJ: The use of Diff-Quik stain in the immediate interpretation of fine-needle aspiration biopsies. *Diagn Cytopathol* 6:366–369, 1990.

general, less cell loss occurs than with the Papanicolaou stain. The staining procedure is also quite simple and rapid. Cytologic advantages include large cell size because shrinkage from immediate fixation does not occur, and easier identification of cytoplasmic granularity and inclusions. Metachromatically staining materials such as mucin, colloid, and mesenchymal or stromal fragments are also better visualized in the Diff-Quik stained smears. Hematologic disorders can be better evaluated than with Papanicolaou staining since lymphoglandular bodies (cytoplasmic cell fragments), a feature of lymphoid lesions, are readily appreciated in Diff-Quik stained material. The presence of lymphoglandular bodies is also quite helpful in the FNA workup of small cell lesions. One major disadvantage of Diff-Quik staining when compared with Papanicolaou stain is that American pathologists and cytopathologists are not as familiar with interpreting Romanovsky-stained smears. In addition, keratinized squamous cells and small cell malignancies are not as well appreciated as in Papanicolaou-stained material. In our experience, Papanicolaou staining is superior in revealing nuclear and nucleolar detail, although nuclear features can also be well demonstrated in a properly done Diff-Quik stain. In infectious cases, bacteria are better appreciated in Diff-Quik stained smears owing to the tinctorial quality of the organisms and their larger size. In general, fungi and intranuclear inclusions of viruses are better identified in Papanicolaou stained material. The Diff-Quik stain identifies the intracystic trophozoites of *Pneumocystis carinii,* while the Papanicolaou stain details the honeycomb cast of the cysts.

We agree with Linsk and Franzen that the "controversy concerning which stain is preferable is irrelevant since cytopathologists use the stain that most easily allows [them] to make a correct diagnosis".[18] However, we favor using both Diff-Quik and Papanicolaou stain in FNA cytology and believe that Diff-Quik stain has special value in the evaluation of infectious and inflammatory cases.

REFERENCES

1. Kun M: A new instrument for the diagnosis of tumours. *Monthly J Med Sci* 7:853, 1847.

2. Greig EDW, Gray ACH: Note on the lymphatic glands in sleeping sickness. *Br Med J* 1:1252, 1904.

3. Cohen MB, Miller TR, Bottles K: Classics in cytology: Note on fine needle aspiration of the lymphatic glands in sleeping sickness. *Acta Cytol* 30:451–452, 1986.

4. Webb AJ: Through a glass darkly. (The development of needle aspiration biopsy). *Bristol Med Chir J* 89:59–68, 1974.

5. Guthrie CG: Gland puncture as a diagnostic measure. *Bulletin of Johns Hopkins Hospital* 32:266, 1921.

6. Frable WJ: Thin-Needle Aspiration Biopsy. Volume 14 in the Series *Major Problems in Pathology*. Philadelphia, W. B. Saunders, 1983, pp. 1–6.

7. Martin HE, Ellis EB: Biopsy by needle puncture and aspiration. *Ann Surg* 92:169–181, 1930.

8. Stewart FW: The diagnosis of tumors by aspiration biopsy. *Am J Pathol* 9:801–812, 1933.

9. Godwin JT: Cytologic diagnosis of aspiration biopsies of solid or cystic tumors. *Acta Cytol* 8:206–215, 1964.

10. Martin HE, Ellis EB: Aspiration biopsy. *Surg Gynecol Obstet* 59:578–589, 1934.

11. Franzen S, Zajicek J: Aspiration biopsy in diagnosis of palpable lesions of the breast. *Acta Radiol* 7:241–262, 1968.

12. Zajicek J: *Aspiration Biopsy Cytology*. 1: Cytology of Supradiaphragmatic Organs. New York, S. Karger, 1974.

13. Soderstrom N: *Fine Needle Aspiration Biopsy*. Stockholm, Almqvist & Wiksell, 1966.

14. Kline TS: *Handbook of Fine Needle Aspiration Biopsy Cytology*, ed 2. New York, Churchill Livingstone, 1988.

15. Silverman JF, Finley JL, O'Brien KF, et al: Diagnostic accuracy and role of immediate interpretation of fine needle aspiration biopsy specimens from various sites. *Acta Cytol* 33:791–796, 1989.

16. Silverman JF, Frable WJ: The use of Diff-Quik stain in the immediate interpretation of fine-needle aspiration biopsies. *Diagn Cytopathol* 6:366–369, 1990.

17. Koss LG, Woyke S, Olszewski W: Aspiration biopsy. Cytologic interpretation and histologic bases. New York, Igaku-Shoin, 1984:15–18.

18. Linsk JA, Franzen S: Clinical aspiration cytology. Philadelphia, JB Lippincott, 1989:1–3.

19. Oertel YC: Fine needle aspiration of the breast. Boston, Butterworths, 1987:8–10.

2

A Clinician's Perspective

Harry G. Adams

Over the past two decades there have been remarkable changes in the field of infectious diseases. New organisms such as *Legionella pneumophila* and human immunodeficiency virus (HIV) have been discovered to be the etiologies of frequently occurring diseases: legionellosis and acquired immune deficiency syndrome (AIDS), respectively. Today, more hospitalized patients are immunocompromised, making them susceptible to infection with a variety of microorganisms. The greater prevalence of the immunocompromised state is related to the prevalence of patients with AIDS, therapy with chemotherapeutic agents and corticosteroids, therapy for solid organ and bone marrow transplantation, aggressive use of surgical and other invasive procedures, extensive use of intensive care units, and the aging patient population. All of the foregoing situations set the stage for infection with gram-negative bacilli, fungi including *Cryptococcus, Aspergillus,* and Zygomycetes; mycobacteria including atypical mycobacteria; viruses including cytomegalovirus, varicella-zoster, and herpes simplex; and parasites such as *Pneumocystis* and *Toxoplasma.* Treatment is available for the majority of these infections, but since therapy is in many cases quite specific, it is becoming more important to identify the infecting microorganism so as to choose the appropriate antibiotic. Fortunately, diagnostic technology has kept pace with the development of these often difficult to diagnose problems. Radiographic imaging techniques such as fluoroscopy, ultrasound, computed tomography (CT), or magnetic resonance imaging (MRI) can be combined with fine-needle aspiration (FNA) biopsy to obtain tissue for identification of the pathologic process and infecting microorganism. This chapter describes some of the more common clinical situations in which FNA can be of value and the clinician's perspective when evaluating possible infectious lesions of the most commonly involved sites, such as lungs, lymph nodes, the central nervous system, the abdomen, or soft tissue.

PULMONARY DISORDERS

It is generally agreed that the treatment of pulmonary infections is simplified and optimized if the specific pathogen(s) can be identified. In general, the etiology of pulmonary infections can be determined by the examination of expectorated sputum with Gram stain and culture. In most cases of pneumonia, if adequate sputum cannot be obtained, antibiotic therapy can be given empirically based on the most likely pathogens. In certain situations the causative organism should be identified so that specific antibiotic therapy can be administered. It is particularly important to identify the pathogen(s) in pneumonia occurring in the immunocompromised patient or in the severe cases when the patient is not responding to antibiotic therapy. In these situations there is controversy as to whether transtracheal aspiration, bronchoscopy, transthoracic FNA, or even open lung biopsy is the preferred procedure. The following guidelines are presented for choosing the most appropriate diagnostic procedures.

The above procedures should be reserved for patients in whom less invasive methods, such as expectorated sputum examination, have failed to reveal the infecting organism.

Smears, stains, and cultures appropriate for the suspected infecting organism(s) should be planned before the procedure is performed and the specimen obtained, and the specimen should be handled very carefully and delivered to the laboratory immediately for processing.

The technical expertise for obtaining and the laboratory ability to process the specimen must be available.

When culture results are available, not only the type of organism but also the concentration is important in interpreting the significance of an isolate. A concentration of 10^5 or more organisms per ml of exudate is present in true infections. However, the number of organisms can be reduced by prior antimicrobial therapy.

Consideration must be given to the diagnostic possibilities so that the proper procedure can be selected. If tissue is thought to be required, a procedure that yields only exudate would be inappropriate.

A critical factor is assessing the significance of the specific organism(s) identified. Certain organisms, such as *Mycobacterium tuberculosis, Legionella,* and most viruses, are always regarded as pathogens. Others, such as *Streptococcus viridans,* coagulase-negative staphylococcus, and *Corynebacteria,* which colonize the oropharynx or skin, more likely represent contamination than actual infection.

Transthoracic FNA biopsy allows collection of uncontaminated specimens (except for possible cutaneous flora) directly from the pulmonary parenchyma and adjacent structures for cytologic and microbiologic studies. Transthoracic FNA guided by fluoroscopy or computed tomography can be an alternative to other invasive procedures such as bronchoscopy or open lung biopsy. In addition, FNA can be employed when inflammatory lesions or masses are inaccessible to other diagnostic procedures. These include lesions of the chest wall, pleura, mediastinum, and lung hilum.

Indications

In the past, FNA has been used most frequently for pulmonary lesions in which malignancy is suspected. In suspected pulmonary infections it has its greatest usefulness in immunocompromised patients with undiagnosed pulmonary infiltrates, in patients with severe, complex pneumonias, and in patients in whom unusual pathogens are likely. FNA can also be used in children with pneumonia since expectorated sputum is very difficult to obtain from pediatric patients.

Types of Pneumonia in Which FNA May Be Considered

Nosocomial Pneumonia

Pneumonia accounts for about 15% of hospital-acquired infections. It is the most common fatal nosocomial infection, with the mortality ranging from 20 to 50%.[2] Patients at greatest risk for hospital-acquired pneumonia include postoperative patients and patients in intensive care units. Tracheal intubation and tracheostomy are particular risk factors for pneumonia. Additional risk factors include older age, severe underlying disease, obesity, and antibiotic use. According to the National Nosocomial Infections Study, over 60% of nosocomial pneumonias are caused by gram-negative aerobic bacilli, with the 1984 survey reporting the organisms and frequencies outlined in Table 2.1.[3]

Other less common causes include anaerobes, *Legionella* sp., *Streptococcus pneumoniae, Aspergillus* sp., and respiratory viruses. Patients at risk for nosocomial pneumonia develop upper airway colonization with gram-negative bacilli, which can infect the lower respiratory tract if aspiration of oropharyngeal secretions occurs. In these patients it can be difficult to determine whether the pulmonary infiltrate is secondary to infection or some other process and frequently impossible to determine whether the bacteria recovered from respiratory secretions represent colonization of the airway or actual infection. If the patient develops a new infiltrate in association with fever, leukocytosis, oxygen desaturation, and purulent sputum production, it is assumed that pulmonary infection is present. Antibiotic therapy is given empirically to "cover" gram-negative bacilli and possibly *Staphylococcus aureus* and is adjusted for the antibiotic sensitivity of bacteria recovered from the sputum culture. If the patient's infection does not respond appropriately to what is usually

TABLE 2.1. Etiologic Agents of Hospital-Acquired Pneumonia

Etiologic Agent	Frequency, %
Pseudomonas aeruginosa	16.9
Staphylococcus aureus	12.9
Klebsiella sp.	11.6
Escherichia coli	6.4
Other Enterobacteriaceae	9.4
Serratia marcescens	5.8
Proteus sp.	4.2

TABLE 2.2. Etiology of Pulmonary Infection in the Granulocytopenic Patient

Pseudomonas aeruginosa	*Escherichia coli*
Klebsiella sp.	*Serratia*
Aeromonas	Other gram-negative bacilli
Staphylococcus aureus	*Aspergillus* sp.
Zygomycetes	

broad-spectrum antibiotic therapy, consideration should be given to an invasive procedure, such as FNA biopsy, to determine whether parenchymal infection is present and to attempt to recover the specific pathogen.

Pneumonia in Association With Granulocytopenia

Most patients who are severely granulocytopenic (absolute granulocyte count < 500/mm^3) have myelo- or lymphoproliferative disorders or solid tumors treated with chemotherapy. Because of both the underlying disease and the presence of granulocytopenia, these patients are very susceptible to infectious processes; pulmonary infections are quite common. The most common infecting organisms are outlined in Table 2.2.[4]

It can be difficult for the clinician to differentiate infectious from noninfectious etiologies of a pulmonary infiltration. Fever is almost always present, but other signs of pneumonia may be absent or subtle. Because of granulocytopenia the cough can be nonproductive or minimally productive of sputum, and infiltrate seen on the chest radiograph may be relatively unimpressive. Rapid institution of broad-spectrum antibiotic therapy selected especially to treat more resistant gram-negative bacilli is imperative, as infection in these patients may rapidly progress if appropriate therapy is delayed. It is important to obtain blood and sputum cultures before beginning antibiotic therapy, but identifying the pathogen can be problematic. If the patient's infection does not respond within 24 to 48 hours after the antibiotic therapy, the clinician may have to perform an invasive procedure in a severely ill and often thrombocytopenic patient. The type of procedure chosen (bronchoscopy with or without transbronchial biopsy, transthoracic aspiration, or open lung biopsy) is controversial, but FNA has its highest yield in the patient with localized consolidation on the chest radiograph.

Pneumonia Associated With Abnormal T-Lymphocyte Function

Conditions that impair T-lymphocyte function include, among others, Hodgkin's and non-Hodgkin's lymphoma, AIDS, organ transplantation, and high-dosage corticosteroid therapy. The most common pulmonary infections related to T-cell dysfunction are outlined in Table 2.3.[4]

It is important to realize that rarely do these patients have a single immune defect that is caused by the underlying disease, its therapy, or both. Defects in antibody production and in the quantity and function of granulocyte's will also be present.

TABLE 2.3 Etiology of Pneumonia in Patients With T-Lymphocyte Dysfunction

Typical and atypical *Mycobacteria*
Fungi (especially *Aspergillus*)
Viruses (especially cytomegalovirus)
Pneumocystis carinii
Nocardia
Legionella sp.
Parasites (*Toxoplasma gondii, Strongyloides stercoralis*)

In the setting of multiple immune defects, the list of possible causes of pneumonia needs to be expanded to include both gram-positive and gram-negative pyogenic bacteria. In these patients the etiology of the pneumonia can usually be established by bronchoscopy with bronchoalveolar lavage (BAL), but occasionally, a more invasive procedure such as FNA may be required.

Pneumonia in Patients With AIDS

The major pathogens causing pneumonia in patients with AIDS are outlined in Table 2.4.[5] Even though the list of potential pathogens is extensive, the most common causes of community-acquired pneumonia in these patients are *Pneumocystis* and pyogenic bacteria. Pneumonia due to pyogenic bacteria can usually be recognized by its acute onset and the production of purulent sputum, from which the causative organism can frequently be isolated. *Pneumocystis* pneumonia has a subacute presentation, and its most prominent symptoms are progressive dyspnea and nonproductive cough. Although others have been able to identify *Pneumocystis* in induced, expectorated sputum in up to 80% of patients, in our medical center this procedure has had a disappointing yield. Our approach is to start empiric antibiotic therapy with trimethoprim/sulfamethoxazole if *Pneumocystis* pneumonia is suspected, adding intravenous erythromycin if infection with Legionella is a possibility, and performing bronchoscopy with bronchoalveolar lavage at the earliest opportunity. Bronchoalveolar lavage has a sensitivity of about 90% for diagnosing *Pneumo-*

TABLE 2.4. Types and Frequency (%) of Pulmonary Infections in 441 Patients With AIDS*

Pneumocystis carinii	84
Cytomegalovirus	16
Mycobacterium avium-intracellulare	18
Mycobacterium tuberculosis	4
Cryptococcus	2
Other fungi	1
Legionella	4
Pyogenic bacteria	2
Miscellaneous others	1

*Since a number of patients had more than one organism identified, the total of the isolates exceeds 100%.

cystis. Rarely will FNA or thoracotomy be necessary, although biopsy may be performed in occasional patients with atypical radiologic presentations.

LYMPH NODES

Enlarged lymph nodes are generally defined as those that are >1 cm in diameter, although hard, fixed nodes of any size are considered abnormal. In normal adults, only the inguinal nodes are palpable. The etiology of lymphadenopathy is extensive[6,7]: primary or metastatic neoplasms, drug reactions, serum sickness, collagen vascular diseases, sarcoidosis, infections, and AIDS. Infections are responsible for the majority of enlarged lymph nodes in a primary care setting. This is especially true in the pediatric age group. In the subset of patients who undergo lymph node biopsy, however, neoplasms are found in a significant proportion (up to 40%).

Indications

It is not necessary to perform a lymph node biopsy in every patient with lymphadenopathy. In a number of cases, the diagnosis can be made by evaluating the extranodal manifestations of the process. In others the lymph nodes will regress during a period of observation and not require biopsy. With biopsy, histologic examination of the node leads to a specific diagnosis in 40 to 63% of cases.[8,9] In most nondiagnostic node biopsies, various forms of nonspecific reactive lymphoid hyperplasia are found.

Lymph node surgical biopsy is diagnostic only about half the time, and the procedure is invasive. In the past, most patients with lymph node enlargement have been observed for several weeks if the initial evaluation does not yield the diagnosis. Lymph node surgical biopsy has been traditionally performed in the following circumstances:

Early in the course in the patient with enlarged supraclavicular lymph nodes, since these are frequently the sites of metastatic tumor

Early in the course of a very ill patient or in the patient whose nodes have rapidly enlarged

Early in the patient with a positive tuberculin skin test reaction

Early if there are other clinical features suggestive of lymphoma, metastatic carcinoma, mycobacterial involvement of the lymph nodes

After a period of observation of no longer than 1 to 2 months in the asymptomatic or mildly symptomatic patient if the lymph nodes have not regressed or have increased in size.

We believe, however, that with FNA biopsy, most patients with significant lymphadenopathy should be biopsied as part of the initial workup, since the procedure is minimally invasive and a delay in obtaining tissue can thereby be avoided.

In a study of 414 patients from the Mayo Clinic, Freidig reported that culture and histopathologic examination of surgical lymph node biopsies revealed the diagnostic categories summarized in Table 2.5.[10] In an FNA lymph node study of 113 patients with AIDS, the following diagnoses were obtained: hyperplasia—60 (50%), non-

TABLE 2.5. Clinical Diagnoses for 414 Patients Undergoing Lymph Node Biopsies

Diagnosis	No. of Patients (%)
Infection	66 (16)
Mycobacterial	24
Mycobacterium tuberculosis	13
Mycobacterium avium-intracellulare	8
Mycobacterium kansasii	3
Fungal	23
Histoplasma capsulatum	18
Blastomyces dermatitidis	2
Other fungi	3
Staphylococcus aureus	2
Other	17
Neoplasm	113 (27)
Lymphoma	86
Carcinoma	17
Other	10
Miscellaneous	240 (57)
Lymphadenopathy of unknown etiology	113
Sarcoidosis	93
Other	34

Hodgkin's lymphoma—24 (19%), mycobacterial infection—21 (17%), Kaposi's sarcoma—12 (10%), and other noninfectious diagnoses—4.[11]

CENTRAL NERVOUS SYSTEM INFECTIONS

Parenchymal brain infection is suspected when a patient presents with fever and headache together with stupor or coma, seizures, or focal neurologic signs. Many patients have much subtler manifestations, and a parenchymal CNS process may not be initially suspected. In these patients the initial diagnostic procedure should be CT scanning of the brain with contrast enhancement. The CT scan is very sensitive for detecting and localizing destructive parenchymal disease. A characteristic appearance of a hypodense center with an outlying ring of enhancement surrounded by a hypodense area of edema can be produced by several different processes, such as brain abscess, herpes simplex encephalitis, primary or metastatic tumor, granuloma, cerebral infarction, or resolving hematoma. Frequently, biopsy is necessary to make a specific diagnosis and thereby enable effective therapy.

Specific Infections

Brain Abscess

Clinical manifestations typical of brain abscess include the combination of raised intracranial pressure, focal neurologic signs, fever and other signs of infection, and

TABLE 2.6. Microorganisms Isolated From Brain Abscesses

Organism	Isolation Frequency, %
Staphylococcus aureus	10–15
Enterobacteriaceae	23–33
Streptococcus pneumoniae	<1
Hemophilus influenzae	<1
Streptococci (*S. milleri* group)	60–70
Bacteroides sp.	20–40
Fungi	10–15
Protozoa, helminths	<1

a subacute course over 2 to 4 weeks. Unfortunately, typical findings are present in only about half the patients. Brain abscess develops in the following clinical settings: (1) secondary to a contiguous focus of infection, especially those involving the paranasal or otogenic region; (2) via hematogenous seeding from a distant focus of infection (most commonly from heart, lungs, or pleural space), (3) after trauma or a neurosurgic procedure, and (4) cryptogenically in 20% of cases. A major predisposing condition continues to be sinusitis. The most common sites for a solitary brain abscess are the frontal or temporal lobes, followed in descending order by the frontoparietal, parietal, cerebellar, and occipital lobes. The most common organisms isolated from brain abscesses are listed in Table 2.6.[12]

Staphylococcus aureus is the most common isolate from abscesses secondary to head trauma, whereas the Enterobacteriaceae are more prevalent in abscesses associated with otogenic infections. It is important to note the increasing frequency of streptococcal and anaerobic isolates from brain abscesses. In immunocompromised patients, fungi may cause brain abscess, whereas parasitic infestations such as cysticercosis are a major cause of brain lesions in developing countries.

Herpes (HSV) Encephalitis

The herpesvirus is probably the most common cause of acute sporadic encephalitis. The syndrome may develop suddenly or several days after an influenza-like prodrome. The manifestations are generally those of any acute severe encephalitis with predilection of the destructive process for the frontal and temporal lobes. The patient may manifest bizarre behavior; disorientation and memory loss; olfactory, gustatory, or auditory hallucinations; aphasia; hemiparesis; and defects in the visual fields.[13] Without therapy, signs of increased intracranial pressure dominate the clinical picture. The mortality is very high (approaching 100% in severely ill patients), and neurologic sequelae are common in survivors including those who are mildly affected. Because of the severity of the disease and the rapidity with which patients can deteriorate, high-dosage intravenous acyclovir should be begun as soon as the diagnosis of HSV encephalitis is seriously considered. Evaluation should initially include electroencephalography (EEG), CT brain scan with enhancement, and possibly magnetic resonance imaging of the brain. In the first few days of illness electroencephalography and magnetic resonance imaging may be more sensitive than the CT scan. None of these studies is specific for HSV encephalitis, and other processes such as other forms of viral encephalitis, brain abscess, granulomas, cerebrovascular accident, and brain tumor can produce similar findings. To make a correct diagnosis and administer specific therapy, CT-guided stereotactic needle biopsy of the affected area is probably indicated in most cases. In addition to morphologic studies, a portion of the specimen should also be sent for viral culture and examined for HSV antigens.

Toxoplasma Encephalitis

This form of toxoplasmosis is rare even in immunocompromised hosts but is the most common cause of intracerebral mass lesions in patients with AIDS. It is estimated that 5 to 10% of AIDS patients in the United States develop Toxoplasma encephalitis. The patient generally presents with a clinical picture consistent with multiple mass lesions. Hemiparesis, seizures, visual defects, confusion, and lethargy are common, but fever and nuchal rigidity are unusual.[14] The diagnostic procedures of choice are CT scan or magnetic resonance imaging of the brain. CT scan typically shows multiple enhancing lesions with preference for white matter and basal ganglia and with diffuse changes of cerebral edema. In non-AIDS patients, needle biopsy with demonstration of the trophozoites of Toxoplasma is essential to a definitive diagnosis. In an AIDS patient with a compatible clinical picture and radiologic findings consistent with Toxoplasma encephalitis, empiric therapy with sulfadiazine and pyrimethamine is begun and biopsy is performed only if the patient deteriorates or fails to respond clinically and radiologically to therapy in about 10 days.

INTRAABDOMINAL ABSCESS

Disease processes that may cause intraabdominal abscess include appendicitis, diverticulitis, biliary tract disease, pancreatitis, perforated peptic ulcers, inflammatory bowel disease, trauma, and abdominal surgery. Abscesses secondary to appendicitis are decreasing in frequency, while those due to diverticulitis, trauma, and surgery are increasing. The location of the abscess is related to the site of the primary process and the direction of dependent peritoneal drainage. In a large series of intraabdominal abscesses, the following locations were found: right lower quadrant in 44%, left lower quadrant in 14%, pelvis in 14%, and the perihepatic area in 20%.[15] Intraabdominal abscesses are usually polymicrobial in nature. Anaerobes (*Bacteroides fragilis,* anaerobic cocci, clostridial species) are found in 60 to 70% of cases, followed by gram-negative aerobes, staphylococci, and enterococci.

An acute clinical course is typical with chills, fever, abdominal pain, and tenderness over the involved area. An intraabdominal abscess may present atypically in the postoperative patient or when the abscess is subphrenic in location. The patient who develops an abscess after abdominal surgery may have a prolonged recovery period, whereas a subphrenic abscess may have an indolent course.

Pancreatic abscess generally occurs after an episode of acute pancreatitis[16] but may also result from a penetrating peptic ulcer, an infected pancreatic pseudocyst or as a complication of endoscopic retrograde cholangiopancreatography. In general, the bacteriology of pancreatic abscess is similar to that of intraabdominal abscesses. Several different clinical presentations are possible, including a prolonged period of acute pancreatitis or initial improvement in the initial manifestations of pancreatitis, followed in 1 to 3 weeks by acute deterioration. Symptoms include fever, abdominal pain radiating to the back, abdominal tenderness, nausea, and vomiting.

Hepatic abscess is most frequently pyogenic (caused by a combination of aerobic gram-negative bacilli and anaerobic bacteria) or amebic (caused by *Entamoeba histolytica*).[17] The sources of pyogenic liver abscess include the following: biliary tract infection, infection in sites drained by the portal vein, infection in structures contiguous to the liver; bacteremia with seeding of the liver via the hepatic artery, infections secondary to trauma to or surgery involving the liver, and cryptogenic. Amebic abscess is usually secondary to colonic infection by *E. histolytica*. Signs and symptoms include fever, right upper quadrant pain, and tender hepatomegaly. An abscess high in the dome of the liver can produce cough, pleuritic pain, and right shoulder pain. The most frequently abnormal liver enzyme test is the serum alkaline phosphatase assay. Amebic and pyogenic abscesses are difficult to differentiate, although blood cultures are positive in about 50% of patients with pyogenic abscess. Plain radiographs can demonstrate the abscess in up to half the cases, but the most sensitive and specific diagnostic methods are abdominal ultrasound and CT. Occasionally, radionuclide scans may be helpful, but false-positive results can occur. It is not unusual to require a combination of methods to make the diagnosis and localize the abscess.

Drainage of the abscess is important both for therapy and for identification and antimicrobial susceptibility testing of the infecting microorganisms. The conventional approach has been to drain the abscess surgically. Successful therapy may also be accomplished using percutaneous drainage. Requirements for percutaneous drainage include (1) an abscess that can be safely approached percutaneously, (2) unilocular abscess, (3) abscess that is not vascular, (4) availability of surgical backup for complications or failure, and (5) possibility of dependent drainage via the percutaneous catheter.

SOFT TISSUE INFECTION

In most cases, the cause of soft tissue infection can be suspected from the appearance of the affected skin and the clinical setting in which the infection occurred. Appropriate antibiotic therapy alone will cure most infections. Needle aspiration of the area of cellulitis with Gram stain and culture is a low-yield procedure that should be reserved for selected situations, such as infections in the immunocompromised patient, clinical situations in which unusual pathogens are suspected, and whenever toxicity from antimicrobial therapy is a concern. If necrotizing infection is suspected, a deep soft tissue biopsy, usually via surgical exploration, is indicated. Clues to necrotizing infection include the following: systemic toxicity more severe than would be suspected from the appearance of the skin infection; dermal gangrene; cyanosis, blistering, or bronzing of the skin; severe pain or dermal anesthesia; crepitus; progressive cellulitis despite antibiotics; and abscess with multiple sinus tracts (Table 2.7). Therapy of this form of soft tissue infection requires surgical debridement of involved tissue and appropriate antimicrobial therapy.[18]

TABLE 2.7. Clues to Necrotizing Dermal Infection

Systemic toxicity more severe than wound appearance would indicate
Dermal gangrene
Dermal cyanosis, blistering, or bronzing
Severe pain or dermal anesthesia
Skin crepitus
Progressive cellulitis despite antibiotics
Cutaneous abscess with multiple sinus tracts

CONCLUSIONS

This chapter has been a clinician's overview of the use of FNA in the diagnosis of infections and identification of the responsible pathogen(s). Concise reviews of the most common clinical situations in which FNA could be of value have been presented. The list of uses previously described is by no means complete, as FNA can be used as a diagnostic tool in a number of other suspected inflammatory and infectious problems. The technique has a very broad range of applications so long as there are available the technical expertise to obtain the specimen, the ability and coordination to process the specimen rapidly and accurately, and, probably the most important of all, an experienced pathologist/cytologist to interpret the prepared slides.

REFERENCES

1. Bartlett JG: Invasive diagnostic techniques in pulmonary infections. In: JE Pennington, ed. *Respiratory Infections: Diagnosis and Management,* 2nd ed. New York: Raven Press; 1988:69–96.

2. Pennington JE: Nosocomial respiratory infection. In: Mandell GL, Douglas RG Jr, Bennett JE, eds. *Principles and Practice of Infectious Diseases.* 3rd ed. New York: Churchill Livingstone; 1990:2199–2205.

3. Centers for Disease Control: National Nosocomial Infection Study Report. Annual Summary. 1984. *MMWR* 35:17SS–29SS, 1986.

4. Wilson WR, Cockerill FR, Rosenow EC III: Pulmonary disease in the immunocompromised host (second of two parts). *Mayo Clin Proc* 60:610–631, 1985

5. Murray JF, Garay SM, Hopewell PC, et al: Pulmonary complications of the acquired immunodeficiency syndrome: An update. Report of the Second National Heart, Lung and Blood Institute Workshop. *Am Rev Respir Dis* 135:504–509, 1987.

6. Kubota TT: The evaluation of peripheral lymphadenopathy. *Prim Care* 7:461–471, 1980.

7. Greenfield S, Jordan MC: The clinical investigation of lymphadenopathy in primary care practice. *JAMA* 240:1388–1393, 1978.

8. Moore RD, Weisberger AS, Bowerfind ES: An evaluation of lymphadenopathy in system disease. *Arch Intern Med* 99:751–759, 1957.

9. Sinclair S, Beckman E, Ellman L: Biopsy of enlarged, superficial lymph nodes. *JAMA* 228:602–603, 1974.

10. Freidig EE, McClure SP, Wilson WR, et al: Clinical–histologic–microbiologic analysis of 419 lymph node biopsy specimens. *Rev Infect Dis* 8:322–328, 1986.

11. Bottles K, McPhaul LW, Volberding P: Fine-needle aspiration biopsy of patients with the acquired immunodeficiency syndrome (AIDS): Experience in an outpatient clinic. *Ann Intern Med* 108:42–45, 1988.

12. Wispelwey B, Scheld WM: Brain abscess. In: Mandell GL, Douglas RG Jr, Bennett JE, eds. *Principles and Practice of Infectious Diseases.* 3rd ed. New York, Churchill Livingstone; 1990:777–788.

13. Barza M, Pauker SG: The decision to biopsy, treat, or wait in suspected herpes encephalitis. *Ann Intern Med* 92:641–649, 1980.

14. Luft BJ, Remington JS: Toxoplasmic encephalitis. *J Infec Dis* 157:1–6, 1988.

15. Altemeir WA, Culbertson WR, Fullen WD, et al: Intra-abdominal abscesses. *Am J Surg* 125:70–79, 1973.

16. Holden JL, Berne TV, Rosoff L, Sr: Pancreatic abscess following acute pancreatitis. *Arch Surg* 111:858–861, 1976.

17. Barnes PF, DeCock KM, Reynolds TN, et al: A comparison of amebic and pyogenic abscess of the liver. *Medicine* 66:472–483, 1987.

18. Simor AE, Roberts FJ, Smith JA: Infections of the skin and subcutaneous tissues. In: Smith JA, ed. *Cumitech 23* (Cumulative Techniques and Procedures in Clinical Microbiology). Washington, DC: American Society for Microbiology 1988:1–14.

3

The Role of the Clinical Microbiology Laboratory

John D. Christie
Donald R. Callihan

INTRODUCTION

Aspiration biopsy was first used to diagnose lesions with an infectious etiology.[1] Aspiration of diagnostic material from the lung has been used primarily by infectious disease specialists in the diagnosis of pneumonia, lung abscess, or other lung lesions.[2-27] However, with few exceptions,[28,29] there has been little interest in standardizing methods for optimal recovery of the numerous types of microorganisms that may be obtained in material from fine needle aspiration (FNA) biopsy of inflammatory lesions. This lack of interest is unfortunate, as isolation of the etiologic agent may be more sensitive than cytopathology for the diagnosis of these pathogens. Furthermore, specific identification of the offending microorganism yields information that can guide specific antimicrobial therapy necessary for optimal management of the disease.

Unfortunately, the tissue obtained by FNA biopsy and submitted for culture often consists of a rinse of the material remaining in the needle after the clinician or cytopathologist has prepared smears for morphologic studies. To obtain the maximum amount of information from a limited amount of tissue, the cytopathologist, who is often the bridge between the patient and the microbiology laboratory, must know the appropriate procedures for triage, transport, and culture of this specimen. In this chapter, we offer several procedures designed to maximize the diagnostic yield of microbiological analysis of FNA biopsy of inflammatory lesions.

Which of these procedures are adopted by the cytopathologist must depend on the resources available in the local clinical microbiology laboratory. We urge that anatomic pathologists of any subspecialty consult with their colleagues in the clinical microbiology laboratory to maximize the results from material obtained in any invasive procedure. Perhaps Stewart's statement about aspiration biopsy of tumors[30] should be modified to state: "Diagnosis of inflammatory masses by aspiration is as reliable as the combined intelligence of the clinician, cytopathologist, and clinical microbiologist makes it."

Theoretical Background for Culture Protocols

Aspirate Volume, Transport Media, and Transport Time

The increasing prevalence of immunosuppression due to organ transplantation, treatment of neoplastic disorders, and the AIDS epidemic has rendered futile any attempt to identify a specific microorganism as the cause of a particular inflammatory lesion on the basis of clinical presentation and anatomic location. Examples include abscesses in the right soleus muscle and dermis of the right thigh of an AIDS patient caused by *Acanthamoeba castellannii,* a free-living ameba more commonly associated with granulomatous meningoencephalitis,[35] and the presence of solitary pulmonary nodules due to replication of cytomegalovirus, which more commonly causes diffuse pneumonia.[36]

The cytopathologic features of organisms seen in aspirates of infectious lesions often correctly identify the offending microbe. In some instances, however, cytology may not accurately identify the types of microorganism that are better diagnosed using microbiologic culture. In a study correlating the microbiologic, clinical, and histologic findings in lymph node biopsies from patients with a high probability of infectious diseases,[37] organisms belonging to the *Mycobacterium avium* complex were isolated from a lymph node in which the primary diagnosis was abscess wall. A second biopsy of the same lymph node revealed granulomata with acid-fast bacilli that were seen in material stained with auramine-rhodamine but did not grow in culture.

In another series of papers,[38,39] aspiration biopsies of lymph nodes, extranodal swellings, and other lesions with granulomatous or necrotizing inflammation revealed no difference in the percentage of specimens containing acid-fast bacteria when aspirates that were caseous and contained granulomata were compared with lesions that were purulent and contained necrotic debris.[38,39] In a separate study, the percentage of specimens that were positive for acid-fast bacilli (as demonstrated by the Ziehl–Neelsen technique) increased as inflammation changed from a predominance of epithelioid and giant cells to those lesions with necrosis, acute inflammation, and a lymphocytic infiltrate.[40] Even acellular aspirates had a higher prevalence of acid-fast bacilli positivity than did those that contained epithelioid and giant cells. A spindle cell reaction to nontuberculous mycobacteria has been found in the skin and lymph nodes of immunosuppressed individuals.[41,42] Few or no inflammatory cells were present in many of these lesions in which the "spindle" cells contained numerous acid-fast bacilli.

The preceding examples demonstrate that triage of FNA biopsies to provide the optimal recovery of the offending infectious agent cannot be based solely on the anatomic site of the lesion or the gross or microscopic appearance of the aspirate. On the other hand, most clinical microbiology laboratories are not able to culture all of the wide variety of microorganisms that can potentially cause any given inflammatory mass. Personnel in the clinical microbiology laboratory should not be expected to culture or to identify certain types of microorganisms unless the laboratory has the resources and expertise to do so competently and with confidence. For example, if the population a laboratory serves does not have a significant prevalence of infections due to species of *Legionella,* the clinician and cytopathologist cannot expect the clinical microbiology laboratory to be able to isolate and to identify bacteria belonging to this genus with any degree of success.

With the exception of lesions that contain a large amount of purulent, exudative, or necrotic material, the limiting factor in determining the number of cultures that can be obtained will be the volume of the sample. Unfortunately, in many centers, the material available for culture and special stains is often limited to that remaining in the needle after preparation of slides for cytologic diagnosis. In an FNA biopsy that yields a large volume of material, specimens for culture can be transported in different media, each of which is optimal for each particular type of organism potentially present in the specimen. On the other hand, if the aspirate is limited in volume, transport will of necessity be in a medium that is less than optimal for all potential microorganisms. Whenever possible, material that may contain members of the genus *Legionella* should be transported in water rather than in saline because salt solutions may be inhibitory to some members of that genus.[43]

We believe that once the presence of an infectious lesion is suspected, a separate aspiration or "pass" should be performed for microbiologic examination. Using the majority of the aspirate for a microbiologic workup is especially appropriate when the clinical history, physical examination, and prior laboratory and radiologic tests suggest an inflammatory, rather than a neoplastic lesion. If available quantity of aspirate is limited, the cytopathologist, clinician, and clinical microbiologist should try to determine a priority for special stains and for inoculation of media for different groups of microbes.

The time that elapses between collection of the aspirate and performance of culture studies may significantly affect results. In sets of duplicate transthoracic aspirates from dogs artificially infected with *Streptococcus pneumoniae,* the cultures done at "dog-side" had a higher percentage of positive results than did cultures performed in the microbiology laboratory after prompt transportation of the aspirate. The only weakness of this study was that the second aspirate was not placed in transport media before being taken to the laboratory.[44] Despite these findings, very few investigators routinely inoculate cultures at the time of aspiration,[45,46,47] a practice that may be impractical in many situations. Similarly, only a few reports delineate a specific upper limit on transport time or state whether the transport media was inoculated at the time of aspiration.[8,18,48-51]

Obviously, culture media should be inoculated as soon as possible after the aspiration is performed. If culture media cannot be inoculated at the time of aspiration, the needle should be flushed with an appropriate transport medium that, after appropriate labeling, is transported immediately (ie, "stat") to the clinical microbiology laboratory.

The person aspirating the lesion should *not* send the needle itself to the laboratory for several reasons. First, resheathing the needle and sending it to the laboratory exposes the collector and others to a risk of needle-stick injury that is inappropriate in this era of universal blood precautions. Second, dehydration of organisms that may be present in the needle during the time required to transport the aspirate to the laboratory may cause loss of viability or misleading culture results (due to survival and overgrowth of a more hardy microorganism present in low numbers in the tissue).

Cytology, Culture, and Special Stains

In most situations, culture is more sensitive than cytologic evaluation for detection and identification of microorganisms (Table 3.1). This difference occurs because 10^4 to 10^5 organisms normally have to be present in a gram of tissue before one organism can be seen in a 5-μm section of tissue, whereas culture will detect the presence of one viable organism in the specimen. A classic example of this phenomenon is seen in subcutaneous infections caused by *Sporothrix schenckii,* a dimorphic fungus. Usually, the organism cannot be found in histologic sections, even with classic stains for fungi, since the yeast form of the organism is present in such low numbers.[52] Additionally, culture provides a specific identity and sensitivity for most bacteria, whereas cytology can provide only the Gram-stain reaction and the shape of the microorganism. On the other hand, many organisms, such as *Treponema pallidum,* cannot be cultured. Still other microbes, such as the gram-negative bacterium causing cat-scratch disease, cannot be isolated in the usual clinical microbiology laboratory. Moreover, by the time the lymph nodes infected by the cat-scratch bacteria are fluctuant and suitable for aspiration, only rare degenerating bacteria can be found.[53]

For other organisms, such as *Haemophilus ducreyi,* that are found in low prevalence in most communities, it may be economically unfeasible to maintain the special media and technical expertise required to isolate these microorganisms.

TABLE 3.1. Culture versus Cytology in Detection of Microorganisms in a Community Hospital Setting

Culture Superior	*Cytology Superior*
Few microorganisms present	Many microorganisms present
Species of microorganisms that appear similar to each other	Species of microorganisms that are morphologically distinct from other species
Most bacteria	Bacteria that are rare or have special culture requirements: *Haemophilus ducreyi* *Chlamydia* *Legionella* sp. "cat-scratch" bacterium
Most *Mycobacteria* sp.	Microorganisms other than bacteria that are rare, have special culture requirements, or cannot be cultured, eg: Viruses Most tissue parasites Rickettsia *Treponema pallidum*
Most fungi	Microorganisms that are dead or dying, eg: Zygomyces Bacteria treated with antibiotics Microorganisms transported under suboptimal conditions

Facilities for isolating viruses and *Chlamydia,* which require tissue culture for diagnosis, are generally found only in larger reference laboratories or tertiary care facilities. Similarly, very few clinical microbiology laboratories attempt to culture protozoan and metazoan parasites. The extent to which anaerobic organisms, fungi, and acid-fast bacilli are cultured and identified is determined to a large measure by the financial resources of the institution or its available expertise.

Circumstances in which cytologic examination may be superior to culture in detecting microorganisms also need to be considered. If the patient from whom an aspirate is obtained is being treated with antibiotics, the cytopathologist may detect a dead or metabolically inhibited bacterium even though culture of the same material will be negative. For example, in a study comparing cytologic and culture diagnosis of tuberculosis in lung aspirates, culture was reported negative in 75 of 88 aspirates in which cytologic findings were compatible with tuberculosis. Although the data are somewhat unclear, approximately one third of these 88 aspirates were positive by Ziehl-Neelsen stain for acid-fast bacilli. However, the authors note that many of these patients either had been treated with antituberculous drugs or the pulmonary infiltrates were radiologically stable or were regressing. Thus, the reader should not be surprised that, in such a group of patients, cytologic examination is superior to culture for diagnosis of tuberculosis.[54] The effect of antibiotics on culture of material from needle aspirates is also demonstrated by a later study in which culture was positive for microorganisms in only 5 out of 12 aspirates from cavitary lesions of the lung. However, 6 of the 7 patients who had culture-negative aspirates were being treated with antibiotics.[55]

Other factors decreasing the effectiveness of culture compared to direct microscopic examination of aspirates include use of inappropriate transport media, delays in transport, and failure to inoculate the proper culture media or to obtain material containing viable organisms. Sometimes the aspirator does not realize that anaerobic bacteria may be an important etiology in certain infectious processes. The specimen may then be submitted in an aerobic transport device or may not be transported expeditiously. In such instances the offending pathogen may be dead by the time the specimen reaches the laboratory. In fungal infections due to members of the class Zygomycetes, appropriate cultures are often negative while direct examination of the aspirates reveal many hyphae which can be seen by the cytologist. This discrepancy occurs because the aspirated tissue is from the center of an abscess containing necrotic tissue with very few living fungi. Because the fungus disseminates hematogenously and kills tissue by thrombosis of vessels supplying the tissue, viable fungi will be found mainly in the living tissue "upstream" from the abscess. Thus, fungal specimens adequate for culture may be found only in tissue that still appears normal by physical or radiologic examination. Inappropriate or suboptimal culture can lead to an inaccurate diagnosis. An example is aspirated material from a nocardial abscess in which the laboratory fails to hold culture media for the requisite length of time or fails to inoculate a chocolate agar plate.

Often, culture may be the only means by which to distinguish two organisms whose identity the microscopist may confuse—especially when one of the microbes is fairly common and the other is fairly rare. This situation is illustrated by a comparison of *Aspergillus* sp. and *Pseudallescheria boydii.* Both fungi are septate, branched, and hematoxylinophilic, and both can invade blood vessels. However, the branching pattern of *P. boydii* is nonprogressive and more haphazard than that of *Aspergillus* sp., and the hyphae of the former genus are narrower than that of the latter species (Fig. 3.1).[56] This identification is of importance in determining medical therapy, as *P. boydii* is resistant to amphotericin and ketoconazole and somewhat sensitive to miconazole. Successful treatment of invasive *P. boydii* infections has required a combination of surgery and antifungal therapy with micronazole has been necessary.

The use of special stains for identification of microbes is crucial in both the cytopathologic and clinical microbiologic laboratories. We believe the cytopathologist should utilize the expertise of the clinical microbiologist as a microscopist. The clinical microbiologist, whether technologist or director, has extensive experience interpreting Gram stains, differentiating the many genera of microorganisms, and distinguishing these organisms from pseudomicrobes.[57] Some air-dried smears made at the time of aspiration from a patient with an inflammatory mass should be sent to the clinical microbiology laboratory for processing and examination.

When examining a smear stained with Gram stain or a Giemsa-based stain such as Diff-Quik, the cytopathologist or clinical microbiologist must be alert for the presence of ghost bacteria which betray the presence of species of *Mycobacterium*. On either type of preparation, mycobacteria may appear as negative images of bacilli.[58-63] On Gram stains, mycobacteria may also appear as "ghost bacilli," staining either gram-neutral or gram-positive depending upon the plane of focus.[64] The discovery of ghost bacilli should alert the person examining the specimen to culture for mycobacteria if such cultures are not already included as part of the routine protocol for aspirates. If the specimen is limited in volume, the presence of ghost bacilli should alert the microbiologist or cytopathologist to triage the aspirate so that the specimen is cultured so as to permit optimal recovery of the various acid-fast organisms.

If specimen volume is sufficient, the microbiologist can stain a smear with auramine–rhodomine, a fluorogenic stain, to verify the presence of acid-fast bacilli. We prefer this stain, which can be adapted to tissue sections, to the routine Ziehl–Neelsen used in most histo- and cytopathology laboratories, the fluorogenic stain is more sensitive than Ziehl–Neelsen in detecting acid-fast bacilli. In a study of lymph node biopsies, a fluorescent stain similar to auramine–rhodamine was found to be twice as sensitive as the Ziehl–Neelsen stain in demonstrating the presence of acid-fast bacilli.[65] The major *advantages* of the auramine–rhodamine stain compared to the Ziehl–Neelsen stain include:[66]

Better contrast between the organism and the background

Increased speed of evaluation as the slide is read at low power using an objective lens of $25 \times$ or greater power

Less dependence on the color acuity of the microscopist

Other advantages include the high specificity of the stain for mycobacteria and the positive staining of dead and dying organisms. *Drawbacks* of the auramine–rhodamine stain are

The requirement for a fluorescence microscope

False positivity of some artifacts

Loss of fluorescence in 3 to 4 days

Difficulty of finding granulomas

In addition, some stains of *M. fortuitum* do not stain well with auramine.

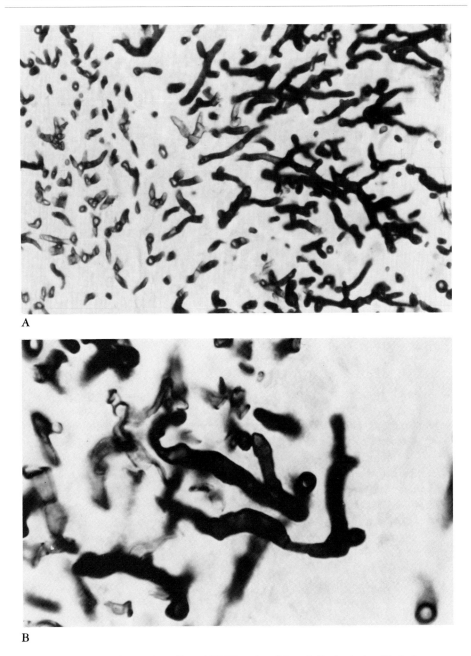

Fig. 3.1. Gomori methenamine silver (GMS) stain of *Pseudallescheria boydii*. **A.** Low-power magnification showing superficial resemblance of *P. boydii* to *Aspergillus* species (GMS stain; × 100). **B.** High-power magnification showing nonprogressive and haphazard branching of *P. boydii* (GMS × 400).

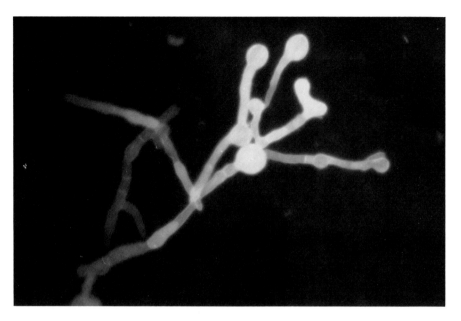

Fig. 3.2. Calcofluor white stain of *Aspergillus* sp. Note the clear staining of the septae of the hyphae (×400).

For staining fungi, a preparation of potassium hydroxide containing calcofluor white, a nonspecific fluorescent dye, can be used with fresh or fixed tissue (Fig. 3.2). This stain offers several advantages over potassium hydroxide alone, lactophenol cotton blue, or Gomori's methenamine silver.[67,68] Potassium hydroxide alone may produce many artifacts as it dissolves any proteinaceous material surrounding the fungi. Additionally, material treated with this stain alone lacks contrast between the dissolved cells and any fungal elements.[69] Staining with calcofluor white takes less time than does staining with Gomori's methenamine silver or lactophenol blue. Lactophenol blue does not stain the cross walls of fungi as well as does calcofluor white. The latter chemical also does not stain the cytoplasmic inclusions of cytomegalovirus as does Gomori's methenamine silver.[70] Moreover, smears stained with calcofluor white can be restained with Gomori's methenamine silver. This stain can also be used to detect the cysts of *Acanthamoeba*.[71,72] Some investigators have found that calcofluor white does not stain *Nocardia, Actinomyces,* or *Streptomyces* well,[68] but we have found the opposite to be true. However, the modified Ziehl)–Neelsen stain is best for differentiating among the variety of branching, gram-positive bacteria. The only drawback of this stain is that the specific illumination requirements are fairly strict.

The fluorescent microscope can also be used to identify those fungi, such as *Aspergillus, Blastomyces, Histoplasma, Cryptococcus* and *Coccidioides,* which autofluoresce in Papanicolaou-stained smears.[73,74] We cannot leave the arena of direct microscopic examination of aspirates for fungi without mentioning the existence of capsule-deficient *Cryptococcus*.[75,76] These forms of *Cryptococcus,* which cannot be detected by the usual mucicarmine stains and thus may be confused with other budding yeasts, can be identified with a modified Fontana–Masson stain.[77]

Immunofluorescent Stains, Monoclonal Antibodies, and In Situ Hybridization

Immunohistochemical staining with polyclonal or monoclonal antibodies and fluorescent or avidin biotin labeled markers has been used to detect a variety of bacterial species including *Mycobacterium,* various genera of fungi, and cysts and trophozoites of free-living amoeba and *Toxoplasma gondii* in tissue sections and other materials.[52,78-85] However, the use of all of these techniques is restricted to large reference or research laboratories. Furthermore, cross-reactions do occur, limiting the usefulness of these staining methods even in the most experienced hands.

Immunofluorescent Staining for Legionella

Perhaps one of the most widespread uses of immunofluorescence techniques in direct identification of organisms in clinical specimens has been in the diagnosis of the several species of *Legionella.* Immunofluorescent assays using a polyclonal antibody, whether direct or indirect, are extremely specific.[43,86,87,88] In laboratories where *Legionella* has a low prevalence, a positive immunofluorescence could be a signal to initiate treatment of the patient and cultures for the organism. However, in comparison to culture, immunofluorescence assays have a low sensitivity owing to the limited number of cross-reactions between different antigenic types and the large number of organisms necessary for visualization by microscopy. Because of this low sensitivity, all specimens submitted to the clinical microbiology laboratory for isolation and identification of *Legionella* should have presumptive *Legionella* identified by both immunofluorescence assay and culture. A positive assay using polyclonal antibodies with a negative culture can mean cross-reaction of the antibody pool with other bacteria such as *Pseudomonas, Bacteroides,* or *Flavobacterium.*[89-92] In such a situation, measurement of specific antibody in acute and convalescent sera from the patient will help distinguish between cross-reaction and a true-positive direct immunofluorescence assay.

The specificity of fluorescence assays in diagnosis of *Legionella* has been increased by the use of monoclonal antibodies directed against a particular *Legionella* species.[92-95] Because 20% of *Legionella* infections are caused by species other than *L. pneumophila,* a pool of monoclonal antibodies will be needed for optimum diagnosis. However, many laboratories have neither the financial resources to maintain a supply of such reagents, which will outdate before they are used; or a technologist who will view enough *Legionella* specimens to maintain competency in discerning false-positive from true-positive results.

Culture and Direct Detection of Viruses

As the population of immunosuppressed patients with viral lesions causing inflammatory masses grows larger and as specific therapy directed against individual viral species becomes available, rapid diagnosis of viral infections becomes more important. Approaches toward increasing the speed and accuracy of diagnosis of a particular viral agent have included (1) the use of improved culture techniques together with identification using antibodies directed against individual viral antigens and (2) the detection of specific viral gene products in tissue or cells with monoclonal antibodies, in situ hybridization, or polymerase chain reaction studies.

Investigators have combined immunofluorescent assays with a monoclonal antibody directed against the early and intermediate (precytopathic effect) nuclear antigens of cytomegalovirus with centrifugation of samples taken for viral culture in attempts to shorten the time required for a culture diagnosis of that virus.[96-111] Generally, the sensitivity·of the immunofluorescence assay and centrifugation culture has been greater than has the sensitivity of recognition of typical cytopathic effect in conventional tissue cell culture in detection of cytomegalovirus. Unfortunately, the meaning of a positive cytomegalovirus culture without specific cytologic findings in patients with clinical and radiologic findings typical of cytomegalovirus disease, especially pneumonitis, remains problematic.[112-117]

Results similar to the work with culture have been found with the use of monoclonal or polyclonal antibodies applied directly to bronchoalveolar lavage and tissue specimens.[118-127] However, confusion still exists about which method (ie, culture with monoclonal antibody detection, observation of cytologic changes in tissue, or immunofluorescent examination of tissue) is most sensitive in detecting infection and not colonization with cytomegalovirus.[97,128,129] The tissue of latent cytomegalovirus infections also confuses the picture.

Differences in the results of the various assays used to diagnose cytomegalovirus pneumonia or colitis may represent differences in the behavior of the virus or the host. For example, in a series of open lung biopsies from patients with bone marrow transplants, those individuals with negative histology and positive immunofluorescence for cytomegalovirus were more likely to have seroconverted before biopsy than were those patients with positive histology and immunofluorescence.[122]

Techniques similar to those used for cultural and immunologic diagnosis of cytomegalovirus have been used for other viruses (eg, adenovirus) with good results.[130] Another promising technique is double-label immunofluorescence. In this method, one culture is inoculated and screened for the presence of two viruses using separate antisera raised in different animals against two different viruses and tagged with two different fluorescent markers. This method has been successful in detecting dual infection with herpes simplex and adenovirus from eye cultures within 48 hours of initiating culture.[131]

The other method used to increase the speed of diagnosis of viral infections applies the techniques of in situ hybridization and polymerase chain reaction to tissue, urine, blood, bronchoalveolar lavage or open lung biopsy specimens.[122,123,129,132-155] Although a great deal of work has been done to detect human papillomavirus by in situ hybridization, we have reviewed only the work performed with cytomegalovirus, adenovirus, and herpes simplex because these viruses are more likely to be detected in aspirates of inflammatory masses. Once again, the results from studies with cytomegalovirus are confusing.[120,122,129,145,149] Perhaps at this time, the proper role of specific monoclonal antibodies and gene probes is to demonstrate the specific cause of lesions in which nonspecific or atypical nuclear and cytoplasmic inclusions are found.[156,157,158] Finally, in ending the discussion on the use of these new techniques for direct identification of viruses in tissues or cytologic preparations, we must point out that some of the conflicting results in these studies may be due to differences in the techniques themselves. Several authors have suggested that because of the great genetic variability in clinical isolates of cytomegalovirus, a pool of monoclonal antibodies must be used to ensure detection of these isolates in different clinical situations.[120,127] The sensitivity of the method used to detect in situ hybridization also differs; at present, radioisotopically labeled probes are more sensitive than are biontinylated probes. This difference may explain the finding that when immunohistochemical and hybridization methods were used concurrently on the same tissue block, the immunohistochemical method was more sensitive than was the hybridization assay.[146,148] Moreover, endogenous avidin binding activity in organs such as the liver may cause false-positive results when biontinylated probes are used. Despite the use of blocking techniques, Niedobitek and colleagues were unable to obtain satisfactory specific labeling of hepatitis B virus DNA in liver sections.[147] We also urge the use of careful technique when working with polymerase chain reaction technology in the laboratory. Cross-contamination of clinical material by minute amounts of nucleic acids may cause false-positive reactions.

Routine Use of In Situ Hybridization in the Clinical Microbiology Laboratory

Although a recent review[159] listed a number of gene probes for the diagnosis of infectious diseases, relatively few suitable for use in the clinical microbiology laboratory are commercially available. At this time, the initial excitement about gene probes, promoted in part by overenthusiasm on the part of basic scientists and overeager sales personnel, has abated.[160] Clinical microbiologists now expect gene probe technology to meet the same standards as any other method used for routine diagnosis.

Commercial gene probes using nonradioisotopic labels are available for direct diagnosis of *Neisseria gonorrhoeae* and *Chlamydia trachomatis* in female genital specimens. At present, however, the probes most useful for diagnosis of microorganisms in FNA biopsy have a radioisotope label with a shelf life of 1 month. The sensitivity of the probe has been optimized by using ribosomal RNA as its target. The limited shelf life of these probes implies that the volume of specimens has to be large enough to make use of the probe economically feasible and that specimens be processed in lots rather than as single samples. This weakness may be eliminated with release of nonradioisotopic versions of the probe accompanied by detection systems currently in development. At present, non-radioactive probes of interest in diagnosis of various species of microbes found in inflammatory masses are undergoing the FDA approval process.

Unfortunately, the two commercially available probes of interest to cytopathologists working with FNA biopsy specimens of inflammatory masses and designed for direct assay of microbes in clinical specimens detect two relatively rare pathogens, namely *Mycoplasma pneumoniae* and *Legionella* sp. Only the probe that detects *Legionella* sp. has been evaluated in any detail.[161-165] These studies prompted improvements in the kit methodology. Nevertheless, a prospective study comparing the gene probe with direct immunofluorescence assay and culture indicated that the probe was comparable to the assay in sensitivity and specificity, but neither the probe nor the fluorescence assay detected *Legionella* in several specimens that were positive by culture.[161] Although these cultures generally had low colony counts, the specimens were obtained from patients with a clinical picture compatible with legionellosis, and the patients responded to erythromycin therapy. The results of all of these studies emphasize that culture is still the gold standard for diagnosis of infections caused by *Legionella* sp.

At this time, commercial gene probes are available for the culture confirmation of *Mycobacterium tuberculosis, M. avium, M. intracellulare,* and *M. gordonae.* A gene probe for culture confirmation of *M. kansasii* is currently undergoing trials and should be available in the near future. A commercially available gene probe for detection of the genus *Mycobacteria* from clinical specimens was withdrawn from the market owing to low sensitivity. The lower limit of sensitivity of direct microscopy is approximately 5,000 mycobacteria/ml of sputum, whereas the lower limit of the gene probe is 50 pg of DNA, which represents the amount of DNA in 10,000 bacterial cells.[166] Thus direct microscopy was more sensitive than was the gene probe in detecting these microbes in sputum.

Studies using the assays for *M. tuberculosis, M. avium,* and *M. intracellulare* have indicated that these tests have very high sensitivity and specificity compared to the use of classic biochemical reactions for identification.[167-172] When combined with the BACTEC radiometric detection system for primary isolation of mycobacteria, the time required for isolation and identification of these microbes can be reduced by 5 to 7 weeks.[173,174] As with the *Legionella* probe, however, use of the kits requires several modifications from the procedures recommended by the manufacturer including adjustment of cutoff range, determination of appropriate growth index in the BACTEC radiometric assay, and determination of cost-efficient testing strategies based on the prevalence of the different species of mycobacteria in a given population.[171,175,176] Although these commercial gene probes represent an exciting advance in the diagnosis of mycobacterial disease, they have not reached a stage of development where their use can be recommended in smaller laboratories.

CULTURE PROTOCOLS

Given the preceding discussion, we submit the following general guidelines for processing FNA biopsy material to ensure maximal recovery of possible infectious agents.

Collection of Specimens

Aspirations Containing a Large Volume (>2 ml) of pus or necrotic Material

1. Express any air from the needle into a sterile gauze pad.
2. If the patient has normal immune status, *immediately* innoculate all of the material into an anaerobic transport vial.
3. If the patient is immunocompromised and the hospital has a virology laboratory, *immediately* inoculate approximately one quarter or 0.5 ml of the specimen, whichever is less, into viral transport medium. The viral transport medium should have been kept in a refrigerator or ice bath until use. The remainder of

the material is then inoculated into an anaerobic transport vial. The clinical microbiology laboratory should provide these vials at regular time intervals or upon request depending upon the number of aspirations performed by the cytopathology team or interventional radiology division.

4. Arrange for "stat" transport of tubes to the clinical microbiology laboratory along with accession forms listing the relevant clinical information. If the viral culture cannot be delivered to the laboratory within 5 minutes of inoculation, it should be kept in a refrigerator until transport and transported in a cup of ice.

5. If possible, notify the clinical microbiologist on call that the aspirate will be arriving in the laboratory. The clinical microbiologist will then be available to make sure that the aspirated material is handled rapidly and appropriately.

Aspirations Yield a Small Volume of Material (<1 ml)

1. Following aspiration and collection of sufficient material for cytologic diagnosis, the operator should make another pass with the needle and then aspirate into the syringe 2 to 4 ml of sterile "degassed" saline or water from tubes supplied by the clinical microbiology laboratory.

   a. Sterile water should be used for aspirates of pulmonary lesions.
   b. Sterile saline should be used for aspirates of other sites.

2. After expressing excess air from the needle into a sterile gauze pad, the cytopathologist should mix the contents of the syringe and dispense the material as follows:

   a. If the patient is immunocompromised or the clinician suspects a viral etiology for the lesion, approximately 0.5 ml of the suspension should be inoculated into viral transport medium and the remainder of the suspension should be inoculated into an anaerobic transport vial.
   b. If the patient is not immunocompromised or a viral lesion is not suspected, the entire suspension may be inoculated into the anaerobic transport vial.

3. The one or two vials along with the relevant requisition slips should then be transported "stat" *directly* to the clinical microbiology laboratory.

4. Again, if possible, notify the clinical microbiologist on call that the aspirate should be arriving at the laboratory. At this time, if a specific group of microbes is suspected as the cause of the lesion, give the clinical microbiologist that information so that triage of the material can be arranged. With a triage procedure, most of the workup and the aspirate volume can be devoted to culture and other procedures designed for optimal recovery of that particular group.

5. Under no circumstances should the needle and syringe be transported to the clinical microbiology laboratory. Not only does this method violate universal biosafety precautions but the material in the syringe is usually a dried clot by the time it reaches the laboratory.

Setting Up Slides and Cultures[177,178,179]

Aspirates With a High Yield of Material

1. The clinical microbiology laboratory should make six slides from the material in the anaerobic transport vial. Two of the slides can be kept in reserve while each of the other four slides can be treated with one of the following stains:

   a. *For bacteria:* Gram stain. If branching, gram-positive bacteria are observed, one of the reserve slides should be used to prepare a modified acid-fast preparation for detection of *Nocardia.*

   b. *For fungi:* Calcofluor white with potassium hydroxide. If fungi are seen by the medical technologist, the same smear can be stained using GMS or periodic acid–Schiff's.

   c. *For mycobacteria:* Auramine-rhodamine stain followed by restaining with Ziehl–Neelsen or Kinyoun acid-fast stain if the auramine–rhodamine stain is presumptively positive for acid-fast bacteria.

   d. *For* Legionella: Direct immunofluorescence assay with polyclonal antibodies if the laboratory handles enough specimens to maintain competency in processing and reading these smears. Otherwise, the slide should be kept unstained in reserve.

2. The clinical microbiology laboratory should inoculate four sets of culture media. Each set is optimal for a group of microbes.

   a. *For aerobic Organisms:*
   Chocolate agar plate
   Sheep blood agar plate
   Enteric agar plate, eg, MacConkey agar, desoxycholate agar, eosin–methylene blue agar

   b. For anaerobic organisms: Reduce all anaerobic plates for ≥ 24 hours prior to use.
   Anaerobic blood agar plate, eg, CDC formulation anaerobic blood agar, brucella 5% sheep blood agar with vitamin K_1 and hemin
   Kanamycin-vancomycin laked blood plate
   Phenylethyl alcohol sheep blood agar plate

   c. *For fungi:*
   Inhibitory mold agar (IMA)
   Brain–heart infusion (BHI) agar with chloramphenicol and Gentamicin
   Sabouraud's 2% dextrose

   d. *For* Legionella:
   —If the clinical microbiology laboratory does not process sufficient *Legionella* cultures to maintain competency in isolation and identification of this group of microorganisms, then this material should be packed in dry ice and sent to a reputable reference laboratory.
   —If the clinical microbiology laboratory does have a history of sufficient volume and positive cultures to maintain competency, then the following plates are appropriate:
   Buffered charcoal yeast extract (BCYE) agar without inhibitory agents

BCYE containing polymyxin B, anisomycin, and
cefamandole
e. *For* Mycobacteria:
—Liquid media: BACTEC 12B Medium or Middlebrook 7H9 broth. Note: The
BACTEC medium is designed for use with the BACTEC culture system only.
—Two solid media
Nonselective, inspissated egg medium, eg, American Thoracic Society,
Lowenstein–Jensen, or Petragnani medium
Nonselective agar medium: Middlebrook 7H11
—If the aspirate is from the skin, a duplicate set of media should be inocu-
lated and incubated at a temperature ≤33°C for isolation of *M. marinum*
f. For viruses (if patient is immunosuppressed and viral transport medium has
been inoculated with aspirate), check with the virology service to see which
medium they recommend for isolation and culture of viruses.

Aspirates With Limited Yield of Material

1. If a definite order of triage has been agreed upon, then the clinical microbiology
laboratory should

a. Make three smears from the tube sent to the laboratory, stain them with
Gram, Calcofluor white in potassium hydroxide and auramine–rhodamine
followed by Ziehl–Neelsen according to 2 above and examine them.
b. Inoculate the full set of cultures for the group of microbes with the highest
priority.
c. Inoculate minimum sets of cultures for the other groups of microbes. These
minimum sets are:
—*For aerobes only:*
Sheep blood agar plate
Chocolate agar plate
—*For anaerobes only:*
Anaerobic blood agar plate
—*For aerobes and anaerobes:*
Chocolate agar plate
Sheep blood agar
Anaerobic blood agar plate
—*For fungi:*
Brain–heart infusion agar with 10% sheep blood
Inhibitory mold agar
—*For mycobacteria:*
If laboratory uses BACTEC culture system:
BACTEC 12B medium
Middlebrook 7H11 medium
If laboratory does not use BACTEC culture system:
Nonselective, egg-based medium
Middlebrook 7H11 medium

2. If an order of triage has not been agreed upon, then the clinical microbiology laboratory personnel should
   a. Make three smears as before, stain, and examine them.
   b. Inoculate a minimum set of cultures for each group of microbes. This set will include those listed above.

CONCLUSIONS

In this chapter, we have tried to give the reader a theoretical background for our approach to the work-up of FNA biopsy of inflammatory masses by the clinical microbiology laboratory. We do not believe that this protocol should be followed blindly without regard for the limitations under which the clinical microbiology laboratory may operate. The extent of identification of each group of microbes may also vary according to the expertise and resources of the laboratory.[177]

The other facet of clinical microbiology that is stressed is the increasing use of the techniques of cellular biology in larger clinical microbiology laboratories. Use of these techniques will provide new information, whose value and benefit to the patient are still unclear at present. In the last analysis, these methods must have the same rigorous quality control standards and expectations that other assays in routine diagnostic use must meet.

Finally, the most important message of the chapter is that a FNA biopsy represents a specimen of limited volume obtained by an invasive technique. If the FNA biopsy is non-diagnostic, the next diagnostic step may be an open biopsy. When the aspiration biopsy is taken from an inflammatory mass, a portion of the specimen or optimally, a separate specimen should be placed in the appropriate transport media and be brought to the laboratory as quickly as possible.

The most vital aspect of the diagnostic work-up of a FNAB of an inflammatory mass is communication between the clinician, cytopathologist, and clinical microbiologist. This dialogue permits triage of the specimen to yield the most appropriate information necessary to help the patient and prevents the aspirate from becoming a dried clot of intermingled blood and tissue which is of little use to anyone.

REFERENCES

1. Frable WJ: Introduction and history. Thin needle aspiration cytology. Philadelphia, W.B. Saunders, 1–6, 1966.

2. Abdel-Khalik AK, Askar AM, Ali M: The causative organisms of bronchopneumonia in infants in Egypt. Arch Dis Child 13:333–342, 1938.

3. Alexander HE, Craig HR, Shirely RG, et al: Validity of etiological diagnosis of pneumonia in children by rapid typing from nasopharyngeal mucus. J Pediatr 18:31–35, 1941.

4. Bandt PD, Blank N, Castellino RA: Needle diagnosis of pneumonitis. Value in high-risk patients. JAMA 220:1578–1580, 1972.

5. Berger R, Arango L: Etiologic diagnosis of bacterial nosocomial pneumonia in seriously ill patients. *Crit Care Med* 13:833–836, 1985.

6. Blacklock JWS, Guthrie KJ: Pneumococcal infections in infancy and childhood. *J Pathol Bacteriol* 36:349–368, 1933.

7. Bullowa JGM, Greenbaum E: The primary pneumonias of infants and children. I. Age distribution, fatality rates, and relation of character of involvement to fatality in 1,000 children. *Public Health Rep* 51:1076–1083, 1936.

8. Castellino RA, Blank N: Etiological diagnosis of focal pulmonary infection in immuno-compromised patients by fluoroscopically guided percutaneous needle aspiration. *Radiology* 132:563–567, 1979.

9. Chaudhary S, Hughes WT, Feldman S, et al: Percutaneous transthoracic needle aspiration of the lung diagnosing *Pneumocystis carinii* pneumonitis. *Am J Dis Child* 131:902–907, 1977.

10. Davidson M, Tempest B, Palmer DL: Bacteriologic diagnosis of acute pneumonia. Comparison of sputum, transtracheal aspirates, and lung aspirates. *JAMA* 235:158–163, 1976.

11. Disney ME, Wolff J, Wood BSB: Staphylococcal pneumonia in infants. *Lancet* 1:767–771, 1956.

12. Ellenbogen C, Graybill JR, Silva J Jr, et al: Bacterial pneumonia complicating adenoviral pneumonia: a comparison of respiratory tract bacterial culture sources and effectiveness of chemoprophylaxis against bacterial pneumonia. *Am J Med* 169–178, 1974.

13. Garcia de Olarte D, Trujillo SH, Uribe A, et al: Lung puncture-aspiration as a bacteriologic diagnostic procedure in acute pneumonias of infants and children. *Clin Pediatr* 10:346–350, 1971.

14. Gherman CR, Simon HJ: Pneumonia complicating severe underlying disease. *Dis Chest* 48:297–304, 1965.

15. Greenman RL, Goodall PT, King D: Lung biopsy in immunocompromised hosts. *Am J Med* 59:488–496, 1975.

16. Hughes JR, Bose SK, Kloene W, et al: Acute lower respiratory tract infections in Calcutta children: an etiologic study. *Indian Pediatr* 3:201–211, 1966.

17. Hughes JR, Sinha DP, Cooper MR, et al: Lung tap in childhood: bacteria, viruses and mycoplasmas in acute lower respiratory tract infections. *Pediatrics* 44:477–485, 1969.

18. Irwin RS, Garrity FL, Erickson AD, et al: Sampling lower respiratory tract secretions in primary lung abscess. A comparison of the accuracy of four methods. *Chest* 79:559–565, 1981.

19. Klein JO: Diagnostic lung puncture in the pneumonias of infants and children. *Pediatrics* 44:486–492, 1969.

20. Lorber G, Swenson RM: Bacteriology of aspiration pneumonia: a prospective study of community- and hospital-acquired cases. *Ann Intern Med* 1974;81:329–331.

21. Mimica I, Donoso E, Howard JE, et al: Lung puncture in the etiological diagnosis of pneumonia. *Am J Dis Child* 122:278–282, 1971.

22. Numiea J: Lung puncture in the etiologic diagnosis of pneumonia. *Am J Dis Child* 122:278–282, 1971.

23. Palmer DL, Davidson M, Lusk R: Needle aspiration of the lung in complex pneumonias. *Chest* 78:16–21, 1980.

24. Sappington SW, Favorite GO: Lung puncture in lobar pneumonia. *Am J Med Sci* 191:225–234, 1936.

25. Schuster CA, Duffau G, Nicholls E, et al: Lung aspirate puncture as a diagnostic aid in pulmonary tuberculosis in childhood. *Pediatrics* 42:647–650, 1968.

26. Schuster CA, Pino CM, Neira SM, et al: La puncion biopsia pulmonar como metodo diagnostico de las neumopatias de la infancia. *Pediatria* (Santiago, Chile) 9:9–12, 1966.

27. Thomas HM Jr, Parker F: Results of antemortem lung punctures in lobar pneumonia: their bearing on the mechanism of crisis. *Arch Intern Med* 26:125–132, 1920.

28. Bottles K, Miller TR, Jeffrey RB, et al: Aspiration cytology characterization of inflammatory masses. *West J Med* 144:695–699, 1986.

29. Layfield LJ, Glasgow BJ, DuPuis MH: Fine-needle aspiration of lymphadenopathy of suspected infectious etiology. *Arch Pathol Lab Med* 109:810–812, 1985.

30. Stewart FW: The diagnosis of tumors by aspiration. *Am J Pathol* 9:801–812, 1933.

31. Abel EA: Cutaneous manifestations of immunosuppression in organ transplant recipients. *J Am Acad Dermatol* 21:167–179, 1989.

32. Isenberg HD, D'Amato RF: Indigenous and pathogenic microorganisms of humans. *In:* EH Lennette, A Balows, WJ Hausler Jr, HJ Shadomy, Eds. *Manual of Clinical Microbiology.* ed. 4. Washington, DC: American Society for Microbiology, 1985, pp 24–35.

33. Rosenow EC III, Wilson WR, Cockerill FR III: Pulmonary disease in the immunocompromised host (first of two parts). *Mayo Clin Proc* 1985;60:473–487.

34. Wilson WR, Cockerill FR III, Rosenow EC III. Pulmonary disease in the immunocompromised host (second of two parts). *Mayo Clin Proc* 60:610–631, 1985.

35. Gonzalez MM, Gould E, Dickinson G, et al: Acquired immunodeficiency syndrome associated with acanthamoeba infection and other opportunistic organisms. *Arch Pathol Lab Med* 110:749–751, 1986.

36. Ravin C, Smith GW, Ahern MJ, et al: Cytomegaloviral infection presenting as a solitary pulmonary nodule. *Chest* 71:220–222, 1967.

37. Freidig EE, McClure SP, Wilson WR, et al: Clinical–histologic–microbiologic analysis of 419 lymph node biopsy specimens. *Rev Infect Dis* 8:322–328, 1986.

38. Bailey TM, Akhtar M, Ali MA: Fine needle aspiration biopsy in the diagnosis of tuberculosis. *Acta Cytol* 29:732–736, 1985.

39. Metre MS, Jayaram G. Acid-fast bacilli in aspiration smears from tuberculous lymph nodes: an analysis of 255 cases. *Acta Cytol* 31:17–19, 1987.

40. Rajwanshi A, Bhambhani S, Das DK: Fine-needle aspiration cytology diagnosis of tuberculosis. *Diagn Cytopathol* 3:13–16, 1987.

41. Brandwein M, Choi H-SH, Stauchen J, et al: Spindle cell reaction to nontuberculous mycobacteriosis in AIDS mimicking a spindle cell neoplasm. *Virchows Arch (A)* 416:281–286, 1990.

42. Wood C, Nikoloff BJ, Todes-Taylor NR: Pseudotumor resulting from atypical mycobacterial infection: a "histoid" variety of mycobacterium avium intracellulare complex infection. *Am J Clin Pathol* 83:524–527, 1985.

43. Edelstein PH. *Legionella, In:* Lennette EH, Balows A, Hausler WJ Jr, et al, *Manual of Clinical Microbiology,* ed 4. Washington, DC, American Society for Microbiology, 1985, pp 373–381.

44. Moser KM, Maurer J, Jassy L, et al: Sensitivity, specificity, and risk of diagnostic procedures in a canine model of streptococcus pneumoniae pneumonia. *Am Rev Respir Dis* 125:436–442, 1982.

45. Conces DJ Jr, Schwenk GR Jr, Doering PR, et al: Thoracic needle biopsy: improved results using a team approach. *Chest* 91:813–816, 1987.

46. Hook EW III, Hooton TM, Horton CA, et al: Microbiologic evaluation of cutaneous cellulitis in adults. *Arch Intern Med* 146:295–297, 1986.

47. Uman SJ, Kunin CM: Needle aspiration in the diagnosis of soft tissue infections. *Arch Intern Med* 135:959–961, 1975.

48. Grinan NP, Lucena FM, Romero JV, et al: Yield of percutaneous needle lung aspiration in lung abscess. *Chest* 97:69–74, 1990.

49. Lee PC, Turnidge J, McDonald PJ: Fine-needle aspiration in diagnosis of soft tissue infections. *J Clin Microbiol* 22:80–83, 1985.

50. Newell PM, Norden CW: Value of needle aspiration in bacteriologic diagnosis of cellulitis in adults. *J Clin Microbiol* 26:401–404, 1988.

51. Valicenti JF Jr, Daniell C, Gobien RP: Thin needle aspiration cytology of benign intrathoracic lesions. *Acta Cytol* 25:659–664, 1981.

52. Russell B, Beckett JH, Jacobs PH: Immunoperoxidase localization of *Sporothrix schenckii* and *Cryptococcus neoformans:* staining of tissue sections fixed in 4% formaldehyde solution and embedded in paraffin. *Arch Dermatol* 115:433–435, 1979.

53. English CK, Wear DJ, Margileth AM, et al: Cat-scratch disease: isolation and culture of the bacterial agent. *JAMA* 259:1347–1352, 1988.

54. Dahlgren SE, Ekstrom P: Aspiration cytology in the diagnosis of pulmonary tuberculosis. *Scand J Resp Dis* 53:196–201, 1972.

55. Zavala DC, Schoell JE: Ultrathin needle aspiration of the lung in infectious and malignant disease. *Am Rev Respir Dis* 123:125–131, 1981.

56. Chandler FW, Watts JC: Pseudallescheriasis, *In:* Pathologic Diagnosis of Fungal Infections. Chicago, ASCP Press, 1987, pp 75–80.

57. Gorelkin L, Chandler FW: Pseudomicrobes: some potential diagnostic pitfalls in the histopathologic assessment of inflammatory lesions. *Hum Pathol* 19:954–959, 1988.

58. Hinson JM, Bradsher RW, Bodner SJ: Gram stain neutrality of mycobacterium tuberculosis. *Am Rev Respir Dis* 123:365–366, 1981.

59. Jannotta FS, Sidaway MK: The recognition of mycobacterial infections by intraoperative cytology in patients with acquired immunodeficiency syndrome. *Arch Pathol Lab Med* 113:1120–1123, 1989.

60. Lawrence C, Schreiber AJ: Leprosy footprints in bone marrow histiocytes. *New Engl J Med* 300:834–835, 1979.

61. Maygarden SJ, Flanders EL: Mycobacteria can be seen as "negative images" in cytology smears from patients with acquired immunodeficiency syndrome. *Mod Pathol* 2:239–243, 1989.

62. Stanley MW, Horwitz CA, Burton LG, et al: Negative images of bacilli and mycobacterial infection: a study of fine-needle aspiration smears from lymph nodes in patients with aids. *Diagn Cytopathol* 6:118–121, 1990.

63. Trifiro S, Bourgault A-M, Lebel F, et al: Ghost mycobacteria on gram stain. *J Clin Microbiol* 28:146–147, 1990.

64. Fisher JF, Ganapathy M, Edwards BH, et al: Utility of gram's and giemsa stains in the diagnosis of pulmonary tuberculosis. *Am Rev Respir Dis* 141:511–513, 1990.

65. Roberts FJ, Linsey S: The value of microbial cultures in diagnostic lymph-node biopsy. *J Infect Dis* 149:162–165, 1984.

66. Sommers HM, Good RC: Mycobacterium. *In:* Lennette EH, Balows A, Hausler WJ Jr, et al, Eds. Manual of Clinical Microbiology, ed 4. Washington, DC, American Society for Microbiology, 1985, pp 216–248.

67. Monheit JG, Brown G, Kott MM, et al: Calcofluor white detection of fungi in cytopathology. *Am J Clin Pathol* 85:222–225, 1986.

68. Monheit JE, Cowan DF, Moore DG: Rapid detection of fungi in tissues using calcofluor white and fluorescence microscopy. *Arch Pathol Lab Med* 108:616–618, 1984.

69. Hageage GJ, Harrington BJ: Use of calcofluor white in clinical mycology. *Lab Med* 15:109–112, 1984.

70. Gorelkin L, Chandler FW, Ewing EW Jr: Staining qualities of cytomegalovirus inclusions in the lungs of patients with the acquired immunodeficiency syndrome: a potential source of diagnostic misinterpretation. *Hum Pathol* 17:926–929, 1986.

71. Marines HM, Osato MS, Font RL: The value of calcofluor white in the diagnosis of mycotic and acanthamoeba infections of the eye and ocular adnexa. *Ophthalmology* 94:23–26, 1987.

72. Wilhelmus KR, Osato MS, Font RL, et al: Rapid diagnosis of acanthamoeba keratitis using calcofluor white. *Arch Ophthalmol* 104:1309–1312, 1986.

73. Graham AR: Fungal autofluorescence with ultraviolet illumination. *Am J Clin Pathol* 79:231–234, 1983.

74. Mann JL: Autofluorescence of fungi: an aid to detection in tissue sections. *Am J Clin Pathol* 79:587–590, 1983.

75. Farmer SG, Komorowski RA: Histologic responses to capsule-deficient *Cryptococcus neoformans.* *Arch Pathol Lab Med* 96:383–387, 1973.

76. Harding SA, Scheld WM, Feldman PS, et al: Pulmonary infection with capsule-deficient *Cryptococcus neoformans.* *Virch Arch (Pathol Anat)* 382:113–118, 1979.

77. Ro JY, Lee SS, Ayala AG: Advantage of fontana-masson stain in capsule-deficient cryptococcal infection. *Arch Pathol Lab Med* 111:53–57, 1987.

78. Barbolini G, Bisetti A, Colizzi V, et al: Immunohistologic analysis of mycobacterial antigens by monoclonal antibodies in tuberculosis in mycobacteriosis. *Hum Pathol* 20:1078–1083, 1989.

79. Conley FK, Jenkins KA, Remington JS: *Toxoplasma gondii* infection of the central nervous system use of the peroxidase-antiperoxidase method to demonstrate toxoplasma in formalin fixed, paraffin embedded tissue sections. *Hum Pathol* 12:690–698, 1981.

80. El Nageeb S, Hay RJ: Immunoperoxidase staining in the recognition of aspergillus infections. *Histopathology* 5:437–444, 1981.

81. Epstein RJ, Wilson LA, Visvesvara GS, et al: Rapid diagnosis of acanthamoeba keratitis from corneal scrapings using indirect fluorescent antibody staining. *Arch Ophthalmol* 104:1318–1321, 1986.

82. Humphrey DM, Weiner MH: Mycobacterial antigen detection by immunohistochemistry in pulmonary tuberculosis. *Hum Pathol* 18:701–708, 1987.

83. Kaplan W, Kraft DE: Demonstration of pathogenic fungi in formalin-fixed tissues by immunofluorescence. *Am J Clin Pathol* 52:420–432, 1969.

84. Moskowitz LB, Ganjei P, Ziegels-Weissman J, et al: Immunohistologic identification of fungi in systemic and cutaneous mycoses. *Arch Pathol Lab Med* 110:433–436, 1986.

85. Tschirhart D, Klatt EC: Disseminated toxoplasmosis in the acquired immunodeficiency syndrome. *Arch Pathol Lab Med* 112:1237–1241, 1988.

86. Brown SL, Bibb WF, McKinney RM: Retrospective examination of lung tissue specimens for the presence of legionella organisms: comparison of indirect fluorescent-antibody testing. *J Clin Microbiol* 19:468–472, 1984.

87. Edelstein PH: Laboratory diagnosis of infections caused by legionellae. *Eur J Clin Microbiol* 6:4–10, 1987.

88. Edelstein PH, Edelstein MAC: Evaluation of the merifluor-legionella immunofluorescent reagent for identifying and detecting 21 *Legionella* species. *J Clin Microbiol* 27:2455–2458, 1989.

89. Benson RF, Malcolm GB, Pine L, et al: Factors influencing the reactivity of *Legionella* antigens in immunofluorescence tests. *J Clin Microbiol* 17:909–917, 1983.

90. Edelstein PH, McKinney RM, Meyer RD, et al: Immunologic diagnosis of Legionnaires disease: cross-reactions with anaerobic and microaerophilic organisms and infections caused by them. *J Infect Dis* 141:652–655, 1980.

91. Orrison LH, Bibb WF, Cherry WB, et al: Determination of antigenic relationships among legionellae and non-legionellae by direct fluorescent-antibody and immunodiffusion tests. *J Clin Microbiol* 17:332–337, 1983.

92. Tenover FC, Edelstein PH, Goldstein LC, et al: Comparison of cross-staining reactions by *Pseudomonas* species and fluorescein-labelled polyclonal and monoclonal antibodies directed against *Legionella pneumophila*. *J Clin Microbiol* 23:647–649, 1986.

93. Cercenado E, Edelstein PH, Gosting LH, et al: *Legionella micdadei* and *Legionella dumoffi* monoclonal antibodies for laboratory diagnosis of *Legionella* infections. *J Clin Microbiol* 25:2163–2167, 1987.

94. Edelstein PH, Beer KB, Sturge JC, et al: Clinical utility of a monoclonal direct fluorescent reagent specific for *Legionella pneumophila:* comparative study with other reagents. *J Clin Microbiol* 22:419–421, 1985.

95. Gosting LH, Cabrian K, Sturge JC, et al: Identification of a species-specific antigen in *Legionella pneumophila* by a monoclonal antibody. *J Clin Microbiol* 20:1031–1035, 1984.

96. Alpert G, Mazeron MC, Colimon R, et al: Rapid detection of human cytomegalovirus in the urine of humans. *J Infect Dis* 152:631–633, 1985.

97. Crawford SW, Bowden RA, Hackman RC, et al: Rapid detection of cytomegalovirus pulmonary infection by bronchoalveolar lavage and centrifugation culture. *Ann Intern Med* 108:180–185, 1988.

98. DiGirolami PC, Dakos J, Eichelberger K, et al: Rapid detection of cytomegalovirus in clinical specimens by immunofluorescent staining of shell vial cultures. *Am J Clin Pathol* 89:528–532, 1988.

99. Gleaves CA, Smith TF, Shuster EA, et al: Comparison of standard T-tube and shell vial cell culture techniques for the detection of cytomegalovirus in clinical specimens. *J Clin Microbiol* 21:217–221, 1985.

100. Gleaves CA, Smith TF, Shuster EA, et al: Rapid detection of cytomegalovirus in MRC-5 cells inoculated with urine specimens by using low-speed centrifugation and monoclonal antibody to an early antigen. *J Clin Microbiol* 19:917–919, 1984.

101. Gleaves CA, Reed EC, Hackman RC, et al: Rapid diagnosis of invasive cytomegalovirus infection by examination of tissue specimens in centrifugation culture. *Am J Clin Pathol* 88:354–358, 1987.

102. Griffiths PD, Stirk PR, Ganczakowski M, et al: Rapid diagnosis of cytomegalovirus infection in immunocompromised patients by detection of early antigen fluorescent foci. *Lancet* 2:1242–1245, 1984.

103. Jesperson DJ, Drew WL, Gleaves CA, et al: Multisite evaluation of a monoclonal antibody reagent (syva) for rapid diagnosis of cytomegalovirus in the shell vial assay. *J Clin Microbiol* 27:1502–1509, 1989.

104. Martin WJ II, Smith TF: Rapid detection of cytomegalovirus in bronchoalveolar lavage specimens by a monoclonal antibody method. *J Clin Microbiol* 21:217–221, 1986.

105. Paya CV, Wold AD, Smith TF: Detection of cytomegalovirus infections in specimens other than urine by shell vial assay and conventional tube cell cultures. *J Clin Microbiology* 25:755–757, 1987.

106. Paya CV, Wold AD, Ilstrup DM, et al: Evaluation of number of shell vial cell cultures per clinical specimen for rapid diagnosis of cytomegalovirus infection. *J Clin Microbiol* 26:198–200, 1988.

107. Rice GPA, Schrier RD, Oldstone MBA: Cytomegalovirus infects human lymphocytes and monocytes: virus expression is restricted to immediate-early gene products. *Proc Natl Acad Sci USA* 81:6134–6138, 1984.

108. Thiele GM, Bicak MS, Young A, et al: Rapid detection of cytomegalovirus by tissue culture, centrifugation, and immunofluorescence with a monoclonal antibody to an early nuclear antigen. *J Virol Methods* 16:327–338, 1987.

109. Woods GL, Johnson AM, Thiele GM: Clinical comparison of two assays for rapid detection of cytomegalovirus early nuclear antigen. *Am J Clin Pathol* 93:373–377, 1990.

110. Woods GL, Young A, Johnson A, et al: Detection of cytomegalovirus by 24-well plate centrifugation assay using a monoclonal antibody to an early nuclear antigen and by conventional cell culture. *J Virol Methods* 18:207–214, 1987.

111. Woods GL, Thiele GM: Rapid detection of cytomegalovirus by 24-well plate centrifugation using a monoclonal antibody to an early nuclear antigen. *Am J Clin Pathol* 91:695–700, 1989.

112. Broaddus C, Dake MD, Stulbarg MS, et al: Bronchoalveolar lavage and transbronchial biopsy for the diagnosis of pulmonary infections in the acquired immunodeficiency syndrome. *Ann Intern Med* 102:747–752, 1985.

113. Golden JA: Cytomegalovirus—infection or disease. *Ann Intern Med* 101:882–883, 1984. Letter.

114. Ruutu P, Ruutu T, Volin L, et al: Cytomegalovirus is frequently isolated in bronchoalveolar lavage fluid of bone marrow transplant recipients without pneumonia. *Ann Intern Med* 112:913–916, 1990.

115. Stover DE, Zaman MB, Hajdu SI, et al: Bronchoalveolar lavage in the diagnosis of diffuse pulmonary infiltrates in the immunosuppressed host. *Ann Intern Med* 101:1–7, 1984.

116. Stover DE, Zaman MB, Hajdu SI, et al: Reply to cytomegalovirus—infection or disease. *Ann Intern Med* 101:883, 1984. Letter.

117. Woods G, Rennard S, Thompson A, et al: Use of bronchoalveolar lavage (bal) cytology and rapid and conventional culture techniques for diagnosis of cytomegalovirus (CMV) *Pneumonia Lab Invest* 60:107A, 1989.

118. Cardonnier C, Escudier E, Nicolas J-C, et al: Evaluation of three assays on alveolar lavage fluid in the diagnosis of cytomegalovirus pneumonitis after bone marrow transplantation. *J Infect Dis* 155:495–500, 1987.

119. Culpepper-Morgan JA, Kotler DP, Scholes JV, et al: Evaluation of diagnostic criteria for mucosal cytomegalic inclusion disease in the acquired immune deficiency syndrome. *Am J Gastroenterol* 82:1264–1270, 1987.

120. Emanuel D, Peppard J, Stover D, et al: Rapid diagnosis of cytomegalovirus pneumonia by bronchoalveolar lavage using human and murine monoclonal antibodies. *Ann Intern Med* 104:476–481, 1986.

121. Goldstein LC, McDougall J, Hackman R, et al: Monoclonal antibodies to cytomegalovirus: rapid identification of clinical isolates and preliminary use in diagnosis of cytomegalovirus pneumonia. *Infect Immunol* 38:273–281, 1982.

122. Hackman RC, Myerson D, Meyers JD, et al: Rapid diagnosis of cytomegaloviral pneumonia by tissue immunofluorescence with a murine monoclonal antibody. *J Infect Dis* 151:325–329, 1985.

123. Masih A, Rennard SI, Binkley LI, et al: Detection of cytomegalovirus in bronchoalveolar lavage specimens by cytology, tissue culture, fluorescent monoclonal antibodies and in situ hybridization. *Acta Cytol* 31:648, 1987.

124. Sacks SL, Freeman HJ: Cytomegalovirus hepatitis: evidence for direct hepatic viral infection using monoclonal antibodies. *Gastroenterology* 86:346–350, 1984.

125. Spector SA, Rua JA, Spector DH, et al: Detection of human cytomegalovirus in clinical specimens. *J Infect Dis* 150:121–126, 1984.

126. Springmeyer SC, Hackman RC, Holle R, et al: Use of bronchoalveolar lavage to diagnose acute diffuse pneumonia in the immunocompetent host. *J Infect Dis* 154:604–610, 1986.

127. Volpi A, Whitley RJ, Ceballos R, et al: Rapid diagnosis of pneumonia due to cytomegalovirus with specific monoclonal antibodies. *J Infect Dis* 147:1119–1120, 1983.

128. Gal AA, Klatt EC, Koss MN, et al: The effectiveness of bronchoscopy in the diagnosis of *Pneumocystis carinii* and cytomegalovirus pulmonary infections in acquired immunodeficiency syndrome. *Arch Pathol Lab Med* 111:238–241, 1987.

129. Myerson D, Hackman RC, Meyers JD: Diagnosis of cytomegaloviral pneumonia by in situ hybridization. *J Infect Dis* 150:272–277, 1984.

130. Shields AF, Hackman RC, Fife KH, et al: Adenovirus infection in patients undergoing bone-marrow transplantation. *New Engl J Med* 312:529–533, 1985.

131. Walpita P, Darougar S: Double-label immunofluorescence method for simultaneous detection of adenovirus and herpes simplex virus from the eye. *J Clin Microbiol* 27:1623–1625, 1989.

132. Allen KA, Markin RS, Rennard SI, et al: Bronchoalveolar lavage in liver transplant patients. *Acta Cytol* 35:539–543, 1989.

133. Brigati DJ, Myerson D, Leary JJ, et al: Detection of viral genomes in cultured cells and paraffin-embedded tissue sections using biotin-labeled hybridization probes. *Virology* 126:32–50, 1983.

134. Chebab FF, Xiao X, Kan YW, et al: Detection of cytomegalovirus infection in paraffin-embedded tissue specimens with the polymerase chain reaction. *Mod Pathol* 2:75–78, 1989.

135. Chou S, Merigan TC: Rapid detection and quantitation of human cytomegalovirus in urine through DNA hybridization. *N Engl J Med* 308:921–925, 1983.

136. Churchill MA, Zaia JA, Forman SJ, et al: Quantitation of human cytomegalovirus DNA in lungs from bone marrow transplant recipients with interstitial pneumonia. *J Infect Dis* 155:501–509, 1987.

137. Clayton F, Klein EB, Kotler DP: Correlation of in situ hybridization with histology and viral culture in patients with acquired immunodeficiency syndrome with cytomegalovirus colitis. *Arch Pathol Lab Med* 113:1124–1126, 1989.

138. Gnann JW Jr, Ahlmen J, Svalander C, et al: Inflammatory cells in transplanted kidneys are infected by human cytomegalovirus. *Am J Pathol* 132:239–248, 1988.

139. Grody WW, Cheng L, Lewin KJ: In situ viral DNA hybridization in diagnostic surgical pathology. *Hum Pathol* 18:535–543, 1987.

140. Haase AT: Analysis of viral infections by in situ hybridization. *J Histochem Cytochem* 34:27–32, 1986.

141. Hilborne LH, Nieberg RK, Cheng L, et al: Direct in situ hybridization for rapid detection of cytomegalovirus in bronchoalveolar lavage. *Am J Clin Pathol* 87:766–769, 1987.

142. Keh WC, Gerber MA: In situ hybridization for cytomegalovirus DNA in AIDS patients. *Am J Pathol* 131:490–496, 1988.

143. Loning T, Milde K, Foss H-D: In situ hybridization for the detection of cytomegalovirus (CMV) infection. *Virchows Arch (Pathol Anat)* 409:777–790, 1986.

144. McDougall JK, Myerson D, Beckman AM: Detection of viral DNA and RNA by in situ hybridization. *J Histochem Cytochem* 34:33–38, 1986.

145. Myerson D, Hackman RC, Nelson JA, et al: Widespread presence of histologically occult cytomegalovirus. *Hum Pathol* 15:430–439, 1984.

146. Niedobitek G, Finn T, Herbst H, et al: Detection of cytomegalovirus by in situ hybridization and immunohistochemistry using new monoclonal antibody cch2: a comparison of methods. *J Clin Pathol* 41:1005–1009, 1988.

147. Niedobitek G, Finn T, Herbst H, et al: Detection of viral genomes in the liver by in situ hybridization using 35S-, bromodeoxyuridine-, and biotin-labeled probes. *Am J Pathol* 134:633–639, 1989.

148. Porter HJ, Heryet A, Quantrill AM, et al: Combined non-isotopic in situ hybridization and immunohistochemistry on routine parafin wax embedded tissue: identification of cell type infected by human parvovirus and demonstration of cytomegalovirus DNA and antigen in renal infection. *J Clin Pathol* 43:129–132, 1990.

149. Roberts WH, Hammond S, Sneddon JM, et al: In situ DNA hybridization for cytomegalovirus in colonoscopic biopsies. *Arch Pathol Lab Med* 112:1106–1109, 1988.

150. Schrier RD, Nelson JA, Oldston MBA: Detection of human cytomegalovirus in peripheral blood lymphocytes in a natural infection. *Science* 230:1048–1051, 1985.

151. Seto E, Yen TSB: Detection of cytomegalovirus infection by means of DNA isolated from paraffin-embedded tissues and dot hybridization. *Am J Pathol* 127:409–413, 1987.

152. Shibata D, Klatt EC: Analysis of human immunodeficiency virus and cytomegalovirus infection by polymerase chain reaction in the acquired immunodeficiency syndrome. *Arch Pathol Lab Med* 113:1239–1244, 1989.

153. Shibata D, Martin WJ, Appleman MD, et al: Detection of cytomegalovirus DNA in peripheral blood of patients infected with human immunodeficiency virus. *J Infect Dis* 158:1185–1192, 1988.

154. Ulrich W, Schlederer MP, Buxbaum P, et al: The histopathologic identification of CMV infected cells in biopsies of human renal allografts: an evaluation of 100 transplant biopsies by in situ hybridization. *Pathol Res Pract* 181:739–745, 1986.

155. Abbondanzo SL, English CK, Kagan E, et al: Fatal adenovirus pneumonia in a newborn identified by electron microscopy and in situ hybridization. *Arch Pathol Lab Med* 113:1349–1353, 1989.

156. Geradts J, Wamock M, Yen TSB: Use of the polymerase chain reaction in the diagnosis of unsuspected herpes simplex viral pneumonia: report of a case. *Hum Pathol* 21:118–121, 1990.

157. Green WR, Williams AW: Neonatal adenovirus pneumonia. *Arch Pathol Lab Med* 113:190–191, 1989.

158. Tenover FC: Diagnostic deoxyribonucleic acid probes for infectious diseases. *Clin Microbiol Rev* 1:82–101, 1988.

159. Zwadyk P Jr: DNA probes—reality or glitter and hype? *Clin Microbiol Newslett* 11:84–86, 1989.

160. Doebbeling BN, Bale MJ, Koonty FP, et al: Prospective evaluation of the gen-probe assay for detection of legionellae in respiratory specimens. *Eur J Clin Microbiol Infect Dis* 7:748–752, 1988.

161. Edelstein PH: Evaluation of the gen-probe DNA probe for the detection of legionellae in culture. *J Clin Microbiol* 23:481–484, 1986.

162. Edelstein PH, Bryan RN, Enns RK, et al: Retrospective study of gen-probe rapid diagnostic system for detection of legionellae in frozen clinical respiratory tract samples. *J Clin Microbiol* 25:1022–1026, 1987.

163. Laussucq S, Schuster D, Alexander WJ, et al: False-positive DNA probe test for *Legionella* species associated with a cluster of respiratory illnesses. *J Clin Microbiol* 26:1442–1444, 1988.

164. Wilkinson HW, Sampson JS, Plikaytis BB. Evaluation of a commercial gene probe for identification of *Legionella* cultures. *J Clin Microbiol* 23:207–220, 1986.

165. Grange JM: The rapid diagnosis of paucibacillary tuberculosis. *Tubercle* 70:1–4, 1989.

166. Drake TA, Herron RM Jr, Hindler JA, et al: DNA probe reactivity of mycobacterium avium complex isolates from patients without AIDS. *Diagn Microbiol Infect Dis* 11:125–128, 1988.

167. Drake TA, Hindler JA, Berlin OGW, et al: Rapid identification of mycobacterium avium complex in culture using DNA probes. *J Clin Microbiol* 25:1442–1445, 1987.

168. Gonzales R, Hanna BA: Evaluation of gen-probe DNA hybridization systems for the identification of mycobacterium tuberculosis and mycobacterium avium-intracellulare. *Diagn Microbiol Infect Dis* 8:69–78, 1987.

169. Kiehn TE, Edwards FF: Rapid identification using a specific DNA probe of mycobacterium avium complex from patients with acquired immunodeficiency syndrome. *J Clin Microbiol* 25:1551–1552, 1987.

170. Peterson EM, Lu R, Floyd C, et al: Direct identification of mycobacterium tuberculosis, mycobacterium avium, and mycobacterium intracellulare from amplified primary cultures in BACTEC media using DNA probes. *J Clin Microbiol* 27:1543–1547, 1989.

171. Roberts MC, McMillan C, Coyle MB: Whole chromosomal DNA probes for rapid identification of mycobacterium tuberculosis and mycobacterium avium complex. *J Clin Microbiol* 25:1239–1243, 1987.

172. Ellner PD, Kiehn TE, Cammarata R, et al: Rapid detection and identification of pathologenic mycobacteria by combining radiometric and nucleic acid probe methods. *J Clin Microbiol* 26:1349–1352, 1988.

173. Musial CE, Tice LS, Stockman L, et al: Identification of mycobacteria from culture using the gen-probe rapid diagnostic system for mycobacterium avium complex and mycobacterium tuberculosis complex. *J Clin Microbiol* 26:2120–2123, 1988.

174. Body BA, Warren NG, Spicer A, et al: Use of gen-probe and BACTEC for rapid isolation and identification of mycobacteria correlation of probe results with growth index. *Am J Clin Pathol* 93:415–420, 1990.

175. Sherman I, Harrington N, Rothrock A, et al: Use of a cutoff range in identifying mycobacteria by the gen-probe rapid diagnostic system. *J Clin Microbiol* 27:241–244, 1989.

176. Gray LD, Roberts GD: Laboratory diagnosis of systemic fungal diseases. *Infect Dis Clin North Am* 2:779–804, 1988.

177. Isenberg HD, Schoenknecht FD, von Graevenitz A: Collection and processing of bacteriological specimens, cumitech 9. Washington, DC: American Society for Microbiology, 1979, p 22.

178. Sutter VL, Citron DM, Edelstein MAC, et al: Wadsworth Anaerobic Bacteriology Manual, ed 4. Belmont, Calif, Star Publishing Company, 1985, p 152.

179. Unger ER, Budgeon LR, Myerson D, et al: Viral diagnosis by in situ hybridization description of a rapid simplified colorimetric method. *Am J Surg Pathol* 10:1–8, 1986.

4

Identification of Infectious Microorganisms

Jamie L. Covell
Philip S. Feldman

A wide variety of infectious microorganisms may be seen in fine-needle aspiration (FNA) smears. Many organisms can be distinguished by their morphologic features in routine Papanicolaou and Romanovsky-type stained smears, whereas others require special stains or culture for precise identification. It is important to remember that more than one type of microorganism may be present in a specimen (especially in immunocompromised patients) and that the presence of an infectious organism does not exclude the possibility of a coexisting neoplasm. The patterns of inflammatory response to the microorganisms described herein are discussed in more detail in other chapters.

BACTERIA

Mycobacteria

Mycobacteria are aerobic, nonsporulating, motile bacilli that can produce infections in many organs and tissues accessible to FNA.[1] FNA smears of infected sites usually show granulomatous inflammation and often necrosis. The bacilli are not visible in Papanicolaou-stained material but can be seen as negative images in Romanovsky-stained (Wright–Giemsa) and Diff-Quik stained smears.[2] Acid-fast staining and culture of aspirated material are needed for specific identification. Acid-fast smears demonstrate slender, slightly curved or straight rods that may appear beaded.[1]

M. tuberculosis is the most commonly occurring species causing pulmonary tuberculosis and extrapulmonary disease involving numerous organs.[3-15] The organism is a slender, curved bacillus averaging four microns in length and less than one micron in diameter (Fig. 4.1).[16]

M. avium-intracellulare occasionally causes pulmonary disease in adults and lymph node infections in children (Fig. 4.2).[1,7,17] Its morphology is indistinguishable from

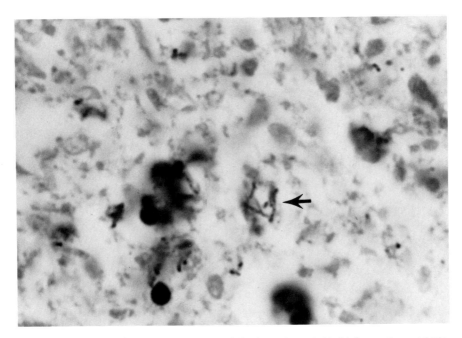

Fig. 4.1. *M. tuberculosis* in FNA smear of the lung (*arrow*) (Acid-fast stain; ×1000).

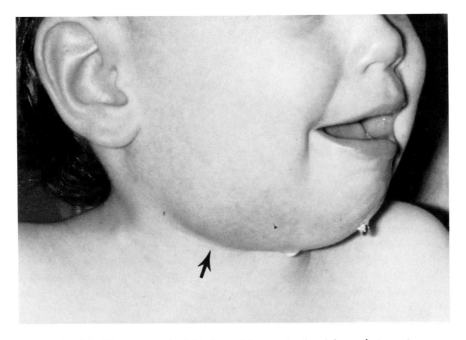

Fig. 4.2. Sixteen-month-old infant with mass in the right neck (*arrow*).

that of the tubercle bacillus (Plate 1). *M. kansaii* can cause pulmonary disease indistinguishable from tuberculosis. This beaded bacillus is longer and broader than the usual *M. tuberculosis.*[18]

M. leprae (Hansen's bacillus) is the causative agent of leprosy, a disease involving the skin and peripheral nerves, as well as other organs.[1] The organisms are morphologically similar to *M. tuberculosis* and are predominantly intracellular. They are typically seen in Fite's acid-fast stained smears as intracellular bundles of bacilli called globi (especially, lepromatous type) but may also be found free in the smear background. Bundles of bacilli are scarce in other mycobacterial infections.[1,19-20]

Legionella

Legionella species are aerobic, motile, pleomorphic gram-negative bacilli that primarily infect the lung.[1,4] The genus was first recognized after its identification as the etiologic agent of the 1976 outbreak of pneumonia known as Legionnaires' disease.[1,21] The original species was named *L. pneumophilia;* however, additional species are now generally accepted within this group.[1]

FNA smears usually demonstrate a marked acute inflammatory exudate with abundant fibrin.[21] The bacilli are not visible in Papanicolaou-stained material. Modified Gram stain, Giemsa, Diff-Quik, Fite's modified acid-fast stain, and Dieterle silver impregnation stain demonstrate the organisms which appear as slender, short rods that tend to cluster in macrophages. Direct fluorescent antibody studies are used to confirm the diagnosis.[1,4,21,22]

L. micdadei acts as an opportunistic pathogen producing pulmonary infection in immunocompromised patients. The bacilli are found within the cytoplasm of neutrophils and macrophages as well as extracellularly with the Fite's acid-fast stain (Plate 2).[23] Direct fluorescent antibody studies are helpful in the specific identification of the organism (Plate 2).

Actinomyces

The actinomyces are members of a genus of gram-positive, non acid-fast bacteria. They produce chronic suppurative inflammatory disease (actinomycosis) that generally involves the head and neck region but may also infect the lungs and other sites accessible to FNA.[1,7,21,24-28] Aspiration smears typically contain an acute and chronic inflammatory exudate with necrosis suggesting abscess formation.[26,27,29]

The microorganisms, as seen in Papanicolaou, Wright-Giemsa, and Diff-Quik stained smears, are fine, straight or wavy filaments. They are approximately 1 to 1.5 microns in diameter but are variable in length (20–70 microns) and degree of branching (Fig. 4.3). Characteristic sulfur granules are identified as round or oval microcolonies, 75 to 160 microns in diameter, composed of finely granular centers surrounded by a radiating fringe of thin bacterial filaments (Fig. 4.4). Occasional filaments show acute angle branching and club-shaped tips.[1,21,24,25,27,28,29]

Gram stain demonstrates the fine detail of pleomorphic branching filaments with diphtheroid-like morphology admixed with coccobacilliary forms giving a beaded appearance.[21] The organisms also stain positively with Gomori's methenamine-silver (GMS) but are not acid-fast.[24,25,27,28] Direct fluorescent antibody studies or

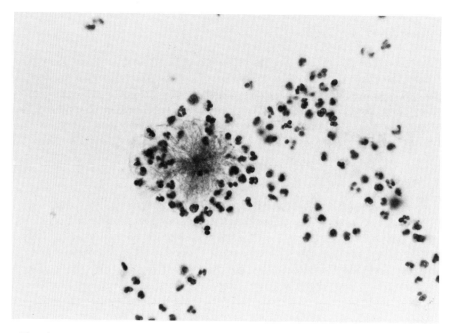

Fig. 4.3. *Actinomyces* in FNA smear of a pelvic mass (Papanicolaou stain; ×400).

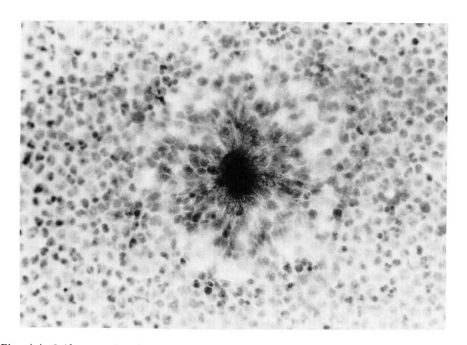

Fig. 4.4. Sulfur granule of *Actinomyces* in FNA smear of a pelvic mass (Wright–Giemsa stain; ×400).

aerobic culture provide precise identification.[21,30] *A. israelii* is the species most frequently reported in the FNA literature.

Nocardia

Nocardia is a genus of gram-positive aerobic bacteria related to Actinomyces.[1] The most common species, *N. asteroides,* is an opportunistic pulmonary infection, often in an immunocompromised host, that has a predilection for spread to the central nervous system. The infection usually produces chronic suppurative disease leading to abscess formation. Although unusual, the presence of granulomas has been described in nocardiosis.[1,21,22]

FNA smears from these lesions contain a marked acute inflammatory exudate and necrotic debris.[31] The microorganisms are not visible with Papanicolaou and H&E stains. However, Gram strains, GMS stain, Fite's acid-fast stain, Gram-Weigert stain, and Giemsa stain can be used to demonstrate their morphology.[21,31] They appear as thin, delicate branching filaments approximately 0.5 to 1 micron in diameter and 10 to 20 microns in length (Plate 3). Branching is extensive and more or less at right angles. The filaments tend to break into bacillary or coccal forms. Sulfur granules are generally absent.[31] Direct fluorescent antibody studies and culture provide specific confirmation of the disease.[30]

Miscellaneous Bacteria

Numerous species of gram-negative and gram-positive bacilli and cocci can infect organs and tissues throughout the body and may cause abscess formation (Fig. 4.5)[4,7,8,9,14,32,33] FNA smears of the infected sites usually contain a marked acute and/or chronic inflammatory exudate. The microorganisms may be visible in Papanicolaou-stained smears but are more clearly seen in Wright, Wright-Giemsa, or Diff-Quik smears (Plate 4). Gram stains may also be used to demonstrate the organisms. Culture of the aspirated material is necessary for precise identification.

Golfo and Galindo reported a rare case of granuloma inguinale diagnosed by FNA.[34] Diff-Quik stained smears revealed acute and chronic inflammation with foamy histiocytes containing typical Donovan bodies (pleomorphic coccobacillary microorganisms) within cytoplasmic vacuoles. Extracellular microorganisms with similar morphology were also observed.

FUNGI

Aspergillus

Aspergillus is one of the more frequently encountered mycotic organisms in needle aspirations.[29] It is an opportunistic pathogen that may produce saprophytic infestations in cavitary lesions or invade the lungs and spread to other organs in immunocompromised patients (systematic or invasive aspergillosis) (Fig. 4.6).[1,8,14,21,35,36,37]

In Papanicolaou or H&E-stained FNA smears, the organism is identified as pale staining, relatively uniform, septate hyphae with parallel walls 3 to 6 microns in diameter and regular dichotomous branching at 45° angles (Plate 5).[1,21,29,31,37] The

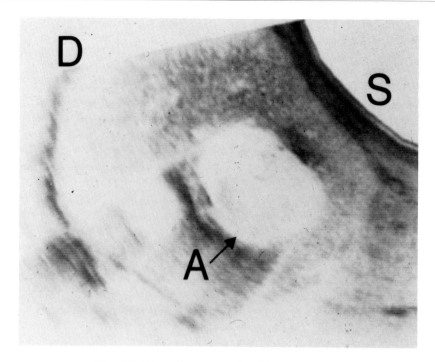

Fig. 4.5. Liver abscess visualized by ultrasound.

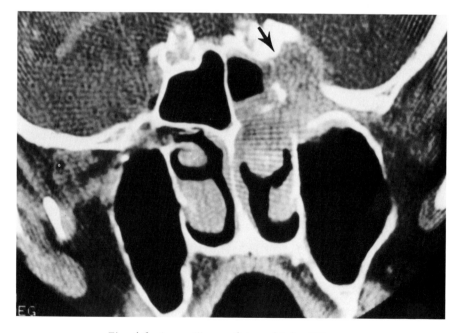

Fig. 4.6. Aspergilloma of the orbit by CT scan.

hyphae may be seen as long strands or in tangled masses. Sporulation with formation of fruiting heads is uncommon but may occur in cavities exposed to air.[21] The fungal forms stain poorly with Wright or Diff-Quik stains but are clearly demonstrated with periodic acid–Schiff (PAS) and GMS stains.[21] Immunoperoxidase staining and culture can be used for specific identification (Plate 5).[1,21,38,39] The smear background usually contains an acute inflammatory exudate with necrosis.[36,37] In extensively necrotic lesions the hyphae may present only in small pieces that are more difficult to identify. Aspiration smears from later stage infections may show a chronic or granulomatous inflammatory response.[37]

Candida

Candida species can act as opportunistic pathogens in immunocompromised patients, causing infections in many body sites.[1] They are identified as hyphae or pseudohyphae showing distinct points of constriction simulating sausage links with budding yeast forms 3 to 4 microns in size.[21] The microorganisms are visible with Papanicolaou, H&E, Wright, or Diff-Quik stains (Figs. 4.7 and 4.8). Their morphology is more clearly demonstrated using the GMS stain. Immunoperoxidase staining and culture may be used for precise diagnosis.[39] The tissue reaction in these infections is usually an acute, purulent inflammatory response in the early stages with some tendency to granuloma formation in chronic disease.[21]

Zygomycetes (Phycomycetes)

Zygomycetes, which include *Mucor, Rhizopus,* and *Absidia,* are opportunistic fungi that can cause infections in a wide variety of organs including the paranasal sinuses, orbit, palate, brain, lung, gastrointestinal tract, and skin of immunocompromised patients.[1,21,29,35,40] FNA smears of these lesions contain acute inflammation with necrotic debris and broad, ribbonlike hyphae devoid of septae (Plate 6).[21,29,31,40] The hyphae range from 3 to 25 microns in width and have nonparallel walls. Branching is common, although the angle and spacing of the branches are irregular. Partially collapsed and distorted hyphae may also be seen. The organisms can be easily seen with the Papanicolaou and H&E stains. However, they can show poor staining with fungal stains (PAS, GMS) and Wright or Diff-Quik stains.[21,31] The FNA diagnosis is based primarily on the morphology of the fungal forms, but culture may be used for confirmation.

Phaeohyphomycosis

Phaeohyphomycosis is an uncommon variety of opportunistic infection in immunocompromised, debilitated patients. It is caused by certain species of dematiaceous or pigmented fungi.[21,41,42] The infections may be localized superficial cutaneous and subcutaneous lesions or a systemic process.[21] FNA of subcutaneous lesions (phaeomycotic cysts) is described in the literature.[41,42] Aspiration smears can contain an admixture of acute and granulomatous inflammation, necrosis, and fungal forms. The fungal elements consist of pseudohyphae composed of round, oval, or rectangular bodies resembling a string of beads (Fig. 4.9). Some show transition from pseudohyphae to true septate hyphae having widths of 2 to 3 microns. The

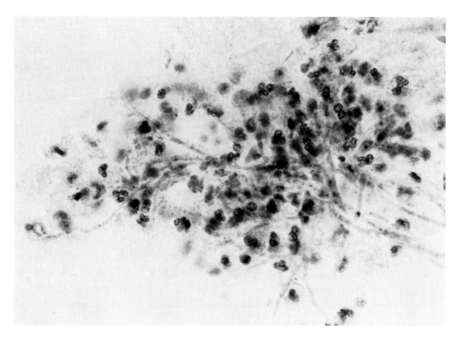

Fig. 4.7. *Candida* species in FNA smear of the lung (Papanicolaou stain; × 400).

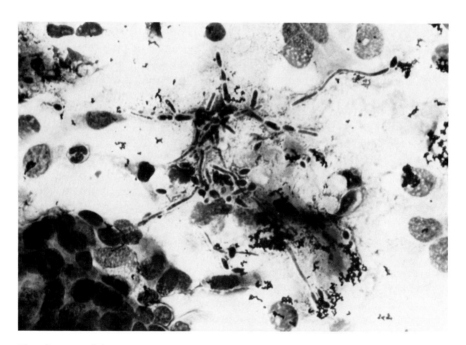

Fig. 4.8. *Candida* species in FNA smear of the lung (Wright–Giemsa stain, × 400).

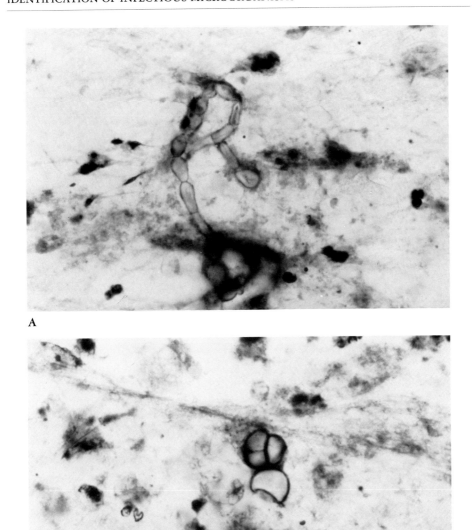

A

B

Fig. 4.9. A. Aspirate of pulmonary phaeohyphomycosis infection demonstrating pseudo-hyphae composed of oval to rectangular bodies resembling string of beads (Papanicolaou stain; ×250) (Courtesy of Dr. Vicki J. Schnadig, University of Texas Medical Branch, Galveston, TX). **B.** Lung aspirate containing true multiseptate body (muriform cell) of phaeohyphomycosis (Papanicolaou stain; ×250). (Courtesy of Dr. Vicki J. Schnadig).

hyphae often demonstrate dichotomous branching. Individual yeastlike cells are approximately 3 microns wide but vary in length and may show budding. Fungal forms are seen within the giant cells and in the smear background. The cell walls range from clear and hyaline to pale yellow-brown or red-brown in color with the Papanicolaou and H&E stains, respectively. GMS stain can also be used to demonstrate the morphologic structure. The exact species of the microorganism is identified by culture.[21]

Blastomyces

Blastomyces dermatitidis is a pathogenic dimorphic fungus that causes chronic granulomatous and suppurative disease (blastomycosis) that usually begins in the lung but may spread to skin, bone, and other organs.[1,21,29,31,32,43] FNA smears will usually demonstrate acute or granulomatous inflammation with relatively large (8–20 microns) yeast forms having thick, refractile, double-contoured walls (Fig. 4.10, Plate 7).[21,29,31] The protoplasm often retracts from the cell wall, leaving a clear space. In Papanicolaou-stained smears the cell wall is blue-green with brown protoplasm. Budding occurs as single buds attached by a broad base (Plate 7). When granulomatous inflammation is present, the organisms may be seen within the cytoplasm of the giant cells as well as in the smear background.[31]

These yeast forms stain poorly with Wright-Giemsa and Diff-Quik stains but are visible in relief against the darker-staining background. GMS stain is excellent for demonstrating the organism.[31] Direct fluorescent antibody studies and culture may be used as confirmatory tests.[1] *B. dermatitidis* is differentiated from other budding yeasts by its overall larger size and characteristic broad-based budding.

Cryptococcus

Cryptococcus neoformans is a pathogenic yeast that causes subacute or chronic fungal disease (cryptococcosis) in the lungs, central nervous system, bone, and other organs (usually in debilitated patients).[1,4,7,18,29,37,44-48] The organisms are round or oval yeasts (5–10 microns) surrounded by a clear, thick mucopolysaccharide capsule. Budding occurs as predominantly single, narrow-based, teardrop-shaped forms.[1,21,29,37,44,45,46,48] In some cases cryptococcus may not be easily seen in Papanicolaou, Wright-Giemsa, or Diff-Quik stained smears but can be identified within macrophages or in relief against a darker-staining background (Plate 8). PAS, mucicarmine, alcian blue, and colloidal iron stains can be used to demonstrate the capsule (Plate 8).[44,45,46,48] GMS stains the organism (Fig. 4.11). Immunoperoxidase and/or immunofluorescent antibody studies and culture can be used for specific identification.[1,39]

FNA smears from early localized lesions may show only scattered organisms, mucoid material, and little inflammation.[45] Aspiration of later lesions may yield an acute inflammatory exudate with necrosis and/or granulomatous inflammation.[21,46] *Cryptococcus* is differentiated from *Blastomyces* by its smaller size, thick capsule, and narrow budding.

Nonencapsulated forms of *Cryptococcus* occur and when seen within the cytoplasm of macrophages, can be confused with *Histoplasma capsulatum*.[21] Positive Fontana–Masson staining helps confirm the diagnosis of nonencapsulated *Cryptococcus*. The

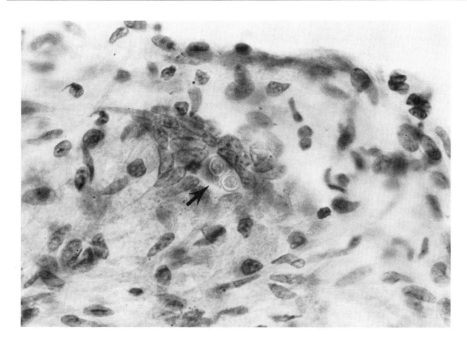

Fig. 4.10. Multinucleated giant cell with blastomyces in FNA smear of the lung (*arrow*).

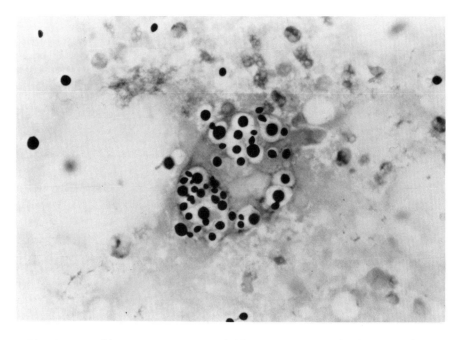

Fig. 4.11. Budding *Cryptococcus* engulfed by a macrophage (GMS stain; ×400).

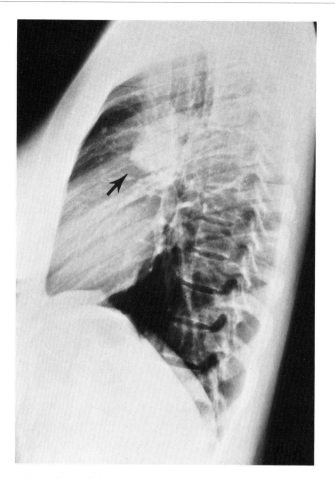

Fig. 4.12. Histoplasmosis. Well demarcated lung mass on chest roentgenogram, lateral view.

cryptococcal organisms can be recognized by their varied sizes, whereas histoplasma yeasts are uniformly small. In difficult cases, especially when only a few organisms are present, culture or immunofluorescent antibody testing is necessary for definitive diagnosis.[1,21]

Histoplasma

Histoplasma capsulatum is a pathogenic dimorphic fungus that can cause systemic infections (histoplasmosis) that begin in the lungs and disseminate via the reticuloendothelial system (Fig. 4.12).[1,4,18,49,50,51] The organisms are identified most often as oval yeast forms 3 to 5 microns in diameter found within the cytoplasm of macrophages. Budding occurs as single buds with a narrow hairlike neck.[21,29,49]

FNA smears usually contain granulomatous inflammation admixed with lymphocytes, neutrophils, and/or necrosis. The macrophages appear to have "bubbly" cytoplasm, and high-power examination reveals that the cytoplasm contains numerous pale-staining microorganisms surrounded by rigid cell walls (Plate 9).[31,50,51] The protoplasm of these organisms may pull away from the wall, producing a clear

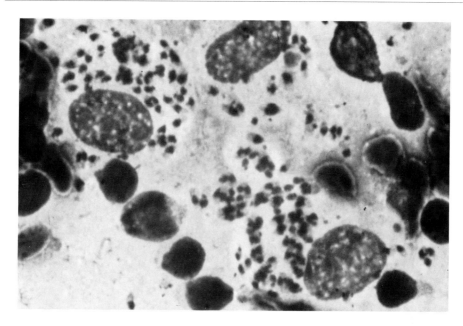

Fig. 4.13. FNA of cutaneous leishmaniasis demonstrating numerous *Leishmania* organisms within histiocytes (Diff-Quik stain; ×1250) (Courtesy of Dr. Miguel Perez-Guillermo, University of Murcia, Faculty of Medicine, Cartagena, Spain).

space, but there is no true capsule.[21] In smears stained with Papanicolaou, H&E, Wright–Giemsa, or Diff-Quik stains, the yeasts are seen almost exclusively within macrophages.[50,51] Their pale staining makes them difficult to appreciate extracellularly. GMS and PAS stains are used to demonstrate the organisms more clearly (Plate 9), and the diagnosis is confirmed by immunoperoxidase staining or culture.[21,39,50,51]

FNA of leishmaniasis can be confused with histoplasmosis, since the *Leishmania* organisms can be found both extracellularly and within histiocytes and are in the size range of 2 to 4 microns (Fig. 4.13). High-power magnification will reveal the nucleus and small paranucleus or kinetoplast of the *Leishmania* organisms. *Leishmania* organisms, in contrast to *Histoplasma,* do not show budding. Perez-Guillermo and associates recently reported the FNA cytologic findings of a case of cutaneous leishmaniasis.[52]

Coccidioides

Coccidioides immitis is a pathogenic dimorphic fungus prevalent in the southwestern United States (especially the San Joaquin Valley), Mexico, and Central America. It is the causative agent of coccidioidomycosis.[1,21] The organism is highly infectious and produces primarily pulmonary disease, but it may involve other organs and tissues.[1,7,9,14,21,29,53,54]

FNA smears contain acute, chronic, or granulomatous inflammation with necrosis.[29,54] *C. immitis* presents as large, thick-walled, nonbudding round structures (spherules) ranging from 5 to 100 microns in diameter with an average size of 10 to 40 microns (Fig. 4.14).[21,29,54] The walls are highly refractile and often double

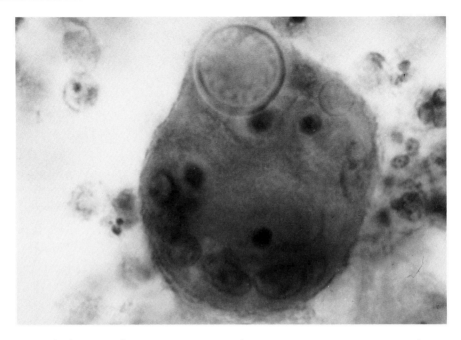

Fig. 4.14. *Cocciciodes* with a multinucleated giant cell (Papanicolaou stain; ×600).

contoured. The spherules contain numerous small endospores 2 to 5 microns in size. Immature spherules, which are small and do not contain endospores, may be confused with *Blastomyces*.[21] Older spherules present as folded, fractured, or collapsed membranes. When the spherules rupture, the endospores may spill out into the smears and resemble *H. capsulatum*.[21] However, these endospores are rarely found in macrophages in contrast to the presentation of the yeast form of *Histoplasma*.

Mycelial forms may also be identified in some cases.[21,54] They present as branched septate hyphae approximately 2 microns thick. Spaced along the hyphae are barrel-shaped arthroconidea 2 to 4 microns in width and 3 to 6 microns in length. These structures are believed to form when the organisms are exposed to air at room temperature.

In Papanicolaou and H&E-stained smears, the organisms are orange to reddish purple. With Wright–Giemsa or Diff-Quik stains, they appear as colorless, highly refractile structures. GMS and PAS stains are used to better demonstrate the fungi.[54] The diagnosis is confirmed by culture.

PARASITES

Pneumocystis

Pneumocystis carinii is an opportunistic parasite of uncertain classification that is one of the most common causes of nonbacterial pneumonia in premature infants, malnourished children, and immunocompromised individuals (especially those with AIDS).[21,55] FNA provides a relatively simple method for evaluating these pneumonias but is seldom used because of the diagnostic accuracy of bronchoalveolar lavage (BAL).[29,35,56,57,58]

The organism occurs in two distinct forms, the cyst (5–8 microns) and the trophozoite (1–2 microns).[55] A number of stains are useful in the identification of pneumocystis. Toluidine blue (fresh material) or GMS and Gram–Weigert stains (fixed material) demonstrate the cyst wall but only sparingly reveal intracystic contents (Plate 10).[29,55,59-62] The cysts appear as rounded, cup-shaped or comma-shaped structures. Wright stain, modified Giemsa stain, or Diff-Quik stain have an affinity for the trophozoites without staining the cyst wall.[37,55,59,60,61] The trophozoites present as 6 to 8 ovoid bodies arranged in a ring pattern within a refractile cyst (Fig. 4.15).

In Papanicolaou and H&E-stained smears, the organisms are most often found within clumps of foamy alveolar exudate.[61,63,64] They appear as colorless round or cup-shaped structures seen in relief against gray-green or pink staining amorphous material (Plate 10). These structures must be identified in order to differentiate the "alveolar casts" from aggregates of hemosiderin or other debris. Although the organisms do not appear to stain by the Papanicolaou method, they exhibit a distinct yellowish-green fluorescence when Papanicolaou-stained material is viewed under ultraviolet light.[61,65] This feature can be used to complement the special stain findings for making the cytologic diagnosis.

P. carinii cannot be routinely cultured; however, immunofluorescent and immunoperoxidase monoclonal antibody techniques can be used as confirmatory tests.[21,66,67]

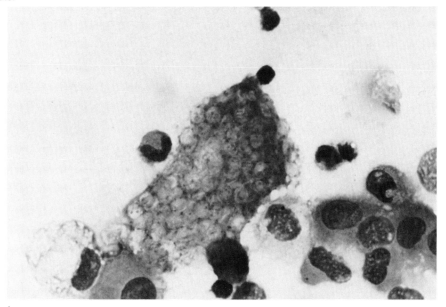

A

Fig. 4.15. A. Clump of nonstaining cysts of *P. carinii* (Diff-Quick stain; ×250). (From Silverman JF: Cytologic Diagnosis In Acquired Immunodeficiency Syndrome. In: *Pathology Of Aids And Other Manifestations Of HIV Infection,* Ed. Joshi VV. New York, Igaku-Shoin, 1990.)

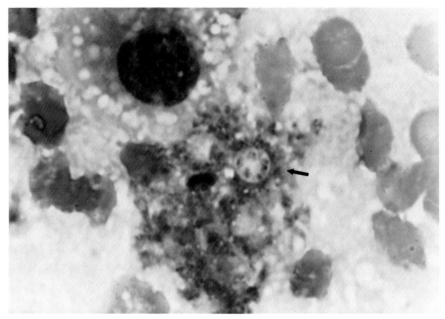

B

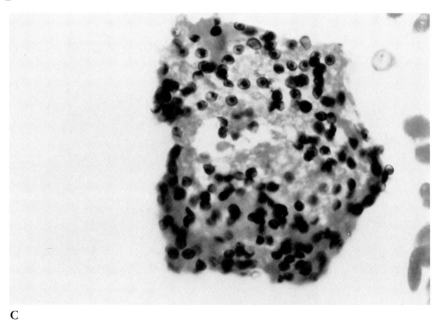

C

Fig. 4.15. B. Trophozoites of *P. carinii* in FNA smear of the lung (Wright–Giemsa stain; ×1000). **C.** (GMS stain; ×400). (From Silverman JF: Cytologic Diagnosis In Acquired Immunodeficiency Syndrome. In: *Pathology Of Aids And Other Manifestations Of HIV Infection,* Ed. Joshi VV. New York, Igaku-Shoin, 1990.)

TISSUE HELMINTHS

Filariae

Filariae include several species of parasitic nematodes that are transmitted to humans by the bite of a mosquito or other arthropod and cause the disease known as filariasis, or elephantiasis.[1,21] The organisms usually inhabit the lymphatic channels and peripheral blood, but they may be found in a variety of other organs accessible to FNA.[1,21,68-72]

The diagnosis is usually made by the identification of the larval forms called microfilaria.[1,21,67-71] Microfilariae are slender, long, ribbonlike organisms measuring up to 200 microns in length and about 7 microns in width. They may possess a sheath. Individual species can be identified by their size ranges and morphology of the tail sections. The background of FNA smears contain chronic and/or granulomatous inflammation with necrosis.

Dirofilaria species usually infects animals but may occasionally be found in humans who serve as accidental hosts.[21] Infection produces granulomatous nodules in the lung or subcutaneous tissues.[21,73,74] The disease is self-limited, since humans are inappropriate hosts and the life cycle of the organism cannot be completed. The nodules contain immature adult worms. Microfilariae are not produced.[21]

Trichinella

Trichinosis is a parasitic disease caused by infection with the nematode *Trichinella spiralis* resulting from the ingestion of raw or poorly cooked meat, especially pork or pork products, containing encysted larvae.[1,21] The larvae are released in the intestines and develop into adult worms. The adult females release numerous larval offspring which then enter the circulation and are deposited throughout the body. Most are killed; however, those that reach skeletal muscle become encysted and survive.[21,75] These larval forms create cystic granulomatous foci within muscle fibers.

We encountered this organism as an incidental finding in the FNA of a pleural-based metastatic carcinoma. In addition to malignant cells, a rare larva was seen. A spiral larval form was also identified in pleural fluid (Fig. 4.16). They were approximately 0.8 to 1.0 mm long and coiled. The infection was subclinical and the organisms were probably released because of the tissue destruction by the metastatic disease.

Diagnosis of *T. spiralis* is primarily based on morphology; however, indirect fluorescent antibody testing can be used for confirmation.[1]

Echinococcus

Echinococcus granulosus, E. multilocularis, and *E. vogeli* are species of tapeworm found in the intestines of dogs and related carnivores whose larval forms produce different types of hydatid disease, echinococcosis.[1,21] Human infection is usually acquired accidentally by close association with dogs. The organisms are ingested, invade the intestinal wall, enter the circulatory system, and are filtered out in various organs.[21] The liver is the most commonly affected site (Fig. 4.17). Depending on the species

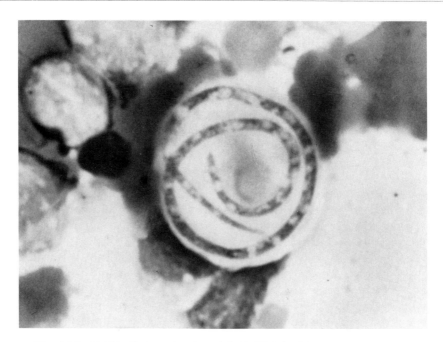

Fig. 4.16. *Trichinella* larva in pleural fluid (Wright-Giemsa stain; × 1000).

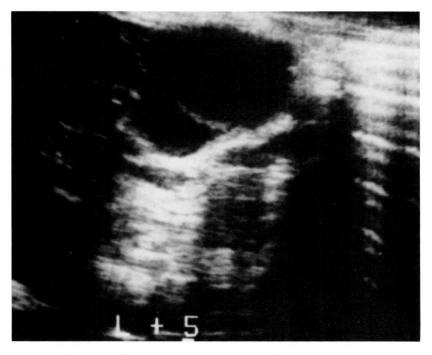

Fig. 4.17. Hydatid cyst of the liver visualized by ultrasound.

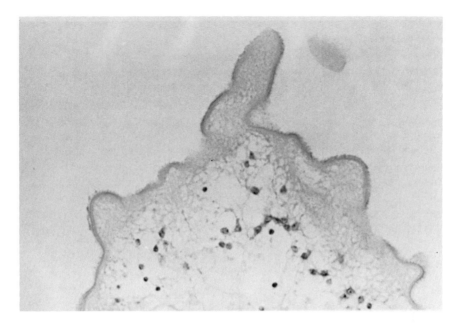

Fig. 4.18. Cell block from FNA of cysticercosis of soft tissue of neck demonstrating wall of worm consisting of thin refractile integument with dome-shaped projection and underlying edematous stroma (H&E; × 500) (Courtesy of Dr. Dick Lee, Royal Columbian Hospital, British Columbia, Canada).

of parasite, infection usually leads to the formation of cystic, polycystic, or proliferative (alveolar) lesions (hydatid cysts).

Needle aspiration is not the preferred method of evaluating these cysts because of the risk of anaphylactic shock secondary to the release of cyst fluid into surrounding tissues.[37,76] However, there are reports in the literature of successful aspiration of these lesions using thin needles without harm to the patients.[7,76,77,78] FNA smears contain invaginated or everted scolices with hooklets (Plate 11). The long oval structures are well defined by both Papanicolaou and Giemsa stains. Detached hooklets and blood capsules may also be seen.[76] The detached hooklets are refractile and are better seen at low illumination.[37] Brood capsules are identified as aggregates of protoscolices. Inflammatory cells, including eosinophils, and/or granulomas compose the smear background.[76]

Cysticercosis

Cysticercosis is a parasitic infection, caused by the larval stage of the pork tapeworm, *Taenia solium*. Muscle is the most frequent site of involvement, but patients are most often seen for cerebral manifestations of the disease. The FNA cytologic findings include the presence of inflammatory cells mixed with spiked spherules[79] and fragments of the body wall of the larvae consisting of integument with fine projections (Fig. 4.18).[79,80,81]

AMOEBA

Entamoeba histolytica is a small parasitic amoeba that causes infections (amoebiasis) most commonly in the intestine but may spread to other organs such as the liver, lungs, brain, spleen, skin and genitourinary tract resulting in abscesses in those sites.[1,21,82] Ameboma, a mass lesion due to this parasite, may be clinically confirmed with neoplasm.

The cytologic diagnosis is based on the demonstration of trophozoites in smears. The trophozoites are round or oval basophilic organisms approximately 20 to 30 microns in diameter with a single round, usually eccentric nucleus and cytoplasm containing phagocytized red blood cells.[82,83] The organisms are PAS positive. The smear background contains acute inflammation and necrotic debris. Specific identification of *E. histolytica* can be confirmed using immunoperoxidase techniques.[83]

VIRUSES

Cytomegalovirus

Cytomegalovirus infections usually occur in immunocompromised patients and may affect a wide variety of organs including the lungs, kidneys, brain, salivary glands, liver, and pancreas (Fig. 4.19).[16] Needle aspiration can be used to obtain material for culture and for cytologic interpretation.[7,29,84] The cytologic diagnosis is based on the identification of infected cells, which may be present only in small numbers. Infected cells are enlarged with a single, large intranuclear inclusion surrounded by a clear space or halo (Plate 12).[1,21,22,29] The inclusions are usually eosinophilic but some may have basophilic staining. Residual nuclear chromatin is condensed at the nucleus periphery. Small cytoplasmic inclusions are seen in some cells (Fig. 4.20).

The cytologic findings can be confirmed by culture, immunoperoxidase staining (Plate 12) or direct in situ hybridization.[1,85]

Herpes Simplex Virus

Systemic herpes simplex virus infections can occur in immunocompetent and immunocompromised or debilitated patients. They tend not to produce mass lesions and are seldom sampled by FNA.[29] However, cellular samples from such lesions might contain infected cells showing the characteristic morphologic features described in other types of cytologic specimens.[1,21,29,86] Typical multinucleated cells have enlarged nuclei with a bland, ground-glass appearance and nuclear molding (Fig. 4.21). Other nuclei may have large, single, eosinophilic intranuclear inclusions surrounded by a clear space. Cytoplasmic inclusions are not found. Single cells showing the same nuclear changes may also be noted.

Culture, immunoperoxidase staining, direct immunofluorescence technique, and direct in situ hybridization can be used as confirmatory tests.[1,87,88,89]

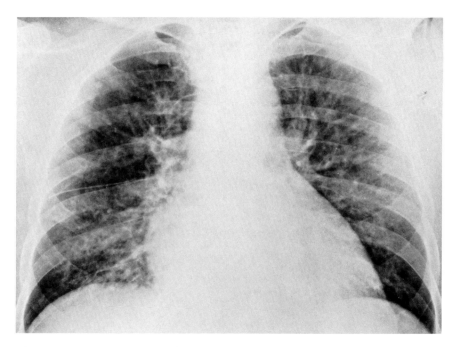

Fig. 4.19. Extensive pulmonary infiltrates on chest roentgenogram in patient with cytomegalic disease.

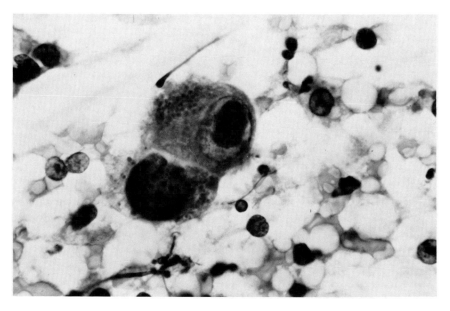

Fig. 4.20. FNA of lung revealing enlarged cells with single intranuclear inclusions and smaller cytoplasmic inclusions consistent with cytomegalovirus infection (Papanicolaou stain; ×250) (Courtesy of Dr. Vicki J. Schnadig, University of Texas Medical Branch, Galveston, TX).

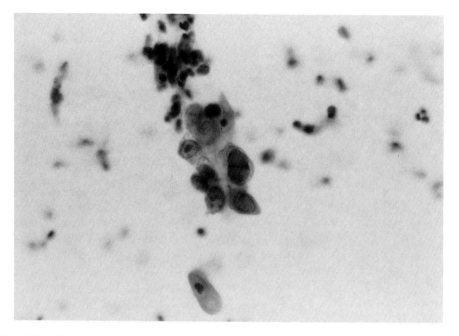

Fig. 4.21. Herpes simplex–infected cells in esophageal brushing (Papanicolaou stain; ×400).

NONMICROBIAL ELEMENTS

Foreign matter, when introduced into body tissues, may induce a tissue response that can mimic infectious disease or neoplasm in its clinical presentation. This material must be recognized and differentiated from pathogenic microorganisms.

Phytopneumonitis (Aspiration Pneumonia)

Aspiration of foreign material into the lung can block small airways and incite an inflammatory response. We have observed one such case that was diagnosed by FNA.[90] Aspiration smears contained chronic inflammation and abundant, variably sized, angulated structures with thick, refractile cell walls (Fig. 4.22). The structures had numerous, basophilic round bodies in their cytoplasm. Their relatively large size, angulated outlines, and thick cell walls indicated the plant origin of this material. The FNA was interpreted as consistent with phytopneumonitis.

Talc Granulomatosis

Talc granulomatosis, a disorder of drug addicts, is caused by the inadvertent intravenous injection of talc into the bloodstream. The talc crystals are filtered out into the lung parenchyma where they cause granulomatous disease.[91] Housini and associates also report a case of talc granulomatosis in a peripheral lymph node.[92]

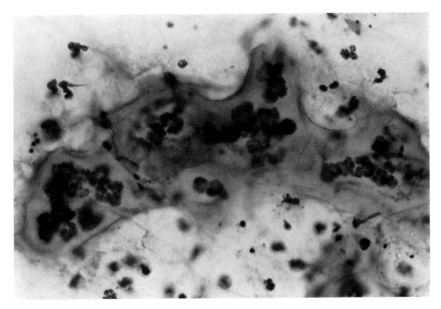

Fig. 4.22. Plant material in FNA smear of the lung (Papanicolaou stain; ×400).

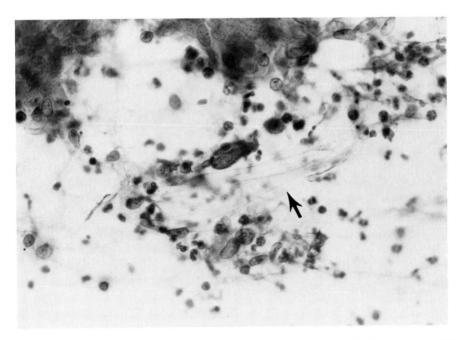

Fig. 4.23. Suture material in FNA smear of the neck (*arrow*) (Papanicolaou stain; ×400).

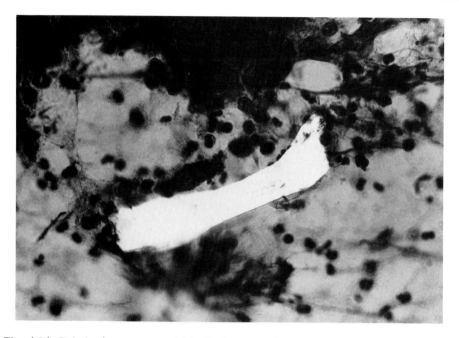

Fig. 4.24. Polarized suture material in FNA smear of neck (Papanicolaou stain; ×400).

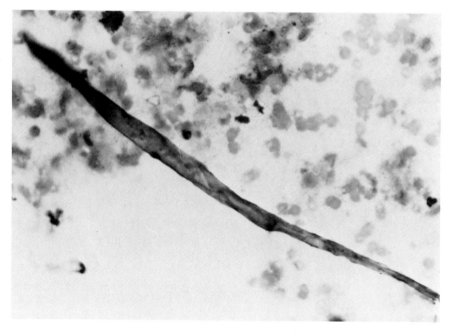

Fig. 4.25. Fiber contaminant in FNA smear (Diff-Quik stain; ×400).

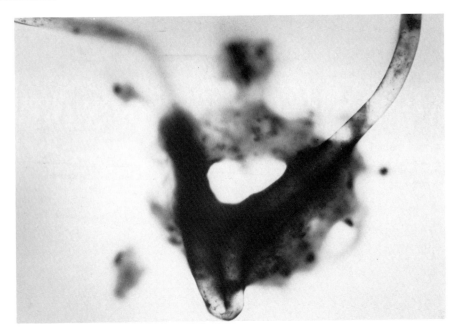

Fig. 4.26. Fiber contaminant in FNA smear (Papanicolaou stain; ×400).

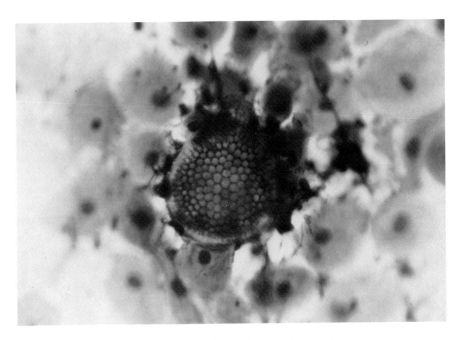

Fig. 4.27. Pollen contaminant (Papanicolaou stain; ×200).

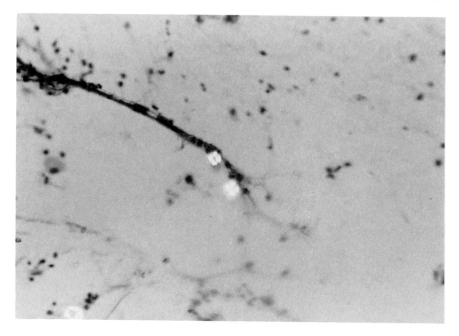

Fig. 4.28. Polarized starch granules in FNA smear of the neck (Papanicolaou smear; ×400).

FNA smears showed chronic and granulomatous inflammation with numerous multinucleated giant cells and occasional fibroblasts. When examined under polarized light, the macrophages and giant cells contained many closely packed, strongly birefringent, platelike crystals compatible with talc.[91]

Suture Material

Retained suture material can provoke a tissue response that may raise the question of recurrent neoplasm at the suture site. The FNA cytologic findings include polymorphonuclear leukocytes, lymphocytes, macrophages, multinucleated giant cells, fibrosis, and/or granulomatous reaction.[93]

We have observed a case of extensive foreign body giant cell reaction to retained suture particles that produced a mass at the suture line that was suspicious for recurrent carcinoma. FNA smears contained marked acute and chronic inflammation with innumerable multinucleated giant cells. Rare aggregates of epithelioid-type cells were observed, but no true granulomas were found. A few small fragments of pale-staining, clear, refractile fibers compatible with suture material were seen (Fig. 4.23). The fragments showed a bluish birefringence under polarized light (Fig. 4.24). There was no evidence of carcinoma.

Contaminants

Contaminants can be introduced into FNA specimens during handling and processing. These materials have no relationship to the disease process seen in smears and must be differentiated from true infectious organisms.

TABLE 4.1. Identification of Bacteria

Microorganism	Morphology	Stains	Organs Affected	Differential Diagnosis*
Mycobacterium tuberculosis	Slender, sometimes slightly curved rods averaging 4 microns in length	Acid-fast stain	Disseminated	Other mycobacteria
Mycobacterium avium-intracellulare	Morphologically indistinguishable from TB	Acid-fast stain	Primarily lungs and lymph nodes	Other mycobacteria
Mycobacterium kansaii	Longer and broader than TB; has beading	Acid-fast stain	Lungs	Other mycobacteria
Mycobacterium leprae	Morphologically similar to TB; usually occurs as intracellular bacilli grouped in bundles; also seen free in smear	Acid-fast stain	Liver, kidneys, subcutaneous tissues, spleen, skin, lymph nodes	Other mycobacteria
Legionella species	Short rods within the cytoplasm of neutrophils; extracellular rods also seen	Fite's acid-fast stain, direct fluorescent antibody stain	Lungs	Mycobacteria
Actinomyces israelii	Delicate, nonseptate filaments 1–1.5 microns in diameter; variable in length and degree of branching; sulfur granules present	Papanicolaou, H&E, Gram stains, methenamine silver	Disseminated	Nocardia, other bacteria
Nocardia asteroides	Delicate, nonseptate filaments 0.5–1.0 microns in diameter and 10–20 microns in length; right-angle branching; sulfur granules usually absent	Gram stains, Fite's acid-fast stain, Gram–Weigert, Geimsa, methenamine silver	Central nervous system, lungs	Actinomyces, other bacteria
Other bacteria	Gram-positive and negative bacilli and cocci	Gram stains	Disseminated	By culture

*Differential diagnosis based on appearance in cytologic preparations.

TABLE 4.2. Identification of Fungi

Microorganism	Morphology	Stains	Organs Affected	Differential Diagnosis*
Aspergillus fumigatus	Septate hyphae 3–6 microns in diameter with uniform, acute-angle, dichotomous branching	Papanicolaou, H&E, PAS, methenamine silver, immunoperoxidase	Disseminated	Candida species
Blastomyces dermatitidis	Spherical organisms (8–20 microns) with sharply defined, thick, refractile cells walls; broad-based budding	Papanicolaou, H&E, PAS, methenamine silver	Lungs, bone, skin, other organs	Cryptococcus, Histoplasma, Coccidioides
Candida species	Pseudohyphae with budding yeast forms (3–4 microns)	Papanicolaou, H&E, Wright, Diff-Quik, methenamine silver, immunoperoxidase	Disseminated	Aspergillus
Coccidiodes immitis	Nonbudding spherules 5–100 microns in diameter with thick refractile walls; contain numerous small endospores (2–5 microns); septate hyphae can also be seen	Papanicolaou, H&E, PAS, methenamine silver	Lungs, bone, skin, subcutaneous tissues, viscera	Pollen grains, parasites, vegetable material, Blastomyces, Cryptococcus

Cryptococcus neo-formans	Round or oval organisms (5–10 microns) surrounded by a clear thick mucopolysaccharide capsule; single, thin-walled, narrow-based budding	PAS, mucicarmine, alcian blue, methenamine silver, immunoperoxidase	Lungs, central nervous system, skin, viscera	*Blastomyces, Histoplasma, Coccidiodes*
Histoplasma capsulatum	Budding oval yeast (2–5 microns) surrounded by rigid cell wall; usually seen within macrophages	PAS, methenamine silver	Disseminated	*Blastomyces, Cryptococcus, Coccidioides*
Phaeohyphomycosis	Pseudohyphae composed of chains of round, oval, or rectangular bodies resembling strings of beads; true septate hyphae, branching, single budding forms also found	Papanicolaou, H&E, methenamine silver	Subcutaneous cysts	Other hyphal fungi
Zygomycetes	Very broad, rarely septate, ribbonlike hyphae that vary greatly in thickness and shape; branching common but angle and shape varied	Papanicolaou, H&E, poor sensitivity to fungal stains	Orbit, nasal sinuses, lungs, central nervous system, GI tract, blood vessels	Other hyphal fungi, contaminants

*Differential diagnosis based on appearance in cytologic preparations.

TABLE 4.3. Identification of Parasites and Viruses

Microorganism	Morphology	Stains	Organs Affected	Differential Diagnosis*
PARASITES				
Pneumocystis carinii	Single round, cup-shaped or comma-shaped organisms; cysts (5–8 microns) with refractile walls containing 6–8 trophozoites (1–2 microns); granular eosinophilic or basophilic background material	Toluidine blue, Wright's, methenamine silver, Gram–Weigert, immunoperoxidase; Papanicolaou, H&E for background material	Lungs	Hemosiderin, cell debris (background material)
Filariae	Slender, long, threadlike nematodes with filiform end (microfilariae)	Papanicolaou, H&E, Wright, Diff-Quik	Disseminated	Other nematodes, contaminants
Trichinella spiralis	Coiled or spiral larval forms 0.8–1.0 mm long	Papanicolaou, H&E, Wright–Giemsa	Muscle	Other nematodes, contaminants
Echinococcus species	Invaginated or everted scolices with hooklets; detached hooklets	Papanicolaou, H&E, Wright–Giemsa	Liver and other organs	Contaminants
Entamoeba histolytica	Round or oval basophilic organisms (18–20 microns) with single, usually eccentric nucleus and cytoplasm containing ingested red cells	Papanicolaou, H&E, PAS, immunoperoxidase	GI tract, liver, disseminated	Contaminants
VIRUSES				
Cytomegalovirus	Enlarged cells with single, large intranuclear inclusion surrounded by halo; small cytoplasmic inclusions	Papanicolaou, H&E, immunoperoxidase	Lungs, kidney, liver, central nervous system, salivary glands, pancreas	Other viruses, degenerative changes in cells
Herpes simplex	Single and multinucleated cells having enlarged nuclei with bland, ground-glass appearance or with large, single intranuclear inclusion surrounded by clear halo; no cytoplasmic inclusions	Papanicolaou, H&E, immunoperoxidase	Lungs, skin, central nervous system, disseminated	Other viruses, degenerative changes in cells

*Differential diagnosis based on appearance in cytologic preparations.

76

Microscopic fibers may mimic hyphal fungi but have more haphazard size, lack internal structure, and are polarizable in contrast to fungi (Figs. 4.25 and 4.26). Some pollen grains may simulate *Coccidiodes,* especially when only rare structures are present (Fig. 4.27). Starch granules, usually from glove powder, are identified by their refractile appearance and characteristic "Maltese cross" configuration under polarized light (Fig. 4.28).

In most cases, careful evaluation of morphology will yield the correct interpretation. Patient history and clinical findings can also contribute to the evaluation process. In more difficult cases, special stains can be used to aid in the differential diagnosis.

CONCLUSIONS

Fine-needle aspiration is a highly effective initial step in the evaluation of many suspected infectious processes. It provides material for cytologic examination as well as for culture and other ancillary studies. In many cases, the diagnosis can be based on the cytomorphology of the microorganism alone, while others require or are enhanced by special stains. The morphologic features of the organisms discussed in this chapter are summarized in Tables 4.1 to 4.3. Rapid evaluation by FNA yields diagnostic information more quickly than culture and can thereby expedite patient treatment.

REFERENCES

1. Bennington JL, Ed.: Dictionary and Encyclopedia of Laboratory Medicine and Technology. Philadelphia: WB Saunders, 1984.

2. Stanley MW, Horwitz CA, Burton LG, et al: Negative images of bacilli and mycobacterial infection: a study of fine needle aspiration smears from lymph nodes in patients with AIDS. *Diagn Cytopathol* 6:118–121, 1990.

3. Dahlgren SE, Ekstrom P: Aspiration cytology in the diagnosis of pulmonary tuberculosis. *Scand J Resp Dis* 53:196–201, 1972.

4. Zavala DC, Schoell JE: Ultrathin needle aspiration of the lung in infectious and malignant disease. *Am Rev Respir Dis* 123:125–131, 1981.

5. Robicheaux B, Moinuddin SM, Lee LH: The role of aspiration biopsy cytology in the diagnosis of pulmonary tuberculosis. *Am J Clin Pathol* 83:719–722, 1985.

6. Bailey TM, Akhtar M, Ali MA: Fine needle aspiration biopsy in the diagnosis of tuberculosis. *Acta Cytol* 29:732–736, 1985.

7. Bottles K, Miller TR, Jeffrey B, et al: Aspiration cytology characterization of inflammatory masses. *West J Med* 144:695–699, 1986.

8. Pontiflex AH, Roberts FJ: Fine needle aspiration biopsy cytology in the diagnosis of inflammatory lesions. *Acta Cytol* 29:979–982, 1985.

9. Layfield LJ, Glasgow BJ, Du Puis MH: Fine needle aspiration of lymph adenopathy of suspected infectious etiology. *Arch Pathol Lab Med* 109:810–812, 1985.

10. Radhika S, Gupta SK, Charkrabarti A, et al: Role of culture for mycobacteria in fine needle aspiration diagnosis of tuberculosis lymphadenitis. *Diagn Cytopathol* 5:260–262, 1989.

11. Metre MS, Jayaram G: Acid-fast bacilli in aspiration smears from tuberculosis of lymph nodes: an analysis of 255 cases. *Acta Cytol* 31:17–19, 1987.

12. Nayar M, Saxena HMK: Tuberculosis of the breast—a cytomorphologic study of needle aspirates and nipple discharges. *Acta Cytol* 28:325–328, 1984.

13. Jayram G: Cytomorphology of tuberculosis mastitis—a report of nine cases with fine needle aspiration cytology. *Acta Cytol* 29:974–978, 1985.

14. Benger SA, Zonszein J, Villamena P, et al: Infectious diseases of the thyroid gland. *Rev Infect Dis* 5:108–122, 1983.

15. Silverman JF, Larkin EW, Carney M, et al: Fine needle aspiration cytology of the lumbar vertebrae (Pott's Disease). *Acta Cytol* 30:538–542, 1986.

16. Robbins SL, Cortan RS: Pathologic Basis of Disease. Philadelphia, WB Saunders, 1979.

17. Feldman PS, Covell JL, Kardos TF: Fine Needle Aspiration Cytology—Lymph Node, Thyroid and Salivary Gland. Chicago, ASCP Press, 1989.

18. Silverman JF, Marrow HG: Fine needle aspiration cytology of granulomatous diseases of the lung including nontuberculous mycobacterium infection. *Acta Cytol* 29:535–541, 1985.

19. Cavett JR, McAfee R, Ramzy I: Hansen's disease (leprosy)—diagnosis by aspiration biopsy of lymph nodes. *Acta Cytol* 30:189–193, 1986.

20. Kaur S, Kumar B, Gupta SK: Fine needle aspiration of lymph nodes in leprosy. A study of bacteriologic and morphologic indices. *Intern J Leprosy* 45:369–372, 1977.

21. Koneman EW, Allen SD, Dowell VR, et al: Color Atlas and Textbook of Diagnostic Microbiology. Philadelphia, JB Lippincott, 1988.

22. Blackmon JA, Paris AL: Infectious diseases of the lung. *Lab Med* 14:77–85, 1983.

23. Walker AN, Walker GK, Feldman PS: Diagnosis of *Legionella micdadei* pneumonia from cytologic specimens. *Acta Cytol* 27:252–254, 1983.

24. Pollock PG, Meyers DS, Frable WJ, et al: Rapid diagnosis of actinomycosis by thin-needle aspiration biopsy. *Am J Clin Pathol* 70:27–30, 1978.

25. Pollock PG, Koontz FP, Viner TF, et al: Cervicofacial actinomycosis—rapid diagnosis by thin-needle aspiration. *Arch Otolaryngol* 104:491–494, 1978.

26. Ramsy I, Aufdemorte TB, Duncan DL: Diagnosis of radiolucent lesions of the jaw by fine-needle aspiration biopsy. *Acta Cytol* 29:419–424, 1985.

27. Shurbaji MS, Gupta PK, Newman MM: Hepatic actinomycosis diagnosed by fine-needle aspiration—a case report. *Acta Cytol* 31:751–755, 1987.

28. Lininger JR, Frable WJ: Diagnosis of pelvic actinomycosis by fine needle aspiration—a case report. *Acta Cytol* 28:601–604, 1984.

29. Bonfiglio RA: Cytopathologic Interpretation of Transthoracic Fine Needle Biopsies. New York, Masson, 1983.

30. Pollack, PG, Valicenti, JF, Meyers DS, et al: The use of fluorescent and special staining techniques in the aspiration of nocardiosis and actinomycosis. *Acta Cytol* 22:575–579, 1978.

31. Feldman PS, Covell JL: Fine Needle Aspiration Cytology and Its Clinical Applications—Breast and Lung. Chicago, ASCP Press, 1985.

32. Arroyo J, Gordan V, Postic B: Transthoracic needle aspiration in the management of pulmonary infections. *J South Carolina Med Assoc* 77:427–432, 1981.

33. Lee P, Turnidge J, McDonald PJ: Fine-needle aspiration biopsy of soft tissue infections. *J Clin Microbiol* 22:80–83, 1985.

34. Golfo EB, Galindo LM: Diagnosis of an unusual presentation of granuloma inguinale by fine needle aspiration cytology. *Acta Cytol* 34:570–572, 1990.

35. Bhatt ON, Miller R, Riche JL, et al: Aspiration biopsy in pulmonary opportunistic infections. *Acta Cytol* 21:206–209, 1977.

36. Austin P, Dekker A, Kennerdell JS: Orbital aspergillosis—report of a case diagnosed by fine needle aspiration biopsy. *Acta Cytol* 27:166–169, 1983.

37. Koss LG, Woyke S, Olszewski W: Aspiration Biopsy—Cytologic Interpretation and Histologic Bases. New York, Igaku-Shoin, 1984.

38. Saeed EN, Hay RJ: Immunoperoxidase staining in the recognition of Aspergillus infections. *Histopathology* 5:437–444, 1981.

39. Moskowitz LB, Ganjei P, Ziegels-Weissman J, et al: Immunohistologic identification of fungi in systemic and cutaneous mycoses. *Arch Pathol Lab Med* 110:433–436, 1986.

40. Bigner SH, Burger PC, Dubois PJ, et al: Diagnosis of cerebral mucormycosis by needle aspiration biopsy—a case report. *Acta Cytol* 26:699–704, 1982.

41. Schnadig VJ, Long EG, Washington JM, et al: *Phialophora verrucosa*-induced subcutaneous phaeohyphomycosis fine-needle aspiration findings. *Acta Cytol* 30:425–429, 1986.

42. Crosby JH, O'Quinn MH, Steele JCH, et al: Fine-needle aspiration of subcutaneous phaeohyphomycosis caused by *Wangiella dermatitidis*. *Diagn Cytopathol* 5:293–297, 1989.

43. Heaston DK, Handel DB, Ashton PR, et al: Narrow-gauge needle aspiration of solid adrenal masses. *Am J Radiol* 138:1143–1148, 1982.

44. Whitaker D, Sterrett GF: *Cryptococcus neoformans* diagnosed by fine needle aspiration cytology of the lung. *Acta Cytol* 20:105–107, 1976.

45. Walts AE: Localized pulmonary cryptococcus: diagnosed by fine needle aspiration. *Acta Cytol* 27:457–459, 1983.

46. Silverman JF, Johnsrude IS: Fine needle aspiration cytology of granulomatous cryptococcus of the lung. *Acta Cytol* 29:157–161, 1985.

47. Szporn AH, Tepper S, Watson CW: Disseminated cryptococcus presenting as thyroiditis-fine needle aspiration and autopsy findings. *Acta Cytol* 29:449–453, 1985.

48. Ganjei P, Evans DA, Fischer ML: Diagnosis of cryptococcal osteomyelitis by fine needle aspiration cytology—a case report. *Acta Cytol* 26:224–226, 1982.

49. Sinner WN: Needle biopsy of histoplasmosis. *ROFO* 133:590–593, 1980.

50. Valente PT, Calafate SA: Diagnosis of disseminated histoplasmosis by fine needle aspiration of the adrenal gland. *Acta Cytol* 33:341–343, 1989.

51. Anderson CJ, Pitts WC, Weiss LM: Disseminated histoplasmosis diagnosed by fine needle aspiration biopsy of the adrenal gland. *Acta Cytol* 33:337–340, 1989.

52. Perez-Guillermo M, Hernandez-Gil A, Bonmati C: Diagnosis of cutaneous leishmaniasis by fine needle aspiration cytology. Report of a case. *Acta Cytol* 32:485–488, 1988.

53. Forseth J, Rohwedder JJ, Levine BE, et al: Experience with needle biopsy of coccidioidal lung nodules. *Arch Intern Med* 146:319–320, 1986.

54. Freedman SI, Ang EP, Haley RS: Identification of coccidioidomycosis by fine needle aspiration biopsy. *Acta Cytol* 30:420–424, 1986.

55. Pifer LL: Pneumocystis. *Carolina Tips* 46:41–42, 1983.

56. Johnson HD, Johnson WW: *Pneumocystis carinii* pneumonia in children with cancer. *JAMA* 214:1067–1073, 1970.

57. Castellino RA: Percutaneous pulmonary needle diagnosis of *Pneumocystic carinii* pneumonitis. *Natl Cancer Inst Monogr* 43:137–140, 1976.

58. Chaudhary S, Hughes WT, Feldman S, et al: Percutaneous transthoracic needle aspiration of the lung-diagnosing *Pneumocystis carinii* pneumonitis. *Am J Dis Child* 131:902–907, 1977.

59. Kim H, Hughes WT: Comparison of methods for identification of *Pneumocystis carinii* in pulmonary aspirates. *Am J Clin Pathol* 60:462–466, 1973.

60. Domingo J, Waksal HW: Wright stain in rapid diagnosis of *Pneumocystis carinii*. *Am J Clin Pathol* 81:511–514, 1984.

61. Guarner J, Robey SS, Gupta PK: Cytologic detection of *Pneumocystis carinii:* a comparison of Papanicolaou and other histochemical stains. *Diagn Cytopathol* 2:133–137, 1986.

62. Paradis IL, Ross C, Dekker A, et al: A comparison of modified methenamine silver and toluidine blue stains for the detection of *Pneumocystis carinii* in bronchoalveolar lavage specimens from immunosuppressed patients. *Acta Cytol* 34:511–516, 1990.

63. Greaves TS, Strigle SM: The recognition of *Pneumocystis carinii* in routine Papanicolaou-stained smears. *Acta Cytol* 29:714–720, 1985.

64. Strigle SM, Gal AA, Koss MN: Rapid diagnosis of *Pneumocystis carinii* infection in AIDS by cytocentrifugation and rapid hematoxylin and eosin staining. *Diagn Cytopathol* 6:164–168, 1990.

65. Ghali VS, Garcia RL, Skolom J: Fluorescence of *Pneumocystis carinii* in Papanicolaou smears. *Hum Pathol* 15:907–909, 1984.

66. Blumenfeld W, Kovacs JA: Use of monoclonal antibody to detect *Pneumocystis carinii* in induced sputum and bronchalveloar lavage fluid by immunoperoxidase staining. *Arch Pathol Lab Med* 112:1233–1236, 1988.

67. Radio SJ, Hansen S, Goldsmith J, et al: Immunohistochemistry of *Pneumocystis carinii* infection. *Mod Pathol* 3:462–468, 1990.

68. Das DK, Khanna CM, Tripathi RP, et al: Microfilaria of *Wucheria bancrofti* in fine-needle aspirate from a colloid goiter. *Diagn Cytopathol* 5:114–115, 1989.

69. Sodhani P, Nayar M: Microfilariae in a thyroid aspirate smear: an incidental finding. *Acta Cytol* 33:942–943, 1989.

70. Jayaram G: Microfilariae in fine needle aspirates from epididymal lesions. *Acta Cytol* 31:59–62, 1987.

71. Arora VK, Bhatia A: Adult filarial worm in fine needle aspirate of an epididymal nodule. *Acta Cytol* 33:421, 1989.

72. Rani S, Beohar PC: Microfilaria in bone marrow aspirate—a case report. *Acta Cytol* 25:425–426, 1981.

73. Hawkins AG, Hsiu J, Smith RM, et al: Pulmonary dirofilariasis diagnosed by fine needle aspiration biopsy—a case report. *Acta Cytol* 29:19–22, 1985.

74. Roussel F, Delaville A, Campos H, et al: Fine needle aspiration of retroperitoneal human dirofilariasis with pseudotumoral presentation. *Acta Cytol* 34:533–535, 1990.

75. Ash LR, Orihel TC: Atlas of Human Parasitology. Chicago, ASCP Press, 1984.

76. Kapila K, Verma K: Aspiration cytology diagnosis of echinococcosis. *Diagn Cytopathol* 6:301–303, 1990.

77. Jacobson E: A case of secondary echinococcosis diagnosed by cytologic examination of pleural fluid and needle biopsy of pleura. *Acta Cytol* 17:76–79, 1973.

78. Epstein NA: Hydatid cyst of the breast: diagnosis using cytologic techniques. *Acta Cytol* 13:420–421, 1969.

79. Vuong PH: Fine needle aspiration cytology of subcutaneous cysticercosis of the breast. Case report and pathogenic discussion. *Acta Cytol* 33:659–662, 1989.

80. Kung ITM, Lee D, Yu H: Soft tissue cysticercosis. Diagnosis by fine-needle aspiration. *Am J Clin Pathol* 92:834–835, 1989.

81. Verma K, Kapila K: Fine needle diagnosis of cysticercosis in soft tissue swellings. *Acta Cytol* 33:663–666, 1989.

82. Walsh TJ, Berkman W, Brown NL, et al: Cytopathologic diagnosis of extracolonic amoebiasis. *Acta Cytol* 27:671–675, 1983.

83. Kobayashi TK, Koretoh O, Kamachi M, et al: Cytologic demonstration of *Entamoeba histolytica* using immunoperoxidase techniques–report of two cases. *Acta Cytol* 29:414–418, 1985.

84. Abdallah PS, Mark JBD, Merigan TC: Diagnosis of cytomegalovirus pneumonia in compromised hosts. *Am J Med* 61:326–332, 1976.

85. Hilborne LH, Nieberg RK, Cheng L, et al: Direct in-situ hybridization for rapid detection of cytomegalovirus in bronchalveolar lavage. *Am J Clin Pathol* 87:766–769, 1987.

86. Vernon SE: Cytologic features of nonfatal herpes virus tracheobraochitis. *Acta Cytol* 26:237–242, 1982.

87. Kapur S, Patterson K, Chandra R: Detection of herpes simplex infection in cytologic smears. *Arch Pathol Lab Med* 109:464–465, 1985.

88. Bedrossian UK, Lozano de Arce EA, Bedrossian CW: Immunoperoxidase method to detect herpes simplex virus in cytologic specimens. *Lab Med* 15:673–676, 1984.

89. Iwa N, Katayama Y, Ito K, et al: Immunoperoxidase staining for the detection of herpes simplex virus antigen in cervicovaginal smears. *Acta Cytol* 29:705–707, 1985.

90. Covell JL, Feldman PS: Fine needle aspiration diagnosis of aspiration pneumonia (phytopneumonitis). *Acta Cytol* 28:77–89, 1984.

91. Tao L, Morgan RC, Donat EE: Cytologic diagnosis of intravenous talc granulomatosis by fine needle aspiration biopsy—a case report. *Acta Cytol* 28:737–739, 1984.

92. Housini I, Dabbs DJ, Coyne L: Fine needle aspiration cytology of talc granulomatosis in a peripheral lymph node in a case of suspected intravenous drug abuse. *Acta Cytol* 34:342–344, 1990.

93. Fechner RE: The surgical pathology of iatrogenic lesions. *In:* Silverberg SG: Principles and Practice of Surgical Pathology. New York, John Wiley and Sons, 1983.

COLOR PLATES

Plate 1. *M. avium-intracellulare* in smear of cultured FNA material (Acid-fast stain; ×1000).

Plate 2. (*Right*) Intracytoplasmic acid-fast bacilli of *L. micdadei* in FNA smear of the lung (Fite's acid-fast stain; ×1000). (*Left*) Direct fluorescent antibody stain for *L. micdadei* (×1000).

Plate 3. *Nocardia* in brain aspiration smear (Fite's acid-fast stain; ×1000).

Plate 4. Bacteria in FNA smear of liver abscess (Diff-Quik stain; ×400).

Plate 5. (*Right*) Branching hyphae of *Aspergillus* in FNA smear of the orbit (Papanicolaou stain; ×400). (*Left*) Immunoperoxidase staining for *Aspergillus* (×400).

Plate 6. Mucor in FNA smear of the lung (Papanicolaou stain; ×400).

82

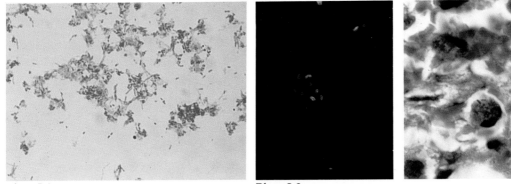

Plate I.1.   Plate I.2.

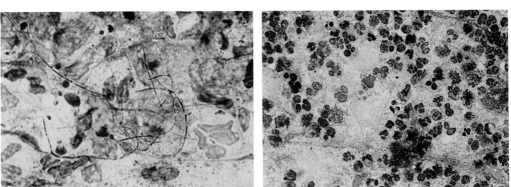

Plate I.3.   Plate I.4.

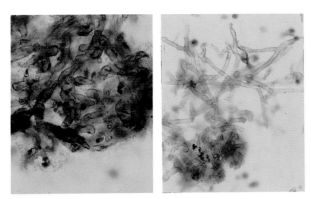

Plate I.5.

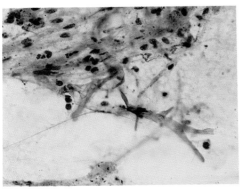

Plate I.6.

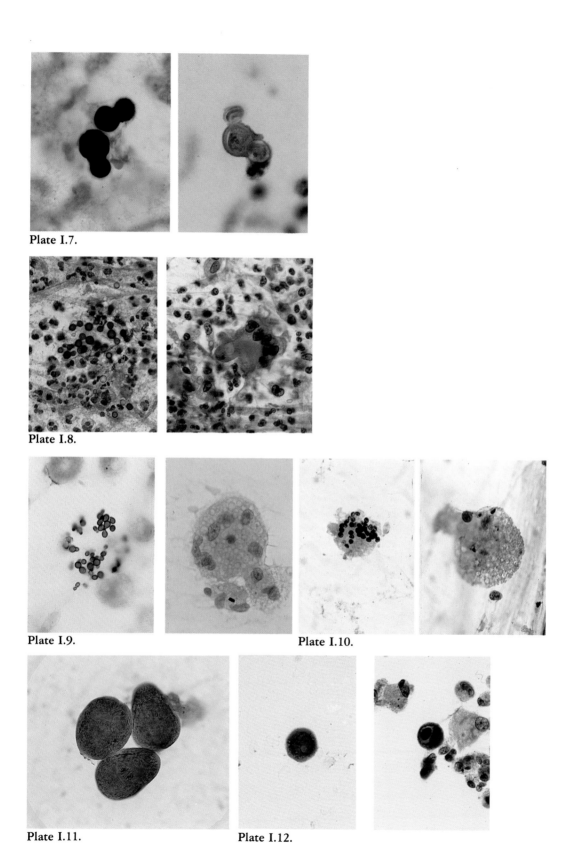

Plate I.7.

Plate I.8.

Plate I.9.

Plate I.10.

Plate I.11.

Plate I.12.

Plate 7. (*Right*) Blastomyces organisms in FNA smear of the lung (Papanicolaou stain; ×1000). (*Left*) Budding blastomyces in FNA smear of the lung (GMS stain; ×1000).

Plate 8. (*Right*) Macrophage containing crypto-coccus organisms in FNA smear of a skin lesion (Papanicolaou stain; ×400). (*Left*) *C. neoformans* in FNA smear of a skin lesion (Mucicarmine stain; ×400).

Plate 9. (*Right*) Macrophage containing *His-toplasma* organisms in FNA smear of the lung (Papanicolaou stain; ×400). (*Left*) *H. capsula-tum* in FNA smear of the lung (GMS stain; ×400).

Plate 10. (*Right*) Alveolar exudate containing *Pneumocystis* organisms in FNA smear of the lung (Papanicolaou stain; ×400). (*Left*) *P. cari-nii* in FNA smear of the lung (GMS stain; ×400).

Plate 11. Scolices with hooklets of *Echinococcus* in liver fluid (Papanicolaou stain; ×200).

Plate 12. (*Right*) Intranuclear and intracy-toplasmic inclusions of cytomegalovirus in FNA smear of the lung (Papanicolaou stain; ×400). (*Left*) Immunoperoxidase staining for cytomega-lovirus (×400).

5

Cytomorphologic Patterns of Inflammatory Aspirates

Jan F. Silverman
Thomas F. Kardos

INTRODUCTION

Inflammatory processes are potentially a more common target of the aspiration needle than are neoplasms. The clinician who requests or performs the aspiration may suspect a tumor or may want to confirm the inflammatory nature of the process and possibly identify pathogens. For the effective use of FNA biopsy, it is important to distinguish inflammatory lesions from malignancy. Unfortunately, the reactive atypias associated with inflammation and repair can be a trap into which unwary and unfamiliar cytologists may sometimes fall. Caution and familiarity with the various patterns seen in inflammatory FNA biopsies will lead you around this trap. An infectious or inflammatory process should be suspected when the smears contain a background of inflammatory cells and/or necrosis. Epithelial and mesenchymal repair along with inflammatory atypia are potential pitfalls for a false-positive diagnosis of malignancy. Recognition of these changes should raise the flag of caution and give cause for careful consideration of the case. Conversely, aspirates of neoplasms that have a prominent inflammatory component can be a pitfall for a false-negative diagnosis if the epithelial cells are obscured by the inflammatory cells or are sparsely present in the smears.

INFLAMMATORY ELEMENTS

Acute Inflammation

Microbes, chemicals, immunologic reactions, and physical causes such as burns, irradiation, and trauma can cause acute inflammation.[1] Clinically, the local signs of acute inflammation include heat, redness, swelling, pain, and loss of function, as classically defined by Celsus and Virchow.[1] Acute inflammation is usually of short duration, lasting from a few minutes to days. It is generally characterized by edema

85

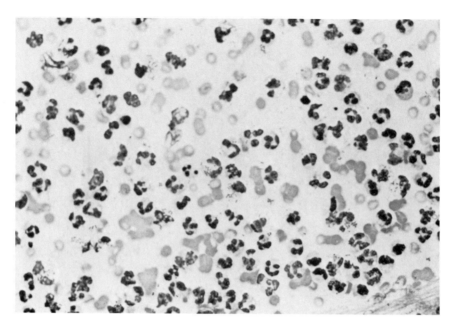

Fig. 5.1. FNA of abscess consisting of numerous neutrophils (Diff-Quik stain; ×200).

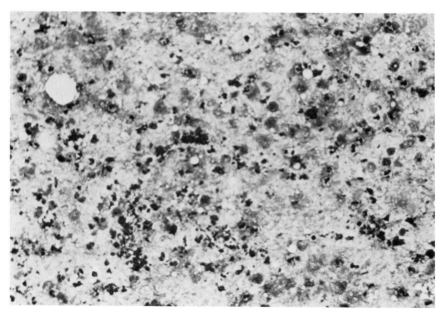

Fig. 5.2. Aspirate of abscess in which there is extensive necrosis in the background along with many degenerating neutrophils (Diff-Quik stain; ×100).

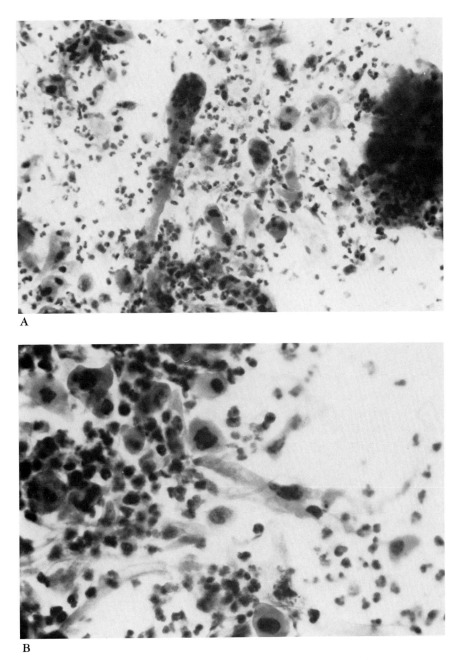

Fig. 5.3. A. Fine-needle aspirate of squamous cell carcinoma metastatic to retroperitoneal lymph node. Scattered neoplastic keratinized squamous cells are present along with numerous neutrophils in the background (Papanicolaou stain; ×200). **B.** High-power view of metastatic keratinizing squamous cell carcinoma showing the presence of bizarre tumor cells and numerous neutrophils (Papanicolaou stain; ×400).

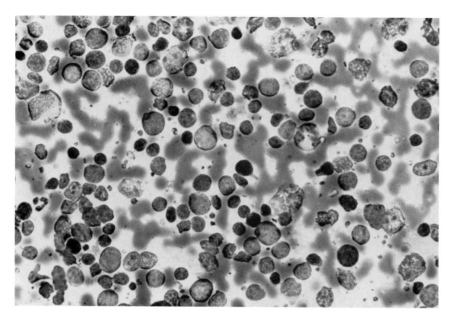

Fig. 5.4. Aspirate of chronic inflammation consisting of a polymorphic population of lymphoid cells including small mature lymphocytes and larger immunoblastic-appearing lymphoid cells. Note the presence of lymphoglandular bodies (cytoplasmic fragments) in the background (Diff-Quik stain; ×200).

and a predominance of neutrophils infiltrating the tissue. The number of inflammatory cells varies, but usually numerous neutrophils and other inflammatory cells will be present (Fig. 5.1). Necrosis is common in this phase of the inflammatory process (Fig 5.2). Epithelial and mesenchymal repair and inflammatory atypia are often more pronounced in acute inflammation than in other inflammatory processes. Occasionally, malignancies can have a prominent associated acute inflammatory response. Metastatic and primary keratinizing squamous cell carcinomas are often associated with varying numbers of neutrophils, foreign-body histiocytes, or both, and in some aspirates the malignant cells may be obscured by the prominent inflammatory process (Fig. 5.3). This phenomenon is discussed and illustrated in Chapter 9. Primary and metastatic colon cancer are also associated with acute inflammation.

Chronic Inflammation

Acute inflammation may have a number of outcomes. These include abscess formation, complete resolution, healing by scarring, or progression to chronic inflammation.[1] Chronic inflammation may be a sequela of acute inflammation caused by a persistence of the inciting stimulus or an interference with the healing process. Occasionally, chronic inflammatory processes are related to repeated bouts of acute inflammation or may represent a low grade smoldering inflammatory process. Chronic inflammation is characterized by varying numbers of mononuclear cells

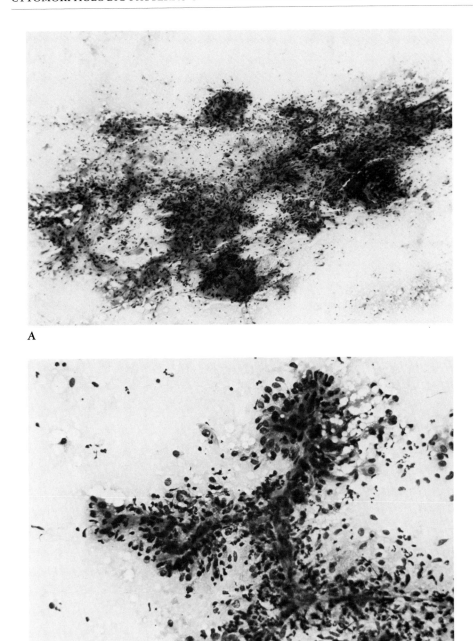

A

B

Fig. 5.5. **A.** Low-power view of aspirate in which there are numerous fragments of granulation-type tissue. The increased cellularity and the presence of reactive-appearing endothelial cells and histiocytes is a potential cause of a false-positive diagnosis of malignancy (Papanicolaou stain; × 100). **B.** Higher-power view of granulation tissue showing crisscrossing capillary network with adherent histiocytes and some inflammatory cells. The nuclear enlargement of endothelial cells and histiocytes which is accentuated in the Diff-Quik stain could be a potential for a false-positive diagnosis of malignancy (Diff-Quik stain; × 200).

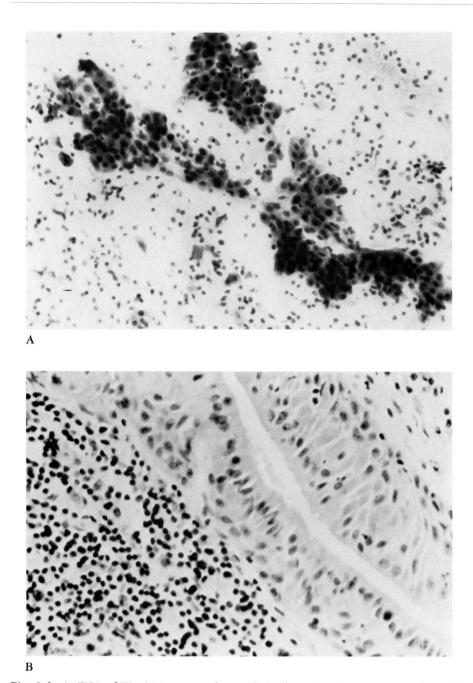

A

B

Fig. 5.6. **A.** FNA of Warthin's tumor of parotid gland in which loose clusters of oxyphilic cells and numerous lymphocytes are present (Papanicolaou stain; ×200). **B.** Resected Warthin's tumor showing histologic correlate of oxyphilic cells and lymphocytes (H&E; ×400).

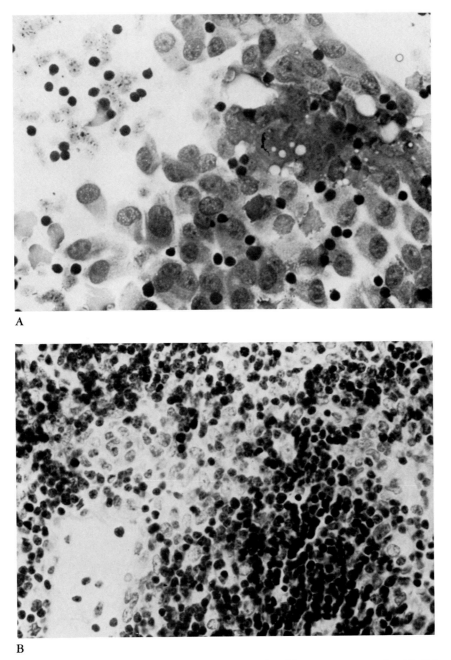

Fig. 5.7. **A.** Aspirate of thymoma showing loose, sheetlike arrangement of epithelial cells with numerous admixed lymphocytes (Papanicolaou stain; ×400). **B.** Resected thymoma demonstrating pale clusters of epithelial cells having bland-appearing nuclei with numerous associated lymphocytes (H&E; ×400).

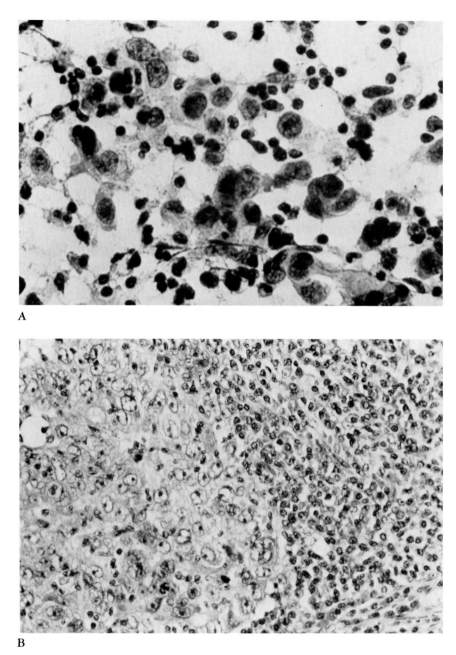

Fig. 5.8. A. Fine-needle aspirate of medullary carcinoma of the breast. Numerous lymphocytes are present along with scattered larger malignant cells. The potential exists for a false-negative diagnosis in those aspirates showing a predominance of lymphoid cells with relatively few malignant cells (Papanicolaou stain; ×400). **B.** Resected medullary carcinoma of the breast demonstrating bimorphic population of poorly differentiating malignant cells arranged in a syncytial fashion along with numerous lymphocytes and some plasma cells (H&E; ×400).

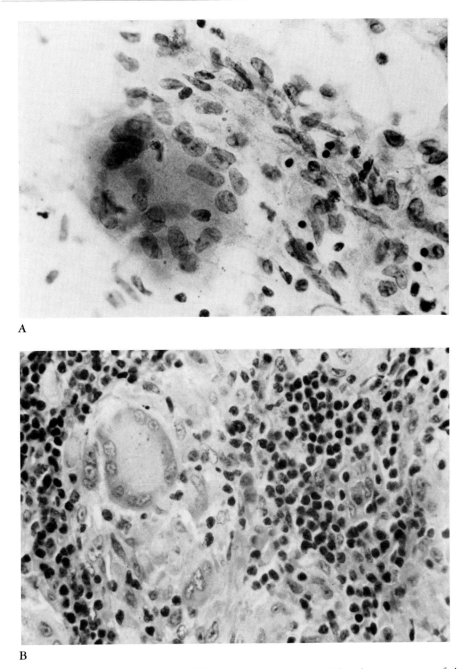

Fig. 5.9. A. Langhans' type giant cell having characteristic peripheral arrangement of the nuclei in an aspirate of tuberculosis (Papanicolaou stain; ×400). **B.** Resected granulomatous lesion containing Langhans' type giant cells (H&E; ×400).

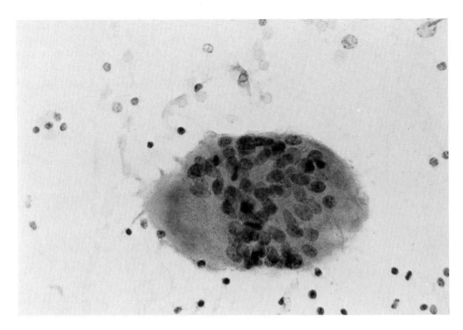

Fig. 5.10. Foreign body–type giant cell having numerous overlapping scattered nuclei (Papanicolaou stain; ×400).

including lymphocytes, plasma cells, and macrophages (Fig. 5.4). The cellularity of the lymphoid infiltrate is variable but most frequently is low. With a more cellular lymphoid infiltrate, a range of smaller, mature and larger, immature lymphoid cells is common.

Proliferation of fibroblasts and small blood vessels may be present along with fibrosis and tissue destruction. Misinterpretation of granulation tissue is a potential for a false-positive diagnosis of malignancy owing to the increased cellularity present and nuclear atypia of endothelial cells and histiocytes [2-5] (Fig. 5.5). The epithelial and mesenchymal repair and atypia associated with chronic inflammation are generally much less pronounced than those occurring with acute inflammation. A chronic inflammatory response can be seen in autoimmune diseases and is associated with benign and malignant nonlymphoid neoplasms. Examples of nonlymphoid neoplasms commonly associated with lymphocytes include Warthin's tumor (Fig. 5.6), lymphoepithelioma, seminoma, thymoma (Fig. 5.7) and medullary carcinoma of the breast (Fig. 5.8). A false-negative diagnosis of these neoplasms may occur if the nonlymphoid elements are overlooked or obscured by the prominent lymphoid population.

Granulomatous Inflammation

Granulomas are generally small collections of modified macrophages called "epithelioid" histiocytes, usually surrounded by a peripheral rim of lymphocytes. Varying numbers of Langhans' or foreign body–type giant cells may be present. The

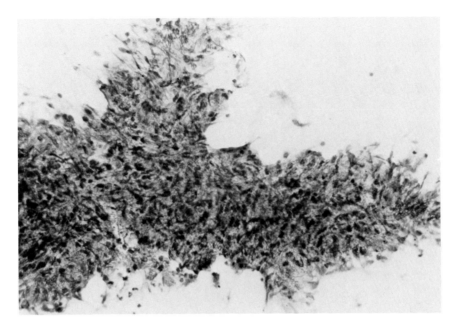

Fig. 5.11. Aspirate of cat-scratch disease showing palisading arrangement of the histiocytes which can be a clue for the correct diagnosis (Papanicolaou stain; × 100).

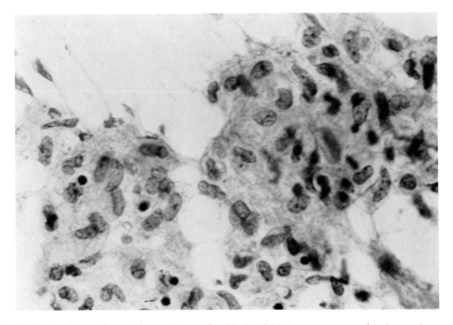

Fig. 5.12. Aspirate of sarcoid consisting of epithelioid histiocytes arranged in loose clusters. The histiocytes have delicate oval to elongated nuclei and surrounding pale greenish-blue to gray cytoplasm (Papanicolaou stain; × 400).

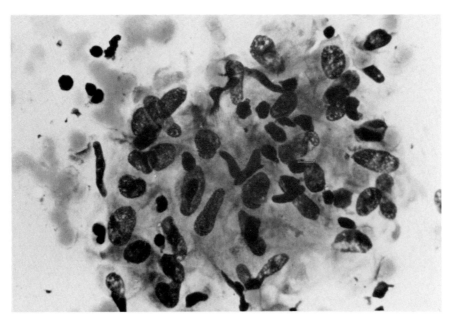

Fig. 5.13. FNA of a sarcoidal-type granuloma in which a cluster of epithelioid histiocytes is present. Note the elongated to bent nature of the nuclei with surrounding cytoplasm arranged in a syncytial fashion (Diff-Quik stain; ×400).

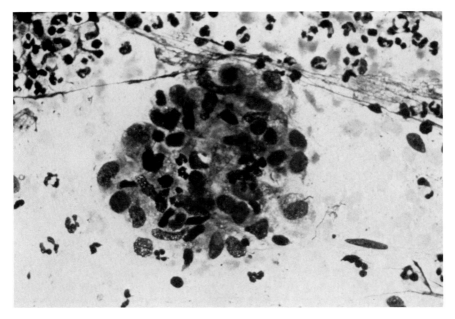

Fig. 5.14. FNA of a granuloma in a case of blastomycosis. The tight clustering of the epithelioid cells in the granuloma along with the enlarged and hyperchromatic nuclei of the cells could be a potential for a false-positive diagnosis of malignancy (Diff-Quik stain; ×200).

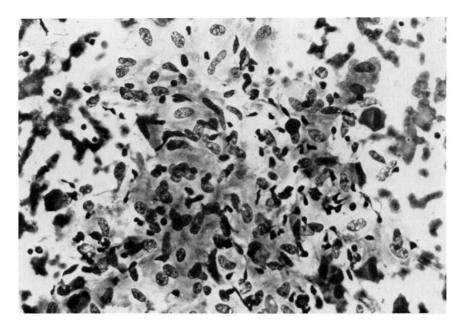

Fig. 5.15. FNA of mediastinal lymph node showing a prominent granulomatous reaction. The aspirate of the lung demonstrated a large cell carcinoma. These findings most likely represent a granulomatous response to the carcinoma in the draining mediastinal lymph nodes (Diff-Quik stain; ×200).

Langhans'-type giant cell contains many nuclei arranged around the peripheral portion of the cytoplasm, in a horseshoe pattern (Fig. 5.9). Foreign body–type giant cells have scattered nuclei and may also demonstrate evidence of cytophagocytosis (Fig. 5.10). Other cellular elements that may be seen in granulomatous inflammation include fibroblasts, plasma cells, and occasional neutrophils. Granulomatous processes can be necrotizing or nonnecrotizing. The morphologic patterns seen in granulomatous diseases may suggest the etiology of the process (Fig. 5.11). Granulomatous inflammation can be seen in bacterial diseases (tuberculosis, leprosy, catscratch disease), parasitic diseases (schistosomiasis), fungal diseases (cryptococcosis, blastomycosis), foreign body reactions to inorganic metals (silicosis, berylliosis), or diseases of unknown etiology such as sarcoidosis.

In FNA specimens, epithelioid histiocytes are arranged individually or in clusters. The epithelioid histiocytes are round, oval, or elongated, with nuclei that are oval, elongated, or bent, resembling boomerangs. With the Papanicolaou stain, the cytoplasm is a pale green-blue; the nucleus is euchromatic with an evenly dispersed granular chromatin and inconspicuous small nucleoli (Fig. 5.12). With the hematoxylin and eosin stain, the cells have a similar appearance, except that the cytoplasm is pale red. With the Diff-Quik stain, the cytoplasm is a pale gray-blue, and the nuclear chromatin is evenly distributed and granular with small blue nucleoli (Fig. 5.13). When the cells are found in aggregate, the cytoplasm may be arranged in a syncytial pattern. Although epithelioid histiocytes are fairly distinctive in the aspirated specimen, other histiocytic cells such as sinus histiocytes, dendritic reticulum

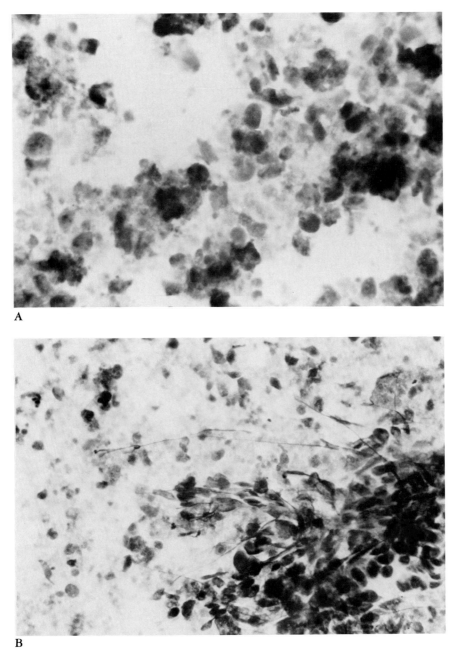

Fig. 5.16. A. Aspirate of poorly differentiated carcinoma of the lung demonstrating extensive coagulative necrosis of the malignant cells. No diagnostic tumor cells are present in this specimen. **B.** An additional aspirate of the peripheral portion of the carcinoma again shows extensive necrosis with a cluster of malignant cells (Papanicolaou stain; × 400).

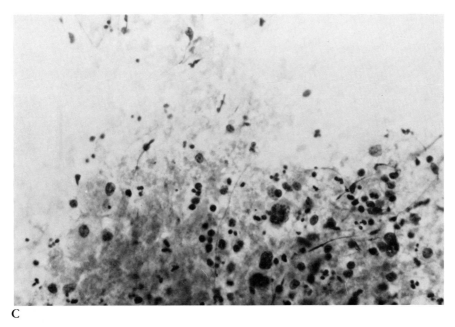

C

Fig. 5.16. C. FNA of Hodgkin's disease in which extensive necrosis is present along with some scattered atypical degenerating cells (Papanicolaou stain; × 100).

cells, interdigitating reticulum cells, and even fibroblasts may share similar features on occasion.

Granulomatous inflammation is one of the leading causes of false-positive diagnosis in FNA biopsy because epithelioid histiocytes tend to aggregate, and the novice or unwary cytologist may therefore confuse them with a clump of tumor (Fig. 5.14). Another cause of a false-positive diagnosis of malignancy is the associated inflammatory atypia of the epithelial cells that may be present in granulomatous inflammation. Moreover, a number of neoplastic lesions are associated with epithelioid histiocytes and granuloma formation. The most common neoplasms to have a granulomatous component include Hodgkin's and non-Hodgkin's lymphoma, seminoma, and thymoma. Occasional cases of carcinoma can be associated with nearby granulomas, or a granulomatous response may be present in the draining lymph nodes (Fig. 5.15).

Whenever granulomatous inflammation is identified, a thorough search for underlying organisms should be undertaken. Preferably, an additional aspirate should be submitted for microbiologic examination and special stains for organisms should be performed on these smears. The smears should also be polarized to identify foreign material.

Necrosis

Necrosis is the change that follows cell death in living tissue or organs and represents the major morphologic manifestation of irreversible cell injury.[1] Several types

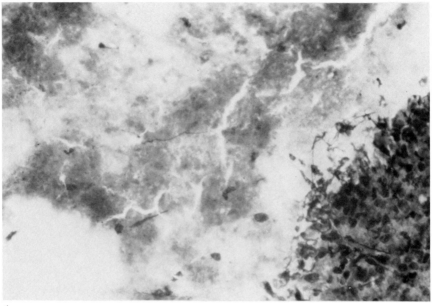

A

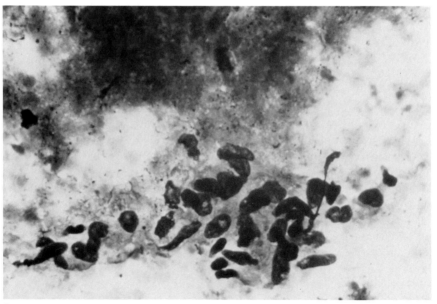

B

Fig. 5.17. **A.** FNA of tuberculosis in which there is extensive caseation necrosis. Note the fluffy granular quality of the caseous material (Diff-Quick stain; ×200). **B.** Another aspirate of tuberculosis in which a cluster of atypical epithelioid histiocytes is present along with caseation-type necrosis in the background (Diff-Quick stain; ×400).

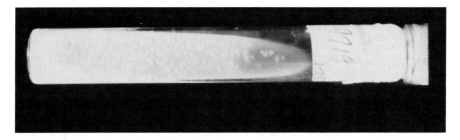

Fig. 5.18. Material cultured from the aspirate revealed a photochromogen which was identified by biochemical tests as *Mycobacterium kansasii*. Ziehl-Neelsen stain performed on the smears demonstrated long and variable length organisms with beadlike crossbanding suggestive of a nontuberculous mycobacterium.

of necrosis exist including coagulation necrosis, liquefactive necrosis, fat necrosis, caseous necrosis, and gangrenous necrosis. The type of necrosis may suggest the cause of cell injury. Coagulative necrosis is present when the cells have lost their nuclei with preservation of the basic shape of the cell. Recognition of these ghost cells may suggest an ischemic origin for the necrosis. Coagulation necrosis is also seen in tumor necrosis (Fig. 5.16). Caseous necrosis represents a combination of coagulative and liquefactive necrosis, converting the cellular material into a distinctive amorphous granular debris. Cytologically, this material takes on a fluffy granular appearance (Fig. 5.17).

Necrosis may be seen in benign or malignant processes. The underlying etiology may be inferred from the nature of the cellular elements associated with the necrosis. Of course, the presence of malignant cells will be diagnostic, although a prolonged search is sometimes required before preserved malignant cells are found. If a lesion is suspected to be neoplastic, reaspiration of the peripheral portion of the mass is recommended to permit a search for more viable cells (Fig. 5.16A & B). Necrosis may also be associated with granulomatous and acute inflammation. In any aspirate consisting predominantly of necrotic material, separate specimens for culture should be obtained and special stains for organisms performed (Fig. 5.18).

Fat necrosis is a specific type of necrosis seen in adipose tissue. Occasional examples may be due to trauma as in fat necrosis of the breast or soft tissue (Chapters 7 and 11). Fat necrosis may also be secondary to acute pancreatitis in which pancreatic enzymes such as lipases are released following necrosis of the pancreatic acinar cells. Fat necrosis may be present not only within the pancreas but in adipose tissue in the region of the pancreas and throughout the peritoneal cavity.[1] We have not encountered examples of enzymatic fat necrosis in our aspirated material.

Necrosis of thyroid neoplasms has been reported following FNA biopsy,[6-10] presumably secondary to biopsy-induced ischemic changes[9] (Fig. 5.19). Other histologic changes noted in thyroid nodules following FNA biopsy include hemorrhage, follicular degeneration, granulation tissue formation, fibrosis, nuclear atypia, and papillary endothelial hyperplasia of blood vessels.[10] The foregoing alterations are potential pitfalls for an incorrect diagnosis in repeat aspiration biopsies or in post-FNA thyroid surgical specimens.

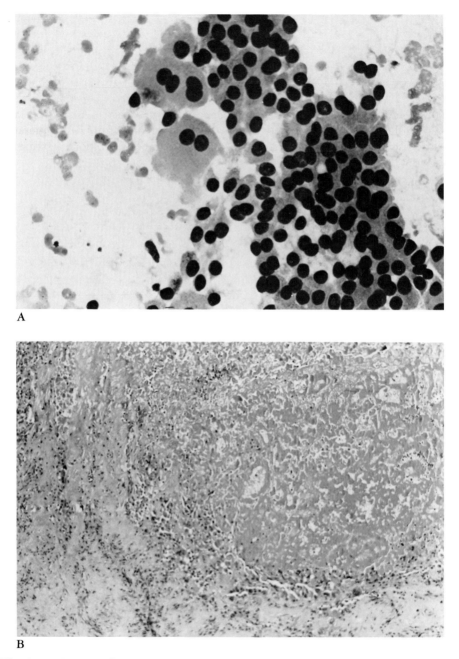

Fig. 5.19. A. FNA of Hurthle cell neoplasm of thyroid in which a loose cluster of Hurthle cells is present along with some nearby single cells demonstrating binucleation (Diff-Quik stain; ×200). **B.** Resected thyroid nodule following the aspiration shows almost complete necrosis of the Hurthle cell neoplasm (H&E; ×200).

Epithelial and Mesenchymal Repair

In conventional gynecologic and nongynecologic cytology, cells derived from epithelial repair and regeneration are quite common, because the cells obtained are from an epithelial mucosal surface. In contrast, the cells derived from aspiration of masses secondary to inflammation and wound healing are more often mesenchymal in origin (Chapter 11). However, when a solid organ is the site of aspiration, significant numbers of atypical epithelial cells may be obtained. This is especially common following a biopsy or surgical procedure, irradiation or chemotherapy, infection, ischemia (ie, pulmonary infarct), or a foreign body reaction to suture or calculus.

Criteria applicable to the recognition of epithelial repair in conventional exfoliative cytology samples are used to diagnose this process in FNA biopsy specimens[11] (Chapter 9). These criteria include appreciation of groups of cells arranged in cohesive flat sheets with distinct cell borders and maintenance of cell polarity. Single cells, when present, are quite few in number. The atypical features of epithelial repair are based mainly on the presence of enlarged nuclei with multiple prominent nucleoli, including macronucleoli. Mitotic figures may also be present. Features favoring a diagnosis of benign epithelial repair include oval or round nuclei with a smooth nuclear border, uniform appearance of the nuclei within the groups, and an evenly distributed chromatin pattern that tends to vary from vesicular to hypochromatic. Mesenchymal repair, in contrast to epithelial repair, tends to be sparsely cellular. However, atypical cytologic features may be present in the aspirate because irregularly shaped and occasional multinucleated cells are present along with loose aggregates and single mesenchymal cells.[2] Examples of epithelial and mesenchymal repair are presented throughout this monograph with a more complete discussion on mesenchymal repair in Chapter 11.

REFERENCES

1. Cotran RS, Kumar V, Robbins SL: *Robbins' Pathologic Basis of Disease,* 4th ed. Philadelphia, W.B. Saunders, 1989, pp 39–86.

2. James LP: Cytopathology of mesenchymal repair. *Diagn Cytopathol* 1:91–104, 1985.

3. Murad TM, August C: Radiation-induced atypia. A review. *Diagn Cytopathol* 1:137–152, 1985.

4. Weidner N, Askin FB, Berthrong M, et al.: Bizarre (pseudomalignant) granulation-tissue reactions following ionizing-radiation exposure: a microscopic, immunohistochemical, and flow-cytometric study. *Cancer* 59:1509–1514, 1987.

5. Silverman JF: Breast. *Comprehensive Cytopathology,* ed. Marluce Bibbo. Philadelphia, W.B. Saunders, 1991, pp 709–713.

6. Bauman A, Strawbridge HTC: Spontaneous disappearance of an atypical Hurthle cell adenoma. *Am J Clin Pathol* 80:399–402, 1983.

7. Jones JD, Pittman DL, Sanders LR: Necrosis of thyroid nodules after fine needle aspiration. *Acta Cytol* 29:29–32, 1985.

8. Jayaram G, Aggarwal S: Infarction of thyroid nodule: a rare complication following fine needle aspiration. *Acta Cytol* 33:940–941, 1989.

9. Merino MJ, LiVolsi VA: Worrisome histologic alterations following fine needle aspiration of thyroid. *Lab Invest* 62:59, 1990 (abstract).

10. Axiotis CA, Merino MJ, Ain K, et al.: Papillary endothelial hyperplasia in the thyroid following fine-needle aspiration. *Arch Pathol Lab Med* 115:240–242, 1991.

11. Bibbo M, Keebler CM, Wied GL: The cytologic diagnosis of tissue repair in the female genital tract. *Acta Cytol* 15:133–137, 1971.

6

Lymph Nodes

Thomas F. Kardos

INTRODUCTION

By definition, lymphadenitis is an acute or chronic inflammation of the lymph node. The inciting agent may be a pathogen (most frequently bacterial, mycobacterial, viral, or fungal) or material foreign to the lymph node such as melanin pigment or silicone. Occasionally, a chronic antigenic stimulus or an abnormal immune response as seen in autoimmune diseases can cause lymphadenitis. The lymphadenites are the most common cause of lymphadenopathy, far outnumbering lymphomas or metastatic malignancies as a cause of lymph node enlargement.

The diagnosis of lymphadenitis is well suited to aspiration biopsy (Table 6.1). The earliest documented application of FNA of lymph nodes was in a lymphadenitis: identifying trypanosomes of sleeping sickness in aspirated material.[1] Early success did not capture the attention or imagination of clinicians, and for years only sporadic reports occurred in which aspiration cytology was applied in the evaluation of lymphadenopathy, including some cases of inflammatory disease.[2,3,4] In recent years however, with expanded interest in FNA cytology of lymph nodes, large series documenting the utility of lymph node aspiration in managing common infectious diseases, as well as isolated reports detailing the appearance of some of the more unusual inflammatory processes are appearing regularly in the medical literature.[5-26]

EXAMINATION OF THE PATIENT

Whenever a patient with lymphadenopathy is evaluated, a number of clinical features need to be considered.

TABLE 6.1. Lymphadenites Diagnosed by FNA Biopsy

Acute suppurative lymphadenitis
Noncaseating granulomatous lymphadenitis
Caseating granulomas
Necrotizing granulomatous lymphadenitis
Granulomas associated with reactive lymphoid cells
Chronic lymphadenitis
Miscellaneous entities

Clinical History

The patient should be questioned regarding such factors as a history of malignancy, autoimmune disease, or drug exposure (eg, diphenylhydantoin, allopurinol), risk factors for AIDS; or a history of recent flulike symptoms.

The age of the patient should be noted. Children and young adults have active immune systems that mount a robust response to stimuli such as infections, with subsequent lymph node enlargement that may persist for some time. It is not at all uncommon to find palpable cervical lymph nodes in children. With increasing age the likelihood that significantly enlarged lymph nodes are benign decreases substantially. Patient age is also important to note because certain types of malignancies have relatively restricted age distributions.

Systemic symptoms such as fever, chills, night sweats, and weight loss should be noted. These symptoms may be associated with inflammatory processes as well as some non-Hodgkin's and Hodgkin's lymphomas.

A number of geographic regions expose individuals to risks of specific infections, including parasitic and fungal diseases. A thorough travel or residence history should alert the pathologist to these possibilities.

Physical Examination

The site of involvement should be noted. Lymphadenopathy may be restricted to a solitary node or to a localized group of nodes draining an anatomic region; or may also be generalized. Both benign and malignant processes may lead to localized or generalized adenopathy. Among the causes of generalized lymphadenopathy are infectious mononucleosis, cytomegalovirus, tuberculosis, infectious hepatitis, bacterial endocarditis, toxoplasmosis, and histoplasmosis, as well as autoimmune diseases. Leukemias and lymphomas (particularly low grade lymphomas) may also lead to systemic lymphadenopathy. Occasionally, patients with carcinoma may even present with diffuse lymphadenopathy.

Lymph nodes are distributed throughout the body. For most purposes the superficial nodes can be divided into five major groups: cervicofacial–supraclavicular, axillary, epitrochlear, inguinal, and femoral. Other superficial nodes that occasionally become pathologically enlarged include the suboccipital, postauricular, suprasternal, and popliteal. These nodes are readily accessible to palpation and aspiration. Deep-seated lymph nodes occur in the mediastinum, abdomen, pelvis, and lower extremities. These nodes usually require radiologic guidance for FNA biopsy.

Palpable lymphadenopathy does not necessarily indicate a pathologic condition.

TABLE 6.2. Drainage Sites of Lymph Nodes

Lymph Node	Region Drained
Submental	Lips, mouth, tongue
Submandibular	Face
Preauricular	Ears, temporal scalp
Postauricular	Scalp
Occipital	Scalp
Superficial cervical	Ears, parotid
Deep cervical	Tongue, larynx, thyroid, trachea, esophagus
Supraclavicular	Neck, axillae, genitourinary and gastro-intestinal tracts (GU and GI involve left supraclavicular lymph node)
Inguinal	Lower extremities, pelvis
Axillary	Chest, upper extremities

Small (<1 cm) inguinal lymph nodes, probably resulting from repeated superficial leg infections are commonplace and are usually not a worthy target for FNA biopsy. Likewise, enlarged but very soft, doughy feeling axillary lymph nodes are found especially in women. These nodes contain only a narrow peripheral rim of lymphoid tissue with a center replaced by fat. Lymphadenopathy of the cervical region is frequent in the pediatric age group, with some children having multiple 1- to 2-cm nodes that may persist in some cases for years. These nodal enlargements are usually caused by infection in sites such as the ear or throat.

To understand the clinical significance of lymphadenopathy resulting from metastatic tumor or infections, it is useful to understand regional drainage patterns (Table 6.2). Isolated occipital, postauricular, or epitrochlear adenopathy is rarely a result of lymphoma, whereas supraclavicular, mediastinal, or abdominal adenopathy generally indicates a serious disease. The region drained by the enlarged lymph nodes should be examined for evidence of inflammation or malignancy.

Lymph node size and contour has some correlation with the cytomorphologic findings seen in the aspirate. A substantially enlarged lymph node (2.5 cm or greater in diameter), to be considered cytologically benign, should have either a characteristic benign polymorphic reactive pattern or evidence of acute lymphadenitis. Otherwise the lymph node should be considered suspicious for malignancy. To gauge its size correctly, a lymph node should be measured with a ruler. Bulging, rounded lymph nodes may be a result of chronic hyperplasia as well as acute lymphadenitis or malignancy in children. However, in older adults they are most often malignant, occasionally secondary to acute lymphadenitis, but only rarely secondary to chronic hyperplasia.

The consistency of the lymph node should be noted. Most acute and chronic lymphadenites are soft to firm in consistency. Hard lymph nodes are only infrequently benign. Malignant processes, although variable in consistency, are generally firm to hard. Fluctuant nodes indicate necrosis related to benign or malignant disease.

Lymph node fixation to surrounding structures occurs in malignant processes including metastatic disease, Hodgkin's disease, and some non-Hodgkin's lymphomas, and, less commonly, in acute lymphadenitis with secondary fibrosis. Acute lymphadenitis may also result in matted, circumscribed, mobile lymph nodes.

Pain or tenderness of an enlarged lymph node generally occurs when the lymph node has rapidly enlarged with stretching of the capsule. Such rapid enlargement is usually associated with a benign infectious process, although rapidly proliferating lymphomas such as Burkitt's and lymphoblastic lymphomas may incite local tenderness or pain. When pain is related to inflammation, the overlying skin may be warm or reddened. A peculiar phenomenon is described in Hodgkin's disease in which tenderness may follow alcohol ingestion.

CHRONIC NONSPECIFIC LYMPHADENITIS

A considerable variety of endogenous or exogenous factors may act on the lymph node, inciting a nonspecific chronic lymphadenitis. Among these causes are inflammation, infection, and autoimmune disease. In most instances the process is a self-limited lymphadenopathy that gradually diminishes and disappears sometime after the offending agent is removed. Reactive hyperplasia of this type is particularly common, and the response is often dramatic in childhood. Lymph nodes may reach prominent proportions and persist for some time. In adulthood the immune response in nonspecific chronic lymphadenitis tends to be more muted with less impressive lymphadenopathy usually the result.

The morphologic appearance of nonspecific chronic lymphadenitis is not uniform; it forms a wide spectrum of histologic patterns. Patterns differ according to the type and the degree of stimulus and the duration of the response. Enlargement of the lymph node may be primarily restricted to expansion of one compartment such as the follicular centers or the paracortical zone. In the great majority of cases, however, all compartments are affected to some degree.

Within compartments the constituent cells vary according to the nature, intensity, and duration of the stimulus. This variability includes both cell size and type. Larger lymphoid cells, both in the germinal centers and the paracortical zones, are the proliferating cells, and the more intense and immediate the stimulus, the greater the percentage of large cells present. However, even with the most intense response, it is rare that smaller lymphocytes are not the dominant cells in terms of total numbers.

When lymphocytes respond to a stimulus, some of the proliferating cells do not survive. Resultant nuclear debris from cell death is engulfed by histiocytes, thereby forming tingible-body macrophages. This process of cell death and nuclear debris engulfment by histiocytes is particularly common in the reactive germinal center. In the aspirate from chronic lymphadenitis, the tingible-body macrophages are often found entrapped in or located near syncytia of histiocytic-appearing cells, dendritic reticulum cells. A range of large and small lymphocytes are also found in and around these syncytia (Fig. 6.1). These tissue fragments represent pieces of reactive follicular centers.[7,27]

A common cellular constituent in chronic lymphadenitis are lymphocytes having an abundant cytoplasm, which stain varying shades of blue from pale to deep in intensity with Romanovsky preparation. This blue cytoplasm imparts a plasmacy-

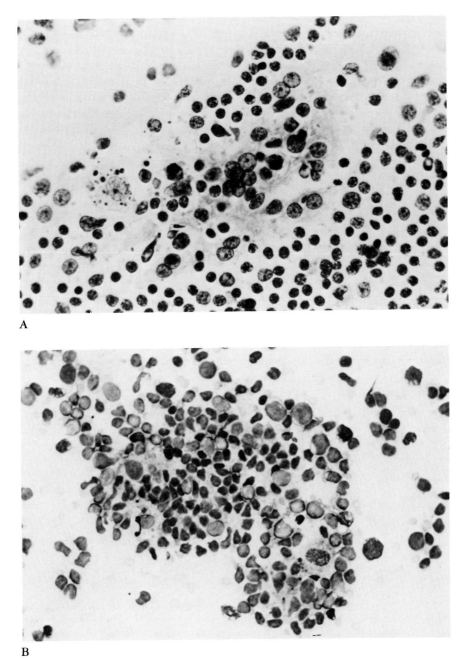

A

B

Fig. 6.1. A. FNA of a reactive lymph node showing a reactive follicular center fragment consisting of a syncytium of dendritic reticulum cells infiltrated and surrounded by reactive lymphocytes of varying size. At the edge of the fragment is a tingible-body macrophage engulfing nuclear debris (Papanicolaou stain; ×100). **B.** Similar fragment containing a syncytium of dendritic cells, reactive lymphocytes, and tingible-body macrophages (Diff-Quik stain; ×100).

toid appearance to the cells. Immunologic studies, however, indicate these cells with abundant cytoplasm may be of either B- or T-cell lineage. These cells range from relatively mature plasmacytoid lymphocytes through more immature plasmablasts to the most immature immunoblasts (Fig. 6.2). Through this transition the cells progressively enlarge, chromatin becomes finer, and nucleoli appear and enlarge with the immunoblasts having a central macronucleolus. In some cases the pattern of more mature plasmacytoid lymphocytes dominates the subpopulation of plasmacytoid cells, whereas in other cases there is a greater shift toward immature plasmablasts and immunoblasts. These cells occupy the paracortical and medullary regions of the lymph node and again the total numbers and percentages of cell types vary from case to case depending on the type, intensity, and duration of stimulus.[27]

The foregoing discussion indicates that the common findings in chronic lymphadenitis with a substantial degree of hyperplasia include:

A range of lymphoid cells with small lymphocytes almost always predominating

A progressive transition in size and other cytologic features from smaller to larger lymphocytes

The presence of tingible-body macrophages, isolated or as part of reactive follicular center fragments

Generally, presence of a subpopulation of plasmacytoid lymphocytes

One striking pattern of chronic lymphadenitis is that in which lymphocytes with abundant cytoplasms dominate. These cells are best seen in the Giemsa-type preparation; the staining intensity ranges from almost clear, pale blue to intense, deep blue with a plasmacytoid appearance. The hallmark disease in which a plasmacytoid pattern is encountered is infectious mononucleosis (Fig. 6.3).[16,17] In most instances this disease has a characteristic and recognizable presentation with patients usually 15 to 30 years old and having sore throat, cervical lymphadenopathy, low grade fever, often a transient rash, and splenomegaly as well as characteristic hematologic and serologic findings. Occasional atypical cases may pose a diagnostic dilemma, and substantially enlarged lymph nodes should be regarded with suspicion. Other viral infections as well as drug-induced lymphadenopathy, angioimmunoblastic lymphadenopathy, and some early-phase necrotizing lymphadenites also present with a pattern in which plasmacytoid lymphocytes are dominant. Drug-induced lymphadenopathy is often accompanied by eosinophils,[28] whereas in angioimmunoblastic lymphadenopathy the specimens may display eosinophils, epithelioid histiocytes, or both.[29]

Some non-Hodgkin's lymphomas also have a plasmacytoid appearance, and this raises diagnostic difficulties in distinguishing these malignancies from reactive plasmacytoid lymphadenites. In some cases distinction based solely on FNA cytologic findings is not possible, but some criteria allow differentiation in many cases (vide infra).[27]

Differential Diagnosis in Chronic Lymphadenitis

The most problematic differential diagnosis of chronic lymphadenitis is lymphoma. Lymphomas, like chronic lymphadenites, can present with a wide spectrum of pat-

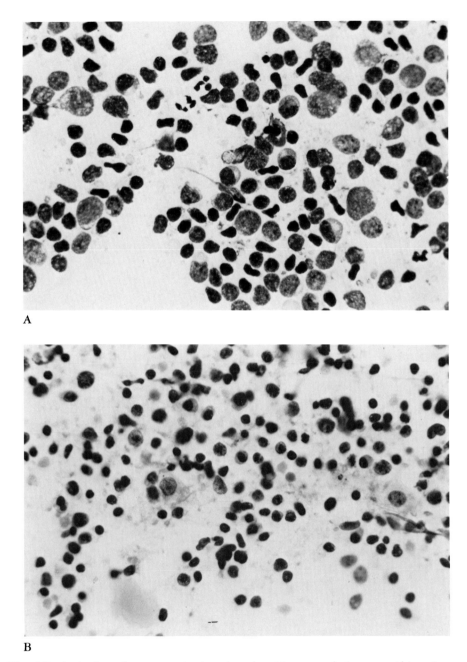

A

B

Fig. 6.2. A. Aspirate from a reactive lymph node with scattered plasmacytoid lymphocytes containing a relative abundance of eccentric blue-staining cytoplasm (Diff-Quik stain; ×200). **B.** The same aspirate as in (A) stained with Papanicolaou stain. Note how the plasmacytoid lymphocytes are much less conspicuous with this type preparation (Papanicolaou stain; ×100).

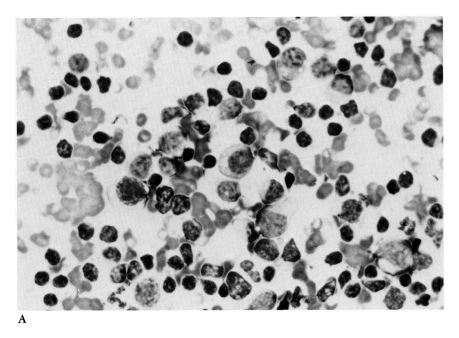

A

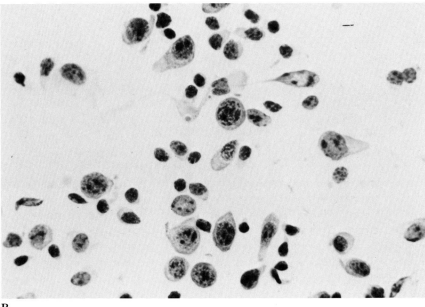

B

Fig. 6.3. A. An aspirate from patients with infectious mononucleosis consisting of various cells ranging from plasmacytoid lymphocytes to immunoblasts, many containing a relative abundance of cytoplasm (Diff-Quik stain; ×200). **B.** The same aspirate as in (A). Numerous cells with plasmacytoid features stained with H&E preparation (Papanicolaou stain; ×400).

TABLE 6.3. Features of Reactive Lymphadenopathy

Variable cellularity; usually moderate to high
Mixed population of lymphocytes
Small lymphocytes almost always predominant
Progressive transformation from small to large lymphocytes
Subpopulation of "plasmacytoid" lymphocytes usually present
Tingible-body macrophages should be present in a mixed population
Reactive follicular center fragments usually present

terns. It is difficult to generalize about distinguishing these processes, but there are a number of features that aid in making a correct diagnosis in FNA specimens (Tables 6.3 and 6.4).

Monomorphism vs. Polymorphism

Classically lymphomas are characterized cytologically as being monotonous in appearance, whereas reactive processes are portrayed as being polymorphous[30] (Fig. 6.4). This is generally true, but there are exceptions. Monotonous populations of small lymphocytes may be obtained from mildly reactive or indolent lymph nodes (Fig. 6.5). These populations may result from prolonged antigenic stimulation of germinal centers or expansion of mantle zones, paracortical zones, or medullary cords. Aspirates from these benign lymph nodes with their monotonous population of small lymphocytes are among the most vexing problems in lymph node aspiration biopsy. On cytologic grounds alone it may be impossible to distinguish these monotonous reactive patterns from some low grade lymphomas. In clinical terms, benign lymph nodes with this pattern are small and isolated and have been present for some time. This clinical setting may assist in correctly identifying this benign monomorphic pattern. Immunologic studies also are often helpful, because the lymphomas with this pattern are almost invariably B cell in type and demonstrate monoclonality, whereas the reactive processes show a mixed immunologic phenotype. In contrast to aspirates with a monotonous population of small lymphocytes, which may occasionally be benign, aspirates composed of monotonous populations of large or intermediate-size cells are almost invariably malignant.

Polymorphous lymph node aspirates are generally benign, but again there are exceptions. Mixed cell lymphomas present a heterogenous population of cells by size and sometimes even by type. Even some large cell lymphomas contain substantial numbers of smaller cells, so they may appear somewhat polymorphic in an aspirate (Fig. 6.6). Hodgkin's disease also may be quite polymorphous. Features noted below allow distinction of polymorphous lymphomas from reactive process in the majority of cases.

TABLE 6.4. Cytologic Features Associated With Neoplastic Lymph Nodes

Low cellularity aspirate in a significantly enlarged lymph node, ie. >2.5 cm
Bizarre enlarged cells
Marked nuclear membrane irregularities
Individual cell necrosis
Lymphoid monomorphism, except in aspirates of indolent lymph nodes

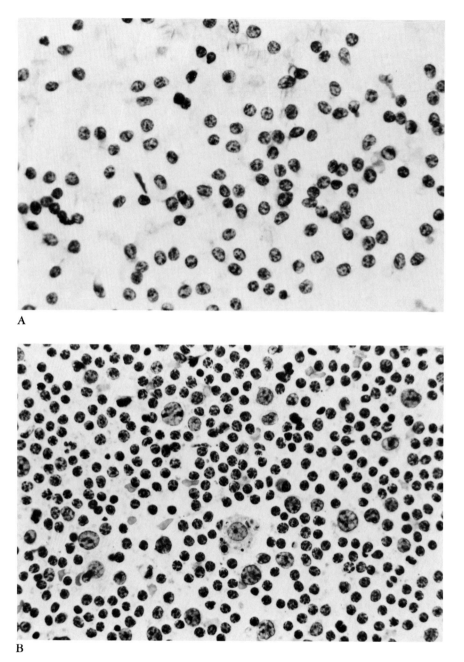

Fig. 6.4. A. Monotonous population of mature-appearing small lymphocytes from a patient with small cell lymphoma (Papanicolaou stain; ×200). **B.** Heterogenuous population of lymphocytes with predominance of small mature-appearing lymphocytes, along with scattered larger forms from a reactive lymph node (Papanicolaou stain; ×200).

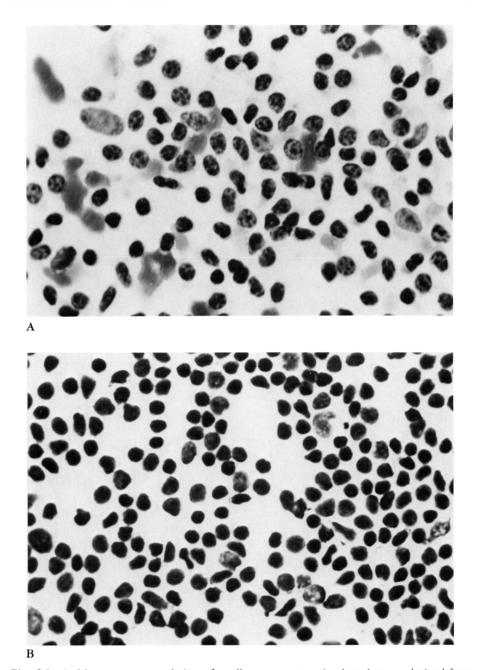

A

B

Fig. 6.5. A. Monotonous population of small, mature-appearing lymphocytes derived from a minimally reactive lymph node (Papanicolaou stain; ×400). **B.** Diff-Quik preparation from the same case as (A). On cytologic grounds, this aspirate cannot be reliably distinguished from a small cell lymphoma (Diff-Quik stain; ×200).

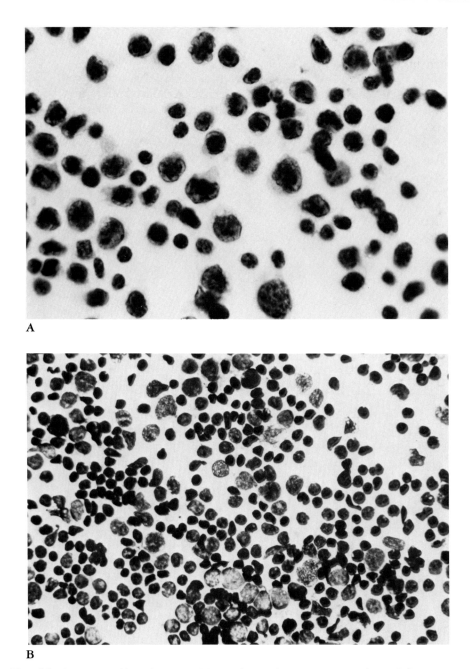

Fig. 6.6. A. Range of lymphocytes with a polymorphous appearance derived from an aspirate of a lymph node involved by a mixed small and large cell lymphoma (Papanicolaou stain; ×400). **B.** Same case as (A) with a range of large and small lymphocytes as well as some transitional forms derived from a mixed small and large cell lymphoma (Diff-Quik stain; ×100).

Tingible-Body Macrophages and Reactive Follicular Center Fragments

As noted previously, tingible-body macrophages in lymph nodes are a result of lymphocyte proliferation, occasional cell death, and engulfment of nuclear debris by histiocytes. In chronic lymphadenitis, reactive germinal centers in particular contribute tingible-body macrophages to the aspirated material. These cells, however, may also be found in high grade lymphomas such as large cell, immunoblastic, lymphoblastic, and small noncleaved cell lymphomas, in which rapid cell proliferation occurs (Fig. 6.7). Fortunately for purposes of identification in aspiration material, reactive lymphadenopathy usually presents as a mixed or occasionally small cell–predominant population in FNA biopsies, whereas high grade lymphomas usually present as a relatively monotonous population of large or intermediate-size lymphocytes. Therefore, a benign process is likely when tingible-body macrophages are found in a mixed cell population either as isolated cells or as part of reactive follicular center fragments. In contrast, when these cells are lacking in a lymph node aspirate with a mixed pattern, the lymph node should be regarded with suspicion.[27]

Bizarre Cells

Scattered bizarre cells in a lymph node should be considered highly abnormal. Bizarre cells are defined as cells that stand out as a distinct second population owing mainly to their relatively large size when an aspirate is scanned with a 10× objective. Rare bizarre cells may represent histiocytes, mesenchymal cells, or lymphoid cells. However, when bizarre cells are seen in substantial numbers, particularly when the cells have prominent macronucleoli or marked irregularities in nuclear contour, the specimen should be suspicious for malignancy. Bizarre cells may be encountered in malignant lymphomas, both non-Hodgkin's and Hodgkin's, as well as metastatic disease (Fig. 6.8).

Nuclear Contours

Aspirates of reactive lymphadenopathies do not yield lymphoid populations in which a substantial subpopulation of the cells have marked nuclear membrane irregularities. Marked irregularities almost always denote a malignant population of cells, either Hodgkin's or non-Hodgkin's lymphoma or a metastatic malignancy. Nuclear membrane irregularities are best appreciated in an alcohol-fixed Papanicolaou or hematoxylin and eosin–stained preparation (Fig. 6.9). With these preparations, the three-dimensional contour of the cells is better preserved. In a Romanovsky-stained preparation, cells are flattened so that internal cleavages are difficult to appreciate. Irregularities are also best evaluated with a 100× lens because cells appearing only mildly irregular at 40× can show profound complexities at high magnification.

Individual Cell Necrosis

With very few exceptions the presence of substantial individual cell necrosis in the absence of acute inflammation is an indication of a malignant process, again representing either lymphoma or metastatic disease (Fig. 6.10). Rare exceptions to

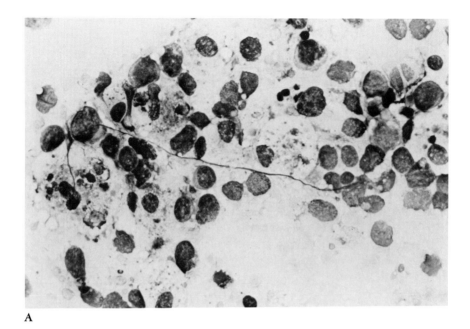

A

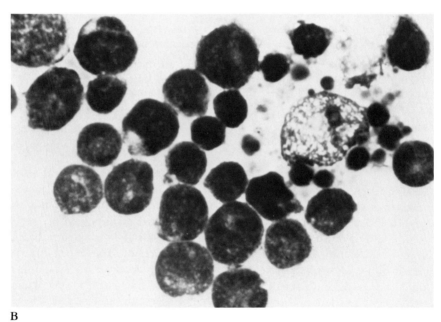

B

Fig. 6.7. A. Tingible body-macrophages in an aspirate of a high grade, large cell lymphoma (Diff-Quik stain; ×400). **B.** Tingible-body macrophage in an aspirate from a lymph node involved by lymphoblastic lymphoma, another high grade lymphoma (Diff-Quik stain; ×600).

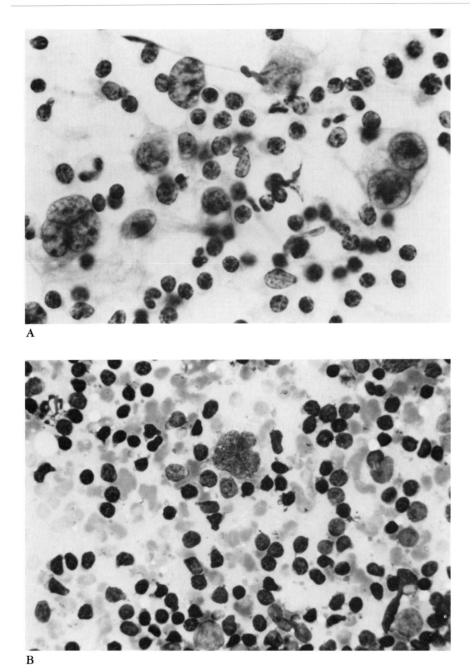

A

B

Fig. 6.8. A. Bizarre cells in an aspirate of Hodgkin's disease. These cells contrast strikingly with the small mature lymphocytes in the same field (Papanicolaou stain; ×400). **B.** Bizarre cell derived from an aspirate of a lymph node involved by a large cell lymphoma which was rich in benign lymphocytes. Bizarre cells are frequently more easily identified in an air-dried Giemsa preparation than in a Papanicolaou-stained preparation (Diff-Quik stain; ×400).

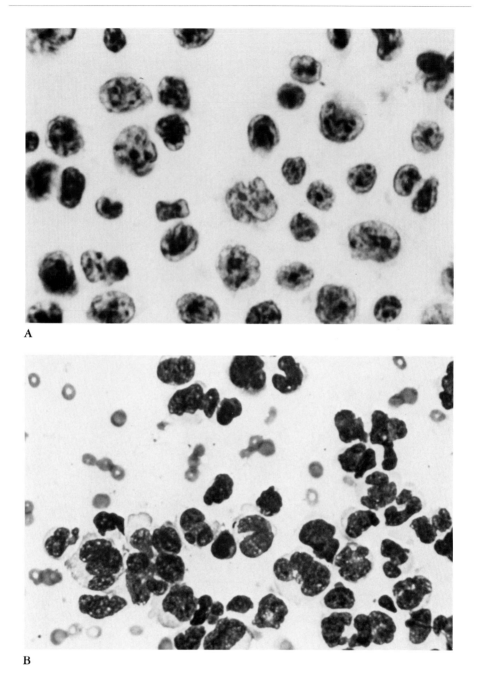

Fig. 6.9. A. Marked cleavages and irregularities of nuclear membrane contour in cells from an aspirate of a lymph node involved by small cleaved cell lymphoma (Papanicolaou stain; ×1000). **B.** Marked nuclear lobations and cleavages in a large cell lymphoma which immunologically was of T-cell type (Diff-Quik stain; ×400). Nuclear membrane irregularities are often best appreciated under oil magnification with a Papanicolaou-stained preparation.

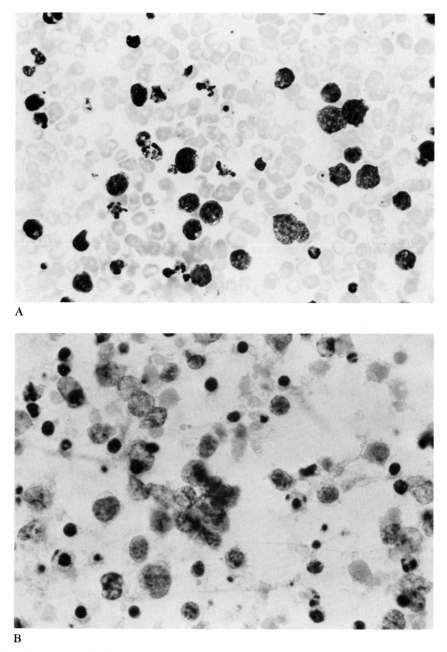

Fig. 6.10. A. Individual cell necrosis in a case of Burkitt's lymphoma (Diff-Quik stain; ×200). **B.** Individual cell necrosis in a case of small cell undifferentiated carcinoma (Papanicolaou stain; ×400).

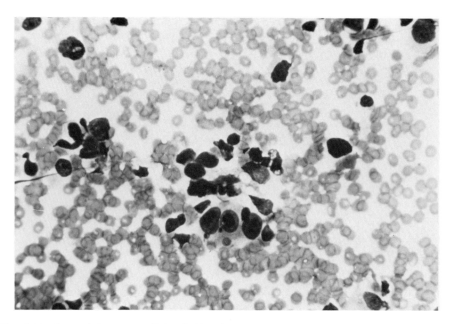

Fig. 6.11. One of the most cellular fields of metastatic adenocarcinoma in an aspirate of a 3.5-cm cervical lymph node. Low cellular aspirates from substantially enlarged lymph nodes almost always indicate a malignant process if the node has been properly aspirated (Diff-Quik stain; ×200).

this include such uncommon conditions as spontaneous infarction of the lymph node, infectious mononucleosis, systemic lupus erythematosus, Kikuchi's lymphadenitis, and Kawasaki's disease.

Cellularity

An adequate sample of a lymph node that is substantially enlarged (2.5 cm in diameter or greater) should yield at least a moderately cellular aspirate. If only very low cellularity is obtained with vigorous sampling, a malignant condition is generally indicated (Fig. 6.11). Rarely, conditions such as sarcoidosis will cause prominent, enlarged lymph nodes although sampling will yield very little material.

As noted earlier, distinction of reactive plasmacytoid processes from plasmacytoid lymphomas may pose considerable problems. Certain features that may be present in an aspirate dominated by plasmacytoid cells are suspicious of malignancy (Table 6.5). These features include a population of cells that is almost exclusively plasmacytoid; a monotypic population of plasmacytoid lymphocytes without some range from plasmacytoid lymphocytes to immunoblasts; numerous multinucleated plasmacytoid cells; prominent nucleoli in small as well as large cells; bizarre cells either by size or nuclear membrane contour; low cellular yield from a substantially enlarged node; numerous eosinophils, fibroblasts or epithelioid histiocytes; or prominent individual cell necrosis.

TABLE 6.5. Features Suspicious for Malignancy in Aspirates Dominated by
Plasmacytoid Lymphocytes

> Vast majority of cells having plasmacytoid feature
> Plasmacytoid cells are monotypic
> Bizarre cells or cells with marked nuclear membrane irregularities
> Numerous multinucleated cells
> Prominent nucleoli in smaller cells
> Numerous eosinophils, fibroblasts, and/or epithelioid histiocytes
> Low cellularity aspirate from an enlarged lymph node

LYMPHADENITIS ASSOCIATED WITH NEUTROPHILS, NECROSIS, AND/OR GRANULOMATA

Acute Suppurative Lymphadenitis

The commonest cause of acute suppurative lymphadenitis is an acute local septic infection such as tonsillitis, cellulitis, facial or oral trauma, or an infected wound or burn. Children are commonly affected, with the most frequent offending organisms being streptococci and staphylococci. Other less common agents causing this process include *Pseudomonas aeruginosa,* as in infections occurring in burns or wounds, and *Escherichia coli* or *Streptococcus faecalis* from localized peritoneal abscesses. *Haemophilus ducreyi,* the etiologic agent of chancroid, and gonococcal infection both can lead to regional suppurative lymphadenitis.[31]

Lymph nodes enlarged as a result of acute suppurative lymphadenitis are generally tender or painful, warm, and fluctuant; they may have overlying erythema. Aspiration often yields gross pus. Microscopic examination reveals neutrophils, histiocytes, and a background of necrosis. Bacteria often may be identified in either the Papanicolaou or the Romanovsky stain-type but are more readily identified in the latter preparation (Fig. 6.12).

Differential diagnosis includes both carcinomas and lymphomas with extensive necrosis and neutrophilic infiltration, inflamed inclusion cyst, congenital cysts, and abscesses. Inflamed branchial cleft and keratinous cysts may overlap cytologically in FNA biopsies when squamous cells are identified. Also, late stages of necrotizing granulomatous lymphadenitis may yield only neutrophils and necrosis (vide infra). Abscesses of soft tissue are cytologically indistinguishable from suppurative lymphadenitis.

Squamous cell carcinomas, particularly those with extensive keratinization, may yield necrosis, neutrophils, and little or no tumor. These specimens can be mistaken for an abscess or suppurative lymphadenitis. Whenever suppurative lymphadenitis is considered in a FNA biopsy of a lymph node, especially in an older individual, a thorough search for tumor cells or even anucleate keratin flakes should be made. In an older individual, several aspirations should be performed with some of the biopsies targeted at the periphery of the mass where viable tumor cells, if present,

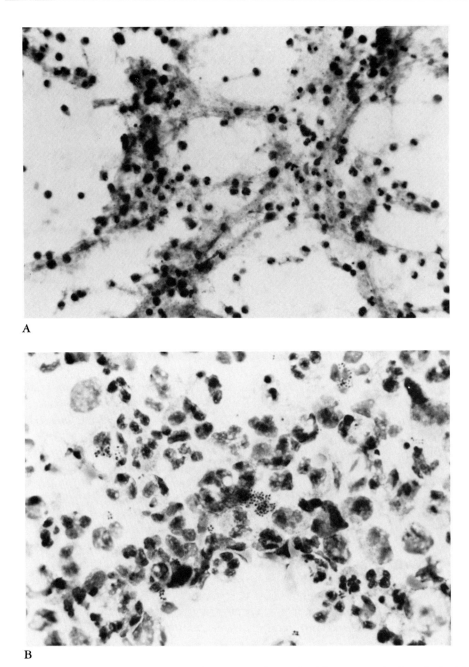

A

B

Fig. 6.12. **A.** Fine-needle aspiration of a lymph node involved by suppurative lymphadenitis secondary to bacterial infection. Aspirate shows numerous neutrophils and histiocytes with a background of granular necrosis (Papanicolaou stain; × 100). **B.** Same case as (A). Neutrophils and histiocytes as well as necrosis are present. Note the presence of cocci within some of the neutrophils (Diff-Quik stain; × 400).

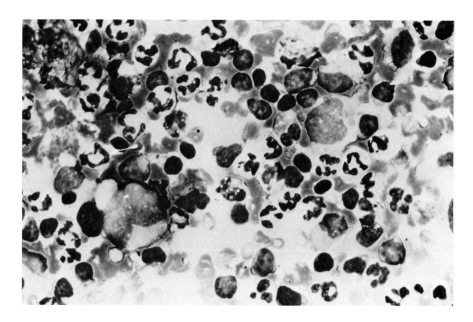

Fig. 6.13. Case of suppurative Hodgkin's disease with numerous neutrophils and large numbers of bizarre cells including Reed–Sternberg cells and Hodgkin's cells (Diff-Quik stain; × 200).

might be found. Other types of carcinoma including adenocarcinoma may occasionally have a necrotizing suppurative pattern.[32]

Hodgkin's disease, usually of nodular sclerosing type, will rarely present with a suppurative lymphadenitis–like pattern (Fig. 6.13). Non-Hodgkin's lymphomas very rarely have a pattern of suppurative necrosis.[33]

Noncaseating Granulomatous Lymphadenitis

Sarcoidosis is the disease most commonly associated with noncaseating granulomas. This is a systemic disease that may involve a number of organ systems and is of uncertain etiology. Although the most commonly involved sites are the lungs, skin, and eyes, in one study 3.5% of patients presented with enlarged superficial lymphadenopathy.[34] Noncaseating granulomas are by no means limited to sarcoidosis, since these structures may also be found in Hodgkin's disease, infrequently in non-Hodgkin's lymphomas, some lymph nodes draining carcinoma (especially breast and stomach), and also in uncommon diseases such as tuberculoid leprosy and berylliosis.[35] Occasionally, granulomatous processes such as tuberculosis, more often characterized by caseating granulomas, will have a dominant pattern of noncaseating granulomas.

Noncaseating granulomas may be sparse or may densely populate the enlarged lymph node. When noncaseating granulomas are numerous, the aspirating needle may encounter a gritty sensation which can also be felt if numerous hard granulomas are spread on a slide. Noncaseating granulomatous processes are among the very few benign processes in which a substantially enlarged lymph node is thoroughly sampled but yields only scant material.

Cytologically, granulomatous processes yield an aspirate containing variable numbers of cohesive or "hard" granulomas, but they are usually relatively limited in number. The background contains variable numbers of mature lymphocytes, possibly a few plasma cells, and some isolated epithelioid histiocytes. Multinucleated giant cells are generally limited in number in sarcoidosis[5] (Fig. 6.14). Other diagnoses should be considered if numerous multinucleated cells are present in the aspirate. Necrosis, although occasionally present as small foci in histologic sections of sarcoid, is very uncommon in FNA biopsies of lymph nodes and if present should suggest other processes. Rarely, nonspecific structures such as asteroid and Schaumann bodies are found in the aspirated material.

The differential diagnosis of noncaseating granuloma is limited. Because granulomas consist of aggregates of epithelioid cells, they have the potential of being mistaken for carcinoma. Experience and care should preclude this possibility.

Caseous Granulomatous Lymphadenitis

Tuberculous lymphadenitis is the most common cause of caseous granulomas in FNA biopsies of lymph nodes. Although tuberculosis has many clinical patterns of presentation, in some instances lymphadenopathy is the initial manifestation. Tuberculous lymphadenopathy may be secondary to spread from pulmonary disease, as part of a virulent tuberculous sepsis, in association with BCG vaccination, or as scrofula (tuberculous cervical lymphadenitis). Scrofula usually presents with an insidious onset of enlarged, matted, painless lymph nodes without fever or other constitutional symptoms. Most frequently this disease is seen in children or in adults from countries where tuberculosis is endemic.

Although caseous necrosis and loose, poorly formed granulomas are the pattern most commonly associated with tuberculous lymphadenopathy (Fig. 6.15), the actual patterns encountered are quite variable.[12,13] Rarely, there may be epithelioid granulomas, with or without giant cells in a milieu of reactive lymphocytes. Exceptionally, the granuloma can be quite cohesive. A more common pattern includes granulomas, sometimes degenerating, and granular necrotic material with some scattered lymphocytes, plasma cells, histiocytes, and neutrophils. Sometimes granulomas are entirely absent, with only necrosis, neutrophils, and histiocytes seen (Fig. 6.15). The patterns of tuberculous lymphadenitis may overlap with noncaseating granulomatous processes, suppurative lymphadenites (although pyogenic bacteria can usually be recognized in Romanowsky-stained preparations), or necrotizing granulomatous lymphadenitis. It is important to recognize this range of patterns and therefore consider the possibility of tuberculosis. Finally, patterns of caseous granulomatous lymphadenitis can also typically be encountered in other fungal infections such as histoplasmosis or coccidiodomycosis. In any specimen suspected to be tuberculous or fungal in origin, additional aspirates for culture and special stains should be obtained.

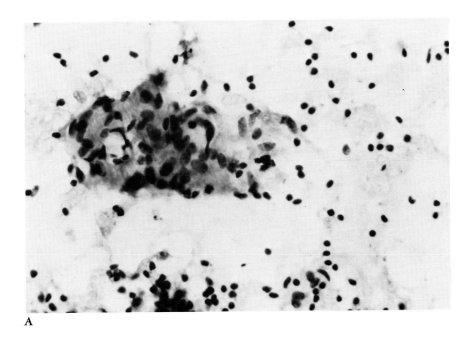

A

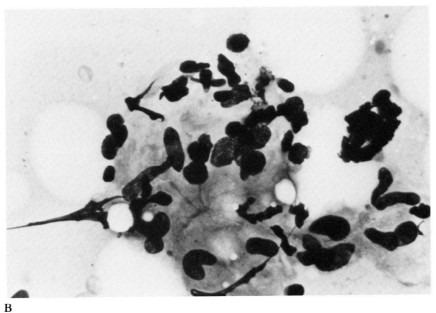

B

Fig. 6.14. A. Noncaseating or hard granuloma in an aspirate from a patient with known sarcoidosis. The background contains only small, mature-appearing lymphocytes (Papanicolaou stain; ×100). **B.** Asteroid body within the cytoplasm of an epithelioid histiocyte (Diff-Quik stain; ×400).

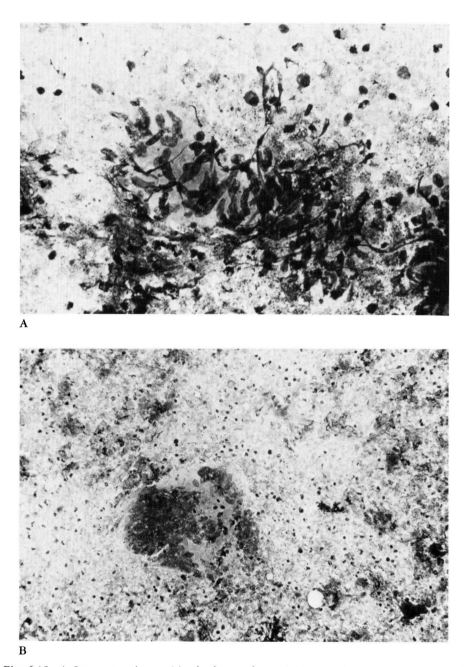

A

B

Fig. 6.15. A. Loose granuloma with a background containing granular necrotic material and plasma cells, a few lymphocytes, and neutrophils. Special stains revealed acid-fast bacilli (Diff-Quik stain; × 200). **B.** Multinucleated giant cell with a background of necrosis (Diff-Quik stain; × 100).

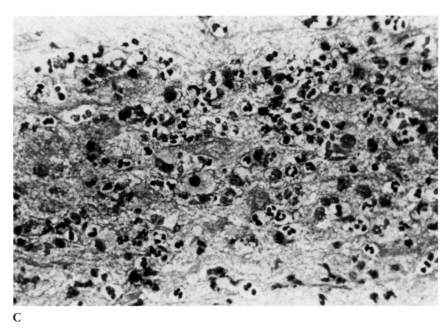

C

Fig. 6.15. C. Neutrophils, histiocytic cells, and necrosis representing a suppurative pattern in a patient with tuberculosis (Diff-Quik stain; × 100).

Acute Necrotizing Granulomatous Lymphadenitis

A wide range of infectious agents involving the lymph node cause a pattern of necrotizing granulomatous lymphadenitis. Diseases to be considered include cat-scratch disease, lymphogranuloma venereum, and uncommon infections such as yersiniosis, listeriosis, tularemia, glanders, meliodosis, and *Pasteurella septica* infection. This pattern is also seen characteristically in some fungal infections, notably blastomycoses.[6,36]

Cat-scratch disease is by far the most common disease that evokes this pattern. This disease is generally a slowly progressive, sometimes chronic process. Lymph nodes are tender, especially when there is extensive suppuration. Fever is present in about one-third of patients. Almost any peripheral lymph nodes may be involved, with axillary nodes being most common followed by cervical lymph nodes. Approximately 90% of patients give a history of contact with a cat. A skin lesion presenting as a small papule or vesicle resembling an insect bite develops at the site of the scratch 7 to 14 days after contact, lasts 1 to 4 weeks, and is often present at the time of lymphadenopathy. The lymphadenopathy usually occurs 1 to 2 weeks after the skin lesion appears.

Necrotizing granulomatous inflammation, regardless of the cause, goes through a relatively constant progression of changes.[36] The initial phase is that of florid hyperplasia. The hyperplasia is mixed follicular and paracortical in nature, often with a relatively pronounced paracortical component. The early phases of necrotizing granulomatous lymphadenitis yield cytologic patterns having a plasmacytoid

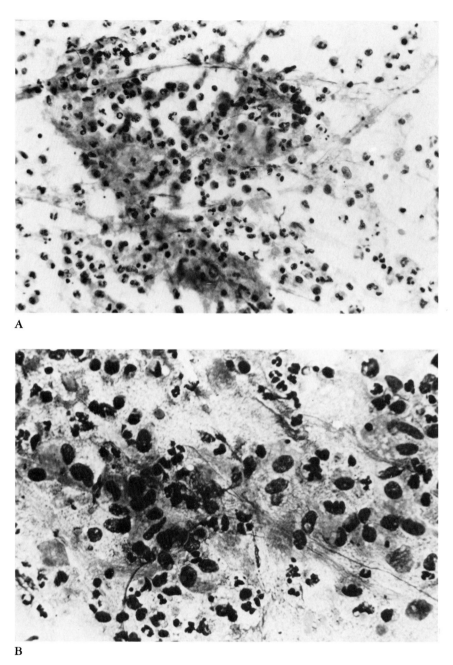

A

B

Fig. 6.16. **A.** Loose granuloma, neutrophils, and necrosis in a patient with a clinical history consistent with cat-scratch disease (H&E stain; × 100). **B.** Loose granuloma, neutrophils, some lymphocytes, and a background of necrosis in a patient with blastomycoses infection (Diff-Quik stain; × 200).

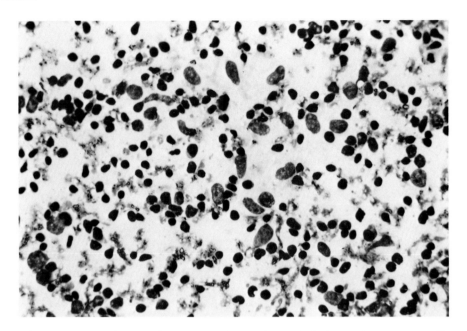

Fig. 6.17. Aspiration biopsy of a patient with toxoplasmosis. Polymorphous pattern of lymphocytes and a small, loose aggregate of epithelioid histiocytes. Serologic studies confirmed diagnosis (Diff-Quik stain; × 100).

component more pronounced than most nonspecific reactive hyperplasias. The next phase is the formation of clusters of epithelioid histiocytes in the paracortex. Aspiration of a node during this phase may yield loose granulomas and isolated epithelioid histiocytes against a reactive lymphoid background. These patterns overlap with granulomatous lymphadenitis with a reactive lymphoid background as encountered in toxoplasmosis and brucellosis. In the third phase, granulomas progressively enlarge and undergo central suppurative necrosis. FNA biopsy at this time should yield reactive lymphoid elements, granulomas, neutrophils, and necrosis in varying degrees (Fig. 6.16). This is the most characteristic finding for this group of diseases. However, as noted earlier, even this pattern is not specific since it may be found in infections more commonly associated with other patterns, such as tuberculosis. The final phase in some lymph nodes is virtually total replacement by necrosis, neutrophils, and histiocytes. Aspiration at this time yields a suppurative pattern of lymphadenitis.

Granulomas Associated With a Reactive Lymphoid Population

Toxoplasmosis and brucellosis are the diseases most characteristically having granulomatous lymphadenitis patterns with a florid reactive lymphoid background.[19] Lymphadenitis is the most common manifestation of symptomatic toxoplasmosis infection in children and adults. The disease may affect lymph nodes in any area, but it most commonly involves the cervical region. Sometimes only a single lymph node is enlarged, but more often groups of nodes are involved. Lymph nodes generally tend to be relatively small, no more than 1.5 to at most 2.5 cm in diameter.

Brucella infection causes lymphadenopathy in the subacute and chronic forms. The classic picture of undulant fever is not always present, and in some cases there may be no fever at all.

The cytologic pattern in lymph node aspirates of toxoplasmosis and brucellosis is that of small loose granulomas or isolated epithelioid histiocytes against a background of reactive lymphocytes with features as described in chronic lymphadenitis (vide supra)[19] (Fig. 6.17). A similar pattern may be encountered in early involvement of lymph nodes by tuberculosis and in earlier phases of necrotizing granulomatous lymphadenitis.

Malignant Processes With Associated Granulomas

Malignant processes that may be associated with granulomas include Hodgkin's and non-Hodgkin's lymphomas and seminoma. Products formed by tumors such as keratin in squamous cell carcinoma or amyloid in medullary carcinoma may also incite a granulomatous response. The most difficult of these processes to recognize as malignant and to distinguish from the lymphadenites are the lymphomas. Hodgkin's disease, in contrast to benign granulomatous lymphadenites, is characterized by scattered bizarre cells, that is, Reed–Sternberg cells and their variants[37] (Fig. 6.18). Non-Hodgkin's lymphomas with granulomas generally lack the spectrum of elements seen in reactive lymphadenites including tingible-body macrophages and reactive follicular center fragments. Cytologic features seen in lymphomas, such as marked irregularities in nuclear membrane contours or bizarre cells, are not present in benign lymphadenopathy. Seminomas are characterized by large germ cells with a moderate amount of cytoplasm and prominent nucleoli, variable numbers of mature lymphocytes, and a peculiar striped or "tigroid" background frequently seen in Romanovsky preparations (Fig. 6.18).

MISCELLANEOUS LYMPHADENITES

One group of uncommon lymphadenites occasionally encountered in lymph node aspiration biopsy share the common feature of proliferation of some form of histiocytes.

Dermatopathic Lymphadenitis

The disorder known as dermatopathic lymphadenites is associated with several skin diseases preceding lymphadenopathy. The subsequently involved nodes present in the drainage area of the affected skin. The most florid form of dermatopathic lymphadenitis is associated with generalized exfoliative dermatitis but may be seen also in localized dermatites, particularly those that cause pruritis or have accompanying hyperemia or desquamation. Cytologic findings include histiocytes, isolated

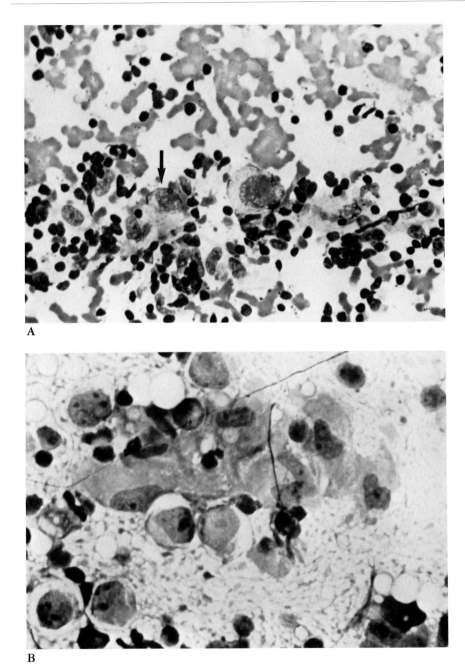

Fig. 6.18. A. Loose granuloma from an aspirate of Hodgkin's disease (*arrow*). There is a Hodgkin's cell present as well as numerous small mature lymphocytes (Diff-Quik stain; ×200). **B.** An aspirate of seminoma containing mature lymphocytes and malignant germ cells. There is a single small granulomatous aggregate. The background contains the "tigroid" pattern characteristic of this neoplasm (Diff-Quik stain; ×630).

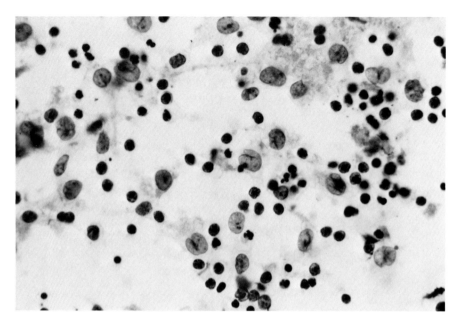

Fig. 6.19. Langerhans' cell histiocytosis (histiocytosis X) involving a lymph node. This aspirate contained numerous isolated histiocytes with abundant cytoplasm, some with linear nuclear grooves, characteristic of Langerhans' cells (Papanicolaou stain; × 200).

or in small sheets, and lymphocytes. Some of the histiocytes may have linear nuclear grooves. Pigment, melanin, or hemosiderin in variable amounts is generally seen in some histiocytes. The dominant lymphocytes are usually small mature forms, although occasionally a more variable lymphoid population is encountered. Occasionally, eosinophils may be conspicuous.

Langerhans' Histiocytosis

Histocytosis of the Langerhans' type is a complex group of diseases with variable clinicopathologic presentations categorized by either localized or generalized presentation and an acute or chronic course. Characteristic cytologic findings in needle aspirates include numerous eosinophils and histiocytes with reniform nuclei. Occasional multinucleated histiocytes may be present. Linear grooves are found in the nuclei of many histiocytes (Fig. 6.19). In a case reported by Layfield,[21] characteristic Birbeck granules could be demonstrated by electron microscopy of the aspirate material.

Histiocytic Necrotizing Lymphadenitis (Kikuchi's Lymphadenitis)

This uncommon disease is generally self-limiting and usually affects young women, who present with cervical lymphadenopathy and often fever. The few investigators encountering Kikuchi's lymphadenitis in needle aspiration biopsy have found it most problematic to distinguish this entity from lymphoma.[23,24] Case descriptions note the presence of both heterogenous and monotonous populations of lymphocytes, individual cell necrosis, and histiocytes, some ingesting nuclear debris.

Sinus Histiocytosis With Massive Lymphadenopathy (Rosai–Dorfman Syndrome)

Although this disease has a broad clinical spectrum, it is usually benign and self-limited; it often affects young, black males who present with massive bilateral cervical lymphadenopathy. A substantial percentage of patients have extranodal disease which may involve a wide range of sites. The syndrome may be associated with fever, leukocytosis, and an elevated erythrocyte sedimentation rate. Cytologic findings include an abundance of lymphocytes, primarily small mature forms, plasma cells, and numerous noncohesive histiocytes with abundant foamy cytoplasm. Many histiocytes contain ingested intact lymphocytes, plasma cells, or red blood cells.[25,26]

Lymphangiogram Effect

A few days after a lymphangiogram is performed for tumor staging, pelvic and abdominal lymph nodes respond by histiocytes ingesting the lipid droplets of contrast material. Foreign body–type giant cells may be present. The cytologic pattern demonstrates the presence of vacuolated histiocytes as well as lymphocytes.

REFERENCES

1. Greig EDW, Gray ACH: Note on the lymphatic glands in sleeping sickness. *Lancet* 1:1570–1573, 1904.

2. Guthrie CG: Gland puncture as a diagnostic measure. *Bull Johns Hopkins Hosp* 32:266–269, 1921.

3. Martin HE, Ellis EB: Biopsy by needle puncture and aspiration. *Ann Surg* 92:169–181, 1930.

4. Lopes-Cardozo P: The cytologic diagnosis of lymph node punctures. *Acta Cytol* 8:194–205, 1964.

5. Frable MA, Frable WJ: Fine needle aspiration biopsy in the diagnosis of sarcoid of the head and neck. *Acta Cytol* 28:175–177, 1984.

6. Silverman JF: Fine needle aspiration cytology of cat-scratch disease. *Acta Cytol* 29:542–547, 1985.

7. O'Dowd GJ, Frable WJ, Behm FG: Fine needle aspiration cytology of benign lymph node hyperplasias. Diagnostic significance of lymphohistiocytic aggregates. *Acta Cytol* 29:554–558, 1985.

8. Bailey TM, Akhtar M, Ali MA: Fine needle aspiration biopsy in the diagnosis of tuberculosis. *Acta Cytol* 29:732–736, 1985.

9. Layfield LJ, Glasgow BJ, DuPuis MH: Fine needle aspiration of lymphadenopathy of suspected infectious etiology. *Arch Pathol Lab Med* 109:810–812, 1985.

10. Cavett JR III, McAfee R, Ramzy I: Hansen's disease (leprosy). Diagnosis by aspiration biopsy of lymph nodes. *Acta Cytol* 30:189–193, 1986.

11. Kumar PV, Hambarsoomina B, Vaezzadeh K: Fine needle aspiration cytology of localized *Leishmania* lymphadenitis. *Acta Cytol* 31:14–16, 1987.

12. Metre MS, Jayaram G: Acid-fast bacilli in aspiration smears from tuberculous lymph nodes. An analysis of 255 cases. *Acta Cytol* 31:17–19, 1987.

13. Radhika S, Gupta SK, Chakrabarti A, et al: Role of culture for mycobacteria in fine-needle aspiration diagnosis of tuberculous lymphadenitis. *Diagn Cytopathol* 5:260–262, 1989.

14. Stani J: Cytologic diagnosis of reactive lymphadenopathy in fine needle aspiration biopsy specimens. *Acta Cytol* 31:8–13, 1987.

15. Lau SK, Wei WI, Hsu C, et al: Fine needle aspiration biopsy of tuberculous cervical lymphadenopathy. *Aust N Z J Surg* 58:947–950, 1988.

16. Kardos TF, Kornstein MJ, Frable WJ: Cytology and immunocytology of infectious mononucleosis in fine needle aspirates of lymph nodes. *Acta Cytol* 32:722–726, 1988.

17. Stanley MW, Steeper TA, Horwitz CA, et al: Fine-needle aspiration of lymph nodes in patients with acute infectious mononucleosis. *Diagn Cytopathol* 6:323–329, 1990.

18. Hidvegi DF, Sorensen K, Lawrence JB, et al: Castleman's disease: cytomorphologic and cytochemical features of a case. *Acta Cytol* 26:243–246, 1982.

19. Christ ML, Feltes-Kennedy M: Fine needle aspiration cytology of toxoplasmic lymphadenitis. *Acta Cytol* 425–428, 1982.

20. Reticuloendotheliosis with eosinophilia (Omenn's syndrome). Findings in fine needle aspirate of a lymph node. *Acta Cytol* 31:20–24, 1987.

21. Layfield LJ, Bhuta S: Fine-needle aspiration cytology of histiocytosis X: a case report. *Diagn Cytopathol* 4:140–143, 1988.

22. Tabatowski K, Elson CE, Johnston WW: Silicone lymphadenopathy in a patient with a mammary prosthesis. Fine needle aspirate cytology, histology and analytical electron microscopy. *Acta Cytol* 34, 10–14, 1990.

23. Moriarty AT, Aust CA, Strate RW, et al: Kikuchi's histiocytic necrotizing lymphadenitis: a pitfall in the diagnosis of lymphadenopathy by fine needle aspiration biopsy (abstract). *Acta Cytol* 33:716–717, 1989.

24. Kung IT, Ng WF, Yuen RW, et al: Kikuchi's histiocytic necrotizing lymphadenitis. Diagnosis by fine needle aspiration. *Acta Cytol* 34:323–328, 1990.

25. Layfield LJ: Fine needle aspiration cytologic findings in a case of sinus histiocytosis with massive lymphadenopathy (Rosai–Dorfman syndrome). *Acta Cytol* 34:767–770, 1990.

26. Pettinato G, Manivel JC, dAmore ES, et al: Fine needle aspiration cytology and immuno-cytochemical characterization of the histiocytes in sinus histiocytosis with massive lymphadenopathy (Rosai–Dorfman syndrome). *Acta Cytol* 34:771–777, 1990.

27. Feldman PS, Covell JL, Kardos TF: *Fine Needle Aspiration Cytology. Lymph Node, Thyroid & Salivary Gland.* Chicago, ASCP Press, 1989, pp 13–95.

28. Saltzstein SL, Ackerman LV: Lymphadenopathy induced by anticonvulsant drugs and mimicking clinically and pathologically malignant lymphomas. *Cancer* 12:164–182, 1959.

29. Frizzera G, Moran EM, Rappaport H: Angioimmunoblastic lymphadenopathy. Diagnosis and clinical course. *Am J Med* 59:803–818, 1975.

30. Pontifex AH, Klimo P: Application of aspiration biopsy cytology to lymphomas. *Cancer* 53:553–556, 1984.

31. Margileth AM: Cervical adenitis. *Pediatr Rev* 7:13–24, 1985.

32. Dejmek A, Lindholm K: Fine needle aspiration biopsy of cystic lesions of the head and neck, excluding the thyroid. *Acta Cytol* 34:443–448, 1990.

33. Fulciniti F, Zeppa P, Vetrani A, et al: Hodgkin's disease mimicking suppurative lymphadenitis: a possible pitfall in fine-needle aspiration biopsy cytology. *Diagn Cytopathol* 5:282–285, 1989.

34. Symmers WSTC: Lymphoreticular system. *Systemic Pathology*. 2nd ed. Vol. 2. New York, Churchill Livingstone, 1978, pp 504–891.

35. Wuketich S: On the epithelioid cellular tuberculoid reactions in the lymph nodes in malignant tumors. *Frankfurt Z Path* 70:187–200, 1959.

36. Campbell JA: Cat-scratch disease. *Pathol Annu* 12:277–292, 1977.

37. Jaffe ES: Surgical pathology of the lymph nodes. *Major Problems in Pathology*. Bennington JL, Ed. Philadelphia, WB Saunders, 1985, pp 228, 254.

7

Breast

Most inflammatory lesions of the breast are secondary to bacterial infections.[1] Tuberculous (TB), fungal, and viral infections are unusual causes of inflammatory breast lesions.[2,3] A listing of inflammatory lesions of the breast that can be diagnosed by FNA cytology is presented in Table 7.1.

ACUTE INFLAMMATION

Breast abscesses are relatively uncommon but typically occur in approximately 1 to 3% of lactating women.[1,4,5] They are quite uncommon in nonlactating premenopausal women and are rare in the postmenopausal age group.[1,5] Suggested pathogenetic mechanisms in lactating women are duct stasis of milk and excessive drying of nipple skin with fissuring and cracking of nipple.[1,3] Occasionally, mastitis in the lactating breast evolves into an obvious abscess with the clinical findings of skin reddening, edema, elevation of temperature, and associated fluctuation. In nonlactating women, nipple inversion, trauma, and augmentation implants, and injections have been cited as causes.[5] Most breast abscesses are due to *Staphylococcus aureus*, although other bacteria such as group B streptococci, coagulase-negative staphylococci, *Proteus* species, and unspecified streptococci have been implicated.[1,3,6,7] Fine-needle aspiration (FNA) biopsy can be readily used to diagnose breast abscesses. In addition, aspiration with drainage is the mainstay of proper treatment along with antibiotic therapy.[1,3]

FNA cytology of acute mastitis with or without breast abscess will reveal increased numbers of neutrophils and foamy macrophages, including evidence of cytophagocytosis and considerable cell debris in the background (Fig. 7.1). Epithelial atypia may be present, especially when the acute inflammatory process is prominent. The atypical epithelial cells may show features of regeneration and repair, including nuclear enlargement and prominent nucleoli (Fig. 7.2). In inflammatory atypia, however, the nuclear:cytoplasmic ratio is usually within normal limits and the atypical cells are arranged in flat, sheetlike groupings. One should suspect in-

139

TABLE 7.1. Nonneoplastic Breast Lesions

Acute mastitis
Breast abscess
Comedomastitis
Subareolar breast abscess
Ruptured epidermal inclusion cyst
Plasma cell mastitis
Fat necrosis
Sarcoid
Infectious granulomatous inflammation
Foreign body reaction
Granulomatous mastitis
Amyloid tumor with foreign body reaction
Radiation atypia of benign breast tissue

flammatory atypia rather than malignancy when there are numerous acute inflammatory cells in the background and neutrophils are found infiltrating the epithelial clusters. Cytologic features not supportive for the diagnosis of carcinoma are relatively limited numbers of epithelial cells and degenerating atypical cells set in an inflammatory background.[8-12]

In comedomastitis, which is part of fibrocystic change, a greater number of ductal cells may be present, including those showing a variable degree of inflammatory atypia[8] (Fig. 7.3). In any process demonstrating inflammatory atypia, the degree of atypia usually appears greater in the Romanovsky-stained air-dried smears (eg, Diff-Quik stain) than in the Papanicolaou-stained alcohol-fixed smears. This difference is due to the greater size of the cells not undergoing initial fixation. When epithelial atypia is present, one should evaluate the background of the smears for an inflammatory process. A more conservative cytologic interpretation based on the findings in the Papanicolaou-stained smears often serves as an important check to avoid a false-positive diagnosis of malignancy.

CHRONIC INFLAMMATION

Plasma cell mastitis is a common chronic inflammatory lesion of the breast characterized by the presence of numerous plasma cells and lymphocytes surrounding ducts filled with inspissated secretion in the acute phase. During the healing stage of the lesion, fibrosis and scar formation occur. The aspiration biopsy cytology (ABC) findings will reflect the stage of the lesion.[13]

Mammary duct ectasia is a benign condition in older women characterized by dilatation of the collecting ducts in the subareolar region with surrounding fibrosis and inflammation.[3] It is important to recognize this lesion cytologically, since it may clinically simulate carcinoma.[3] Pathologically, mammary duct ectasia begins with dilatation of the terminal collecting ducts beneath the nipple and areola, which

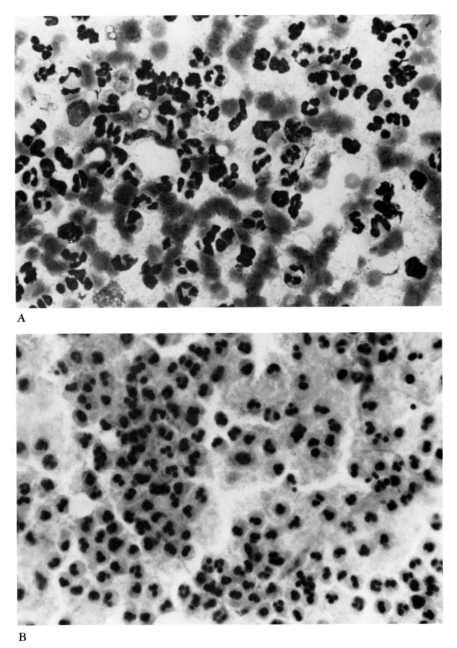

A

B

Fig. 7.1. A. FNA of breast abscess showing numerous neutrophils and a few mononuclear cells (Diff-Quik stain; ×200). **B.** Aspirate of breast abscess showing sheets of neutrophils including some undergoing liquefactive necrosis (Papanicolaou stain; ×200).

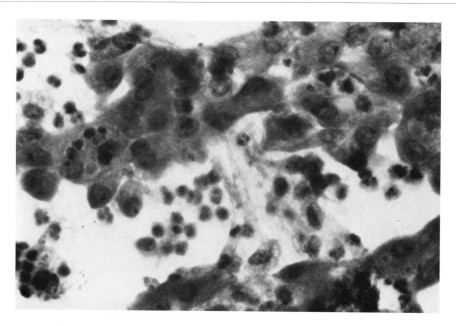

Fig. 7.2. Aspirate of breast abscess in which atypical epithelial cells are present showing features of regeneration and repair including sheetlike groupings showing no loss of polarity and consisting of cells having unremarkable nuclear:cytoplasmic ratio with somewhat enlarged nuclei possessing prominent nucleoli. Numerous associated neutrophils are present (Papanicolaou stain; ×400).

become distended with cellular debris and lipid-containing material[3] (Fig. 7.4). As the disease progresses, the dilatation of the duct extends peripherally with the duct wall becoming thickened by chronic inflammation and fibrosis. The ductal epithelium shows atrophy rather than proliferation or hyperplasia. When the intraluminal material extends into the periductal soft tissue, an intense inflammatory reaction ensues with fat necrosis, foreign body reaction to lipid material, and numerous histiocytes, lymphocytes and neutrophils along with a zone of granulation tissue.[3] In some patients, a low-grade inflammatory process consisting predominantly of plasma cells is seen, which accounts for the diagnostic term of plasma cell mastitis.

The extremely rare extramedullary *plasmacytoma of the breast* is cytologically differentiated from plasma cell mastitis by the monomorphic proliferation of atypical plasma cells, including many demonstrating binucleation and prominent nucleoli.[2,3]

FAT NECROSIS

Fat necrosis occurs following trauma or foreign body reaction, or as a secondary response to a breast malignancy, especially if tumor necrosis is present. It is important to recognize fat necrosis since it can clinically simulate carcinoma.[3] Although microscopic fat necrosis is fairly frequent, fat necrosis producing a breast mass is

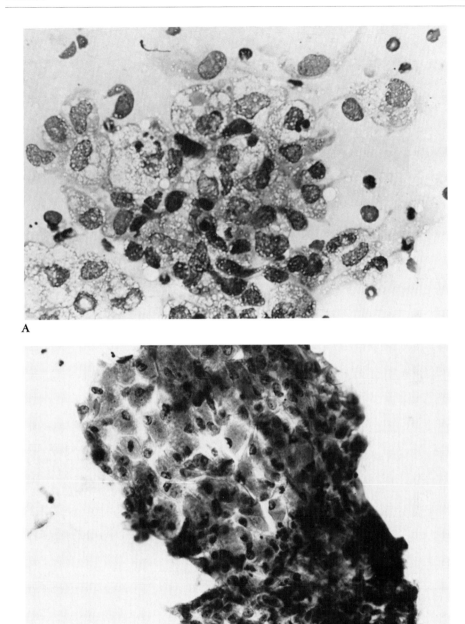

Fig. 7.3. A. Cluster of vacuolated histiocytes and some atypical ductal cells along with a few scattered inflammatory cells in an aspirate of comedomastitis (Diff-Quik stain; ×400). **B.** Comedomastitis consisting of sheet of ductal cells showing some apocrine features associated with scattered neutrophils. Note the loosely cohesive nature of the sheet along with the presence of some small nucleoli in a few of the cells (Papanicolaou stain; ×400).

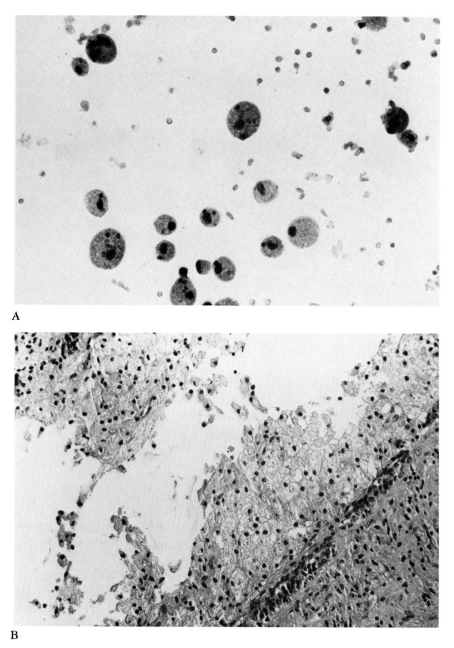

Fig. 7.4. A. Scattered histiocytes having a finely vacuolated cytoplasm with some phago-cytosed material in an aspirate of mammary duct ectasia (Papanicolaou stain; ×200). **B.** Resected mammary duct ectasia showing marked dilatation of collecting duct which contains numerous lipid-laden macrophages and cellular debris (H&E stain; ×200).

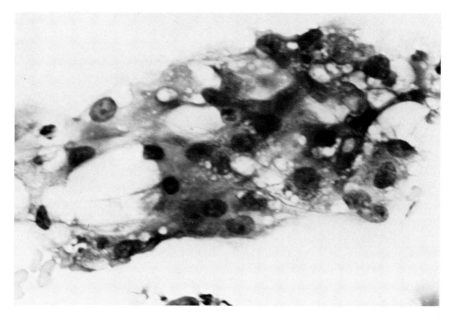

Fig. 7.5. Fat necrosis consisting of fat vacuoles and surrounding histiocytes, some of which have slightly enlarged nuclei with nucleoli (Diff-Quik stain; ×400).

relatively uncommon.[3] In Haagensen's series, the mean age of patients with fat necrosis was approximately 52 years, with an age range of 27 to 80 years. The predominance of older women may be due to the greater tendency of older women to fall and injure their breasts.[3] Fat necrosis can radiologically, grossly, and histologically (especially at frozen section) mimic malignancy.

The ABC cytologic features of fat necrosis will reflect the stage of the lesion. Initially there is hemorrhage and necrosis of the adipocytes with fusion of individual fat cells into larger vacuoles. Between the vacuoles, fibroblasts, lipoblasts, and histiocytes are present including many foam cells which are engulfing the fatty debris (Fig. 7.5). Therefore, the ABC will demonstrate fat; amorphous debris (degenerating fat); inflammatory cells including neutrophils, plasma cells, and lymphocytes; and numerous lipid-laden macrophages (foam cells or lipophages) having abundant vacuolated cytoplasm (Fig. 7.6). Multinucleated macrophages and spindle-shaped fibroblastic cells can also be present.

Clinically, the patient may give a history of trauma to the breast with subsequent development of ecchymosis and a mass. The clinician may assume that the lesion is entirely due to fat necrosis and therefore believe there is no need for a biopsy. Haagensen reported that he has seen several patients in whom a history of trauma and subsequent ecchymosis first called attention to an associated carcinoma.[3] FNA biopsy is a readily available technique to confirm the presence of fat necrosis. However, one should also be aware that fat necrosis can coexist with breast carcinoma. If only the areas of fat necrosis are sampled, then a false-negative diagnosis of malignancy will occur.

Hashimoto and Cobb[14] recently reported the cytologic features of a hibernoma which can potentially occur in the breast. Cytologic examination revealed moderately cellular smears in which fragments of large round to oval cells having abundant, multivacuolated cytoplasm and moderately defined cytoplasmic borders were present. The differential diagnosis of hibernoma includes granular cell tumor of the breast, which is also an uncommon breast lesion.[15,16] Granular cell tumors are frequently found in black patients and are often multifocal. Granular cell tumors of the breast can closely simulate scirrhous carcinoma, both clinically and at gross examination. ABC examination will generally reveal a cellular specimen consisting of scattered groups of cells with abundant granular cytoplasm and indistinct cell borders with the Romanovsky stains,[17] in contrast to the coarsely vacuolated hibernoma cells[14] (Fig. 7.7). In addition, a fat stain (oil red-O) performed on an air-dried smear will be positive in hibernoma and negative in granular cell tumors. Granular cell tumors have cells with uniform oval to round nuclei with an evenly dispersed chromatin pattern. With the Papanicolaou stain, the cytoplasm takes on a reddish granular appearance, and the granules are accentuated with the periodic acid–Schiff (PAS) stain. Immunoperoxidase stains on cytologic material would demonstrate S-100 and carcinoembryonic antigen (CEA) positivity,[14] although the S-100 staining intensity may be decreased in alcohol-fixed smears.[18] Electron microscopic examination demonstrates granules resembling autophagosomes and angulate bodies.[15]

SUBAREOLAR ABSCESS

Subareolar abscess of the breast is a specific clinicopathologic entity well known to surgeons but, until recently, not well described in the pathology or cytology literature.[12,19] The lesion is a specific type of low grade infection occurring in the subareolar region of the breast. It often begins as a localized area of inflammation beneath the nipple, which then progresses to form an abscess. This is often followed by subsequent cycles of sinus tract formation, drainage, partial healing, and then recurrences.[12]

Clinically, subareolar abscess can simulate breast neoplasms such as an adenoma of the nipple or even a breast carcinoma because of the presence of nipple retraction and a mass. We have encountered a number of examples of subareolar abscess of the breast and reported our initial experience of eight cases diagnosed by FNA biopsy.[12] A spectrum of cytomorphologic findings was appreciated including the presence of diagnostic anucleated squamous cells which Galblum and Oertel called the hallmark of the lesion[19] (Fig. 7.8). The numerous associated neutrophils, keratinous debris, cholesterol crystals, parakeratosis, and strips of squamous epithelium along with the anucleated squamae may give the lesion a "starry sky" appearance[12,19] (Fig. 7.8). A foreign body reaction with sheets of histiocytes and multinucleated foreign body type giant cells may be present in some of the cases (Fig. 7.9).

The cytologic findings are similar to the features seen in a ruptured epidermal inclusion cyst. However, the characteristic subareolar location, coupled with the cytologic findings, will permit a definite diagnosis of subareolar abscess to be made. Similarly, a ruptured epidermal inclusion cyst arising in the skin of the breast will share cytologic and histologic features with subareolar abscess, but the peripheral

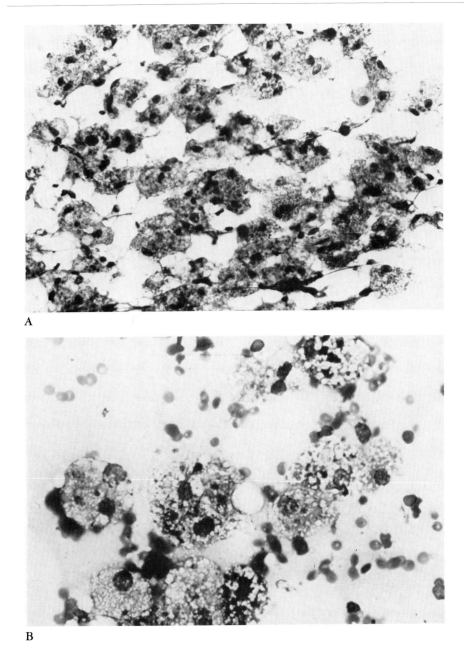

A

B

Fig. 7.6. A. Loose sheets of vacuolated histiocytes in an aspirate of fat necrosis (Papanicolaou stain; ×400). **B.** Scattered vacuolated histiocytes in aspirate of fat necrosis associated with a breast abscess (Diff-Quik stain; ×200). (From Silverman JF: Breast. In Bibbo M (ed): *Comprehensive Cytopathology.* Philadelphia, W.B. Saunders, 1991.)

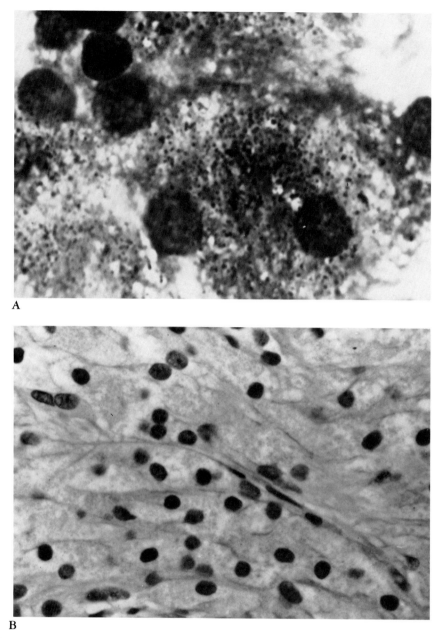

Fig. 7.7. A. Granular cell tumor of the breast consisting of loose cluster of polygonal to spindle-shaped cells having prominent cytoplasmic granularity (Diff-Quik stain; ×630). **B.** Granular cell tumor of the breast consisting of polygonal to spindle-shaped cells having prominent eosinophilic granules (H&E stain; ×100).

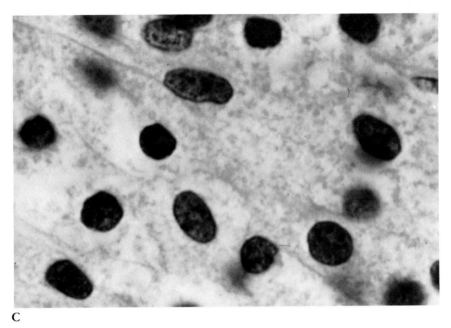

C

Fig. 7.7. C. High-power view of granular cells showing uniform oval to slightly elongated nuclei with surrounding prominent cytoplasmic granularity (H&E stain; × 400).

location of the epidermal inclusion cyst should clearly differentiate this lesion from a central subareolar abscess (Fig. 7.10).

Proposed theories concerning the pathogenesis of subareolar abscess include the lesion being part of comedomastitis, squamous metaplasia of columnar epithelium of large lactiferous ducts, or a congenital anomaly of the ductal system.[12,20] The most likely explanation for the pathogenesis of subareolar abscess is squamous metaplasia of the epithelium of the lactiferous duct, which then fills the lumen of the duct with abundant keratinous debris (Fig. 7.11). The duct or milk sinus dilates and is plugged with keratin. The duct then ruptures and an ensuing inflammatory cell reaction occurs in the surrounding periductal soft tissue, including a foreign body reaction to keratinous type material[12] (Fig. 7.12). The FNA biopsy can influence the management of the patient, since chronic subareolar abscess requires complete surgical excision of the abscess, sinus tract, and dilated duct, whereas the early lesions may be treated adequately by aspiration of the gross purulent material and institution of appropriate antibiotic therapy.[12,21] FNA cytology will clearly differentiate subareolar abscess from other lesions that occur in this locale, including lactational mastitis, breast abscess, tuberculosis, sarcoid, fat necrosis, and neoplastic conditions such as adenoma of the nipple and carcinoma.[3,8,19,22]

Subareolar abscess of the breast can demonstrate some of the potential diagnostic pitfalls for a false-positive diagnosis of malignancy that can occur in inflammatory processes of any site, including those involving the breast. These diagnostic pitfalls include the presence of groups of atypical ductal cells, squamous atypia, and fragments of exuberant granulation tissue (Figs. 7.13 and 7.14). In our study of subareolar abscess of the breast, four of our initial eight cases demonstrated some of these

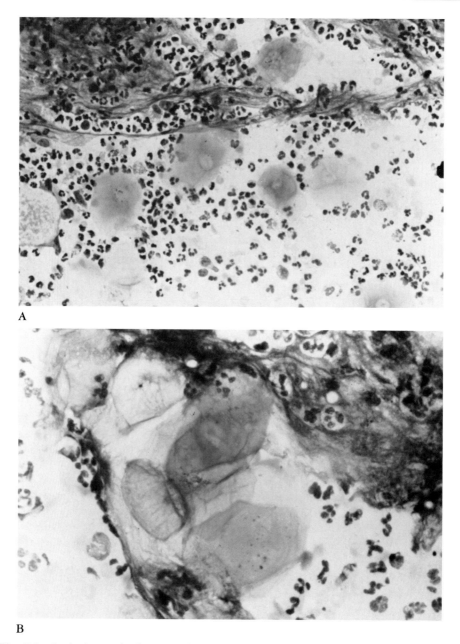

A

B

Fig. 7.8. A. Aspirate of subareolar abscess showing the presence of diagnostic anucleated squamous cells associated with numerous neutrophils (Diff-Quik stain; ×100). **B.** High-power view of anucleated squamae (Diff-Quik stain; ×400).

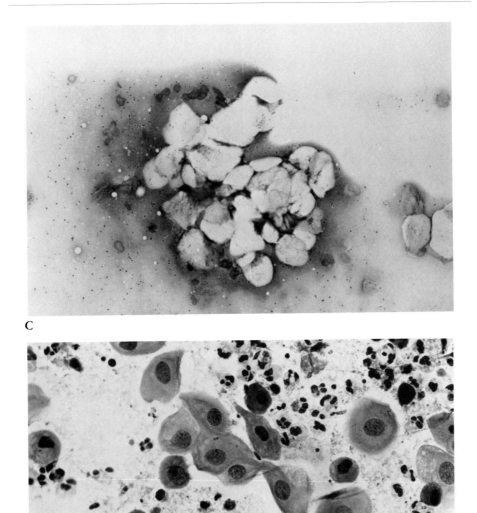

C

D

Fig. 7.8. C. Clump of anucleated squamous cells undergoing degeneration with formation of cholesterol crystals (Papanicolaou stain; ×100). **D.** Parabasal and polygonal squamous cells in aspirate of subareolar abscess associated with numerous neutrophils in the background (Papanicolaou stain; ×630).

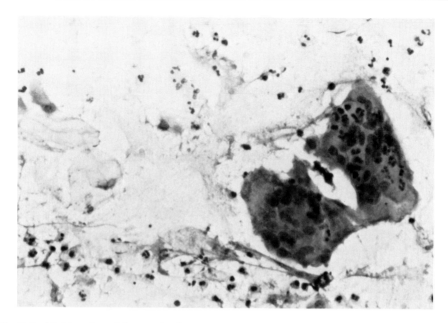

Fig. 7.9. Multinucleated foreign-body type giant cells in aspirate of subareolar abscess (Papanicolaou stain; ×400).

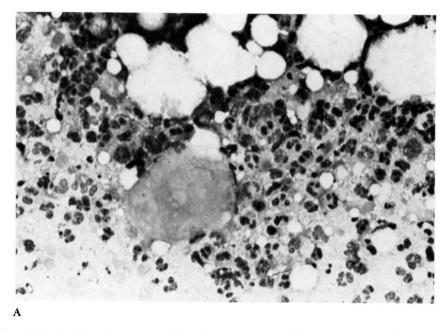

A

Fig. 7.10. A. FNA of ruptured epidermal inclusion cyst of breast showing single anucleated squamous cells and numerous neutrophils with abundant debris in the background (Diff-Quik stain; ×200).

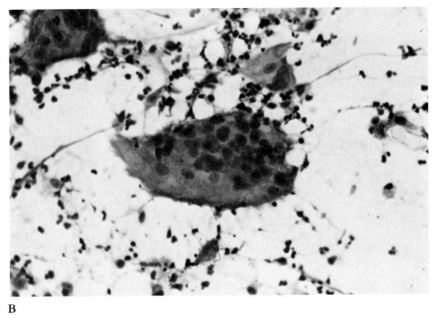

B

Fig. 7.10. B. Scattered multinucleated foreign-body type giant cells reacting to the keratinous debris in an FNA of epidermal inclusion cyst of the breast (Papanicolaou stain; ×400).

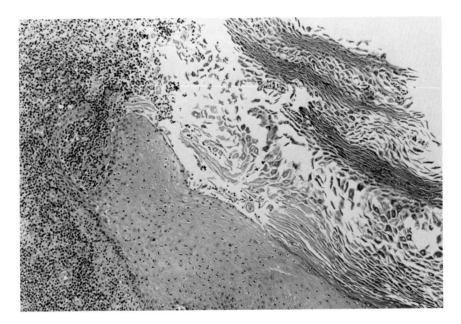

Fig. 7.11. Resected subareolar abscess of the breast demonstrating squamous lining of the duct with desquamation of anucleated squamae in the lumen. Note rupture of the duct with surrounding severe chronic inflammation (H&E stain; ×100). (From Silverman JF: Breast. In Bibbo M (ed): *Comprehensive Cytopathology.* Philadelphia, W.B. Saunders, 1991.)

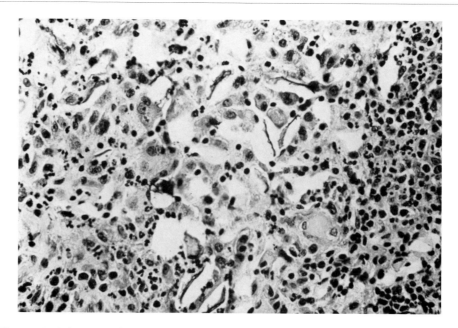

Fig. 7.12. Subareolar abscess demonstrating surrounding inflammation in the periductal parenchyma. Note the linear fragments of keratinous material engulfed by multinucleated histiocytes. Admixed acute inflammation is also seen (H&E stain; ×400). (From Silverman JF: Breast. In Bibbo M (ed): *Comprehensive Cytopathology*. Philadelphia, W.B. Saunders, 1991.)

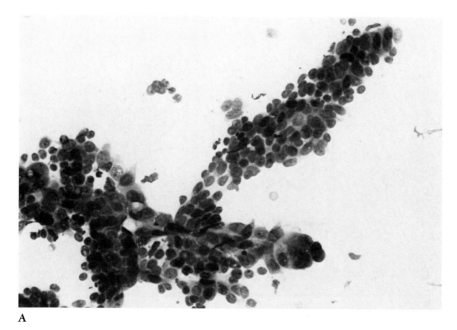

A

Fig. 7.13. A. Atypical ductal cells in an aspirate of subareolar abscess. Note loosely cohesive nature of the fragment along with some anisonucleosis of the ductal cells (Diff-Quik stain; ×200).

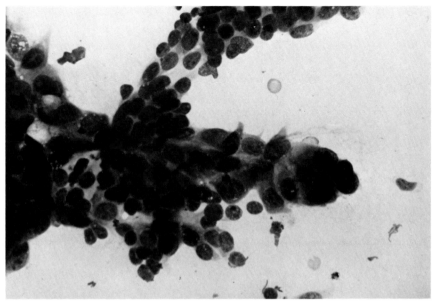

B

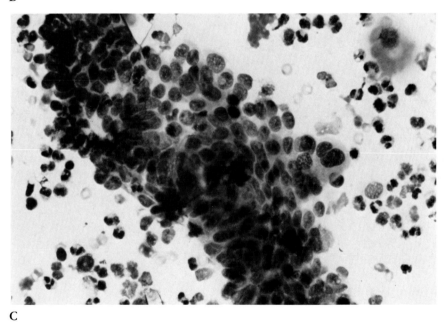

C

Fig. 7.13. **B.** High-power view of group of ductal cells showing anisonucleosis of the ductal cells along with the presence of one or more nucleoli in many of the nuclei (Diff-Quik stain; ×630). **C.** Sheet of ductal cells in subareolar abscess having a loosely cohesive arrangement with prominent anisonucleosis. Many of the ductal cells show some mild nuclear irregularity and hyperchromasia with small nucleoli. Numerous neutrophils are present in the background along with infiltration of the groups (Diff-Quik stain; ×200).

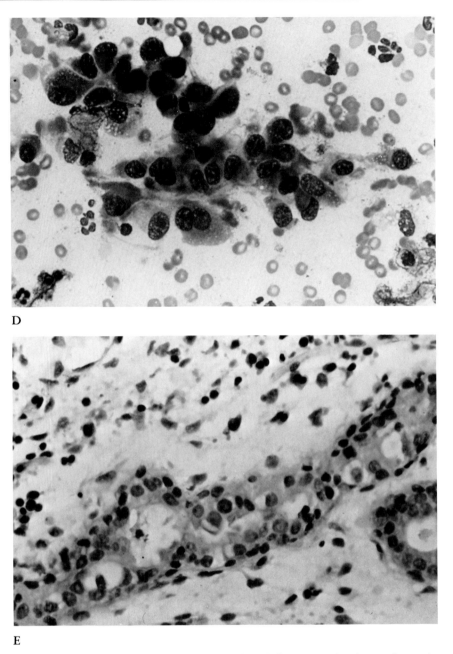

D

E

Fig. 7.13. **D.** Loose cluster of atypical ductal cells including some showing nuclear enlargement, binucleation, and presence of prominent nucleoli in aspirate of subareolar abscess. (From Silverman JF: Breast. In Bibbo M (ed): *Comprehensive Cytopathology.* Philadelphia, W.B. Saunders, 1991.) **E.** Ductal group in a resected subareolar abscess showing some hyperplasia with slight nuclear enlargement and presence of small nucleoli (H&E stain; ×400).

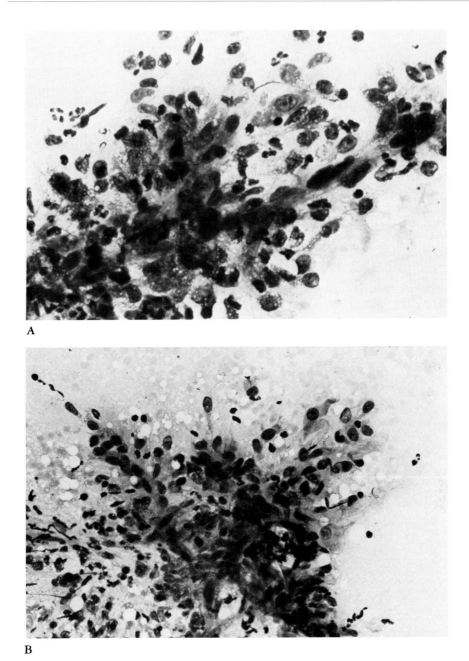

Fig. 7.14. A. Fragment of granulation tissue consisting of transversing capillaries and nearby histiocytes and neutrophils. The endothelial cells of the capillaries show some nuclear enlargement and irregularity. Some of the histiocytes also demonstrate nuclear enlargement with the presence of small nucleoli (Diff-Quik stain; ×400). **B.** Fragment of granulation tissue consisting of blood vessels with associated histiocytes and some neutrophils (Diff-Quik stain; ×100).

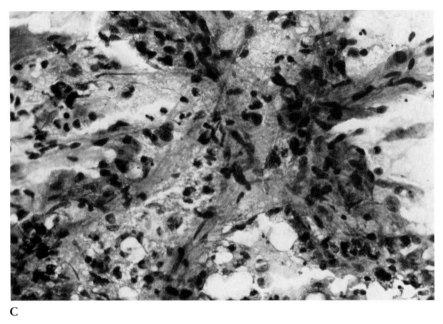

C

Fig. 7.14. C. Granulation tissue consisting of background matrix in which some delicate capillaries are present along with scattered histiocytes and neutrophils (Papanicolaou stain; ×400).

findings, which could potentially lead to a false-positive diagnosis of malignancy if the other characteristic cytologic features of subareolar abscess were not appreciated.[11,12,23,24] In Kline's review of 3,809 benign breast lesions, 69 cases were interpreted as suspicious for malignancy.[11] Six of these cases were overdiagnosed as malignant, based on misinterpretation of granulation tissue and fat necrosis.

GRANULOMAS

Sarcoid of the breast is quite rare. Whenever noncaseating granulomas are appreciated cytologically, the differential diagnosis should include infectious granulomas secondary to tuberculosis, fungi, leprosy, or brucellosis. Granulomas can also be present as a reaction to malignancy[25] or as a component of fat necrosis or foreign body reaction. In Gansler and Wheeler's literature review of mammary sarcoidosis, they noted that the lesion can clinically mimic carcinoma.[26] Doria and associates, in a letter to the editor of *Acta Cytologica,* reported the ABC findings of sarcoidosis presenting initially as a breast mass.[27] FNA biopsy of a breast nodule in a 72-year-old woman revealed cellular smears consisting of clusters of epithelioid histiocytes, multinucleated giant cells, lymphocytes, and plasma cells with no evidence of necrosis. The epithelioid histiocytes were elongated with ill-defined cytoplasm and folded nuclei. Several giant cells of the Langhans' type were found. Since mammary sarcoid can be clinically confused with carcinoma, ABC will correctly diagnose the lesion as a benign granulomatous process. However, other granulomatous lesions must be considered in the differential diagnosis, since the diagnosis of sarcoid should be one of exclusion when no organisms are identified or cultured from the aspirated material.

Tuberculosis of the breast was more frequent in the past when tuberculosis was generally more prevalent.[3,28] Haagensen adopted the classification of others which divides tuberculous breast lesions into primary and secondary types.[3] The primary lesions are those in which the breast lesion is the only manifestation of tuberculosis, whereas patients with secondary lesions have extramammary tuberculosis. Young, pregnant women are predisposed to tuberculosis of the breast, which may present as an abscess or poorly defined mass with skin retraction that can clinically resemble carcinoma. Purulent discharge from the nipple may be present along with fistulous tracts.

Jayaram reported the cytologic features of 15 cases of tuberculous mastitis diagnosed by FNA biopsy.[29] In her series three of the patients clinically were thought to have carcinoma. Epithelioid cell granulomas were found in all cases along with Langhans' giant cells and occasional foreign body giant cells. The presence of a necrotic background with numerous degenerating neutrophils was a helpful cytologic feature. The diagnosis was confirmed by demonstrating acid-fast bacilli with Ziehl–Neelsen staining performed on the smears. Aspirated material should be submitted for culture in all cases cytologically demonstrating a granulomatous reaction.

Recently, Macansh and associates reviewed the pathology literature and reported a case of granulomatous mastitis diagnosed by FNA biopsy.[30] The cytologic findings are similar to those of other granulomatous processes, although certain cytologic features will aid in the differential diagnosis of granulomatous lesions of the breast. An increase in plasma cells is associated with plasma cell mastitis. Collection of lipophages is seen in fat necrosis, whereas sarcoidosis should not demonstrate necrosis or neutrophilic inflammation. Exclusion of infective granulomatous processes requires culture, special stains, and/or serologic tests. Material such as silicone or paraffin can cause a foreign body reaction[31] (Fig. 7.15). Anucleated squamous cells and/or keratinous material are present in subareolar abscess and ruptured epidermal inclusion cysts.[12,30]

LOCALIZED AMYLOID TUMOR OF THE BREAST

Localized amyloid tumor of the breast is an exceedingly uncommon lesion with only five cases previously encountered in the surgical pathology literature.[32] We performed FNA on two patients with examples of this entity including one patient with metachronous bilateral lesions.[32] This rare lesion occurs predominantly in elderly females and can be clinically and mammographically confused with carcinoma.[32,33] FNA biopsy can be an extremely useful procedure for diagnosing amyloidosis, when amyloid is appreciated in the cytology smears. Cytomorphologic findings of amyloid include the presence of irregular clumps of metachromatically

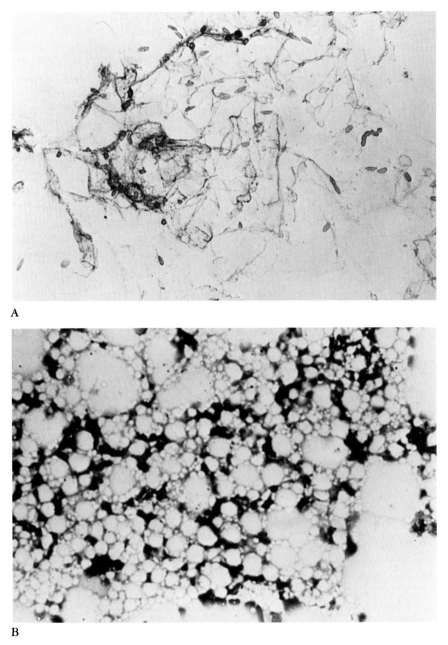

Fig. 7.15. **A.** Linear fragments of silicone material in aspirate of ruptured silicone implant causing a mass lesion (Papanicolaou stain; × 200). **B.** Microvesicular pattern of fat in ruptured silicone implant.

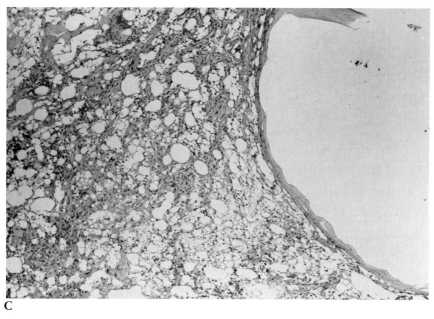

C

Fig. 7.15. C. Resected lesion showing fibrous wall if implant with surrounding microvesicular pattern of fat due to extravasation of the implant material (H&E stain; × 100).

staining homogeneous material in the modified Wright stain (Diff-Quik) and irregular cylindrical fragments of refractile to glassy eosinophilic material in the Papanicolaou-stained smears[32] (Fig. 7.16). Some interspersed spindle-shaped stromal cells can be present at the periphery and within the substance of the amyloid material.[32] Congo red staining with prior potassium permanganate incubation confirmed the AL type of amyloid in both of our cases. Immunofluorescent studies performed on the smears demonstrated IgA with kappa and lambda light chain deposition within the amyloid foci in one case and intracytoplasmic IgG with both light chains within plasma cells and amyloid deposits in samples from the second patient. Ultrastructural confirmation of one of the cases showed the characteristic straight, nonbranching fibrils of amyloid measuring 4 to 9 nm in diameter.

Amyloid tumors of the breast can occur in three settings. These include involvement of the breast by secondary amyloidosis, systemic- or multiple myeloma–associated amyloid, and the uncommon localized benign primary tumor.[32] Localized amyloid deposition is rare, occurring most frequently in the larynx, trachea, and bronchi.[34] Other sites include the nasal cavity, skin, cornea, vaginal mucosa, and urogenital organs with special predilection for the seminal vesicle.[34] In Kyle's series of 236 cases of amyloidosis, 22 cases (9%) had localized lesions.[35,36] The bladder, lungs, skin, and larynx accounted for more than half of the cases with no examples involving the breast. FNA biopsy has been advocated as a useful technique to document the presence of amyloid in other locations.[33,37,38] In our experience, ABC is also a useful technique to diagnose this unusual nonneoplastic breast lesion.[30] Amyloid must be differentiated from fragments of skeletal muscle, especially in the

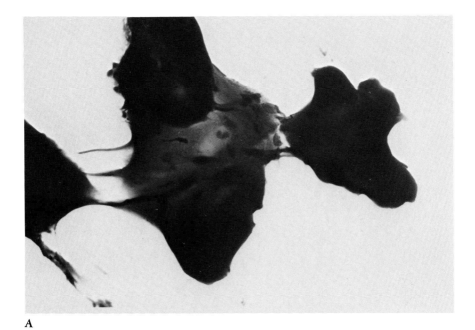

A

B

Fig. 7.16. **A.** Aspirate of amyloid tumor of the breast showing metachromatically staining homogeneous material in the Diff-Quik stain (×100). **B.** High power view of aspirate of amyloid tumor of the breast demonstrating smudged quality of the amyloid with some interspersed spindle-shaped stromal cells (Diff-Quik stain; ×630). (From Silverman JF: Breast. In Bibbo M (ed): *Comprehensive Cytopathology*. Philadelphia, W.B. Saunders, 1991.)

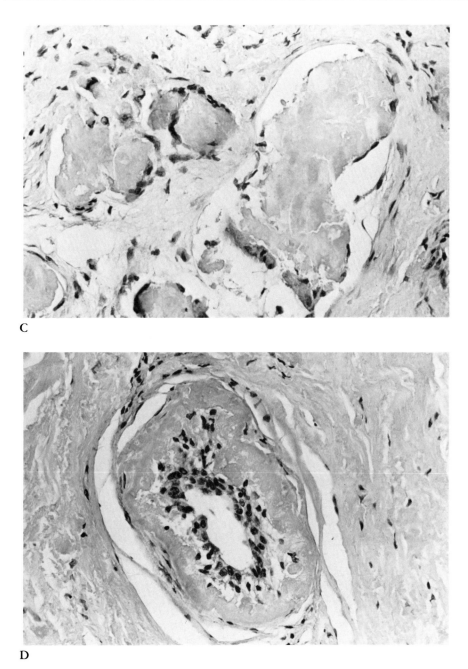

C

D

Fig. 7.16. C. Resected amyloid tumor of the breast in which clumps of amyloid are present in the stroma. Note the characteristic cracked-glass quality of the amyloid along with the presence of some surrounding spindle-shaped cells and multinucleated histiocytes (H&E stain; × 100). (From Silverman JF: Breast. In Bibbo M (ed): *Comprehensive Cytopathology.* Philadelphia, W.B. Saunders, 1991.) D. Amyloid deposition in wall of ductule of the breast (H&E stain; × 400).

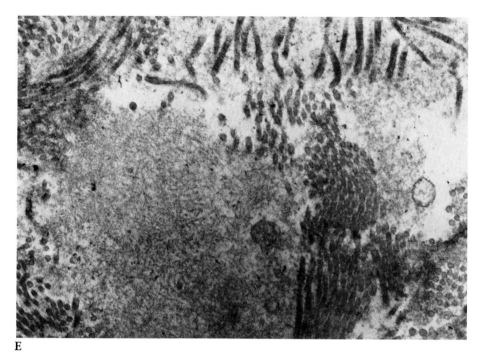

E

Fig. 7.16. E. Ultrastructure of amyloid consisting of straight, nonbranching fibrils measuring 4 to 9 nm in diameter surrounded by thick collagen bundles.

Papanicolaou-stained smears. Skeletal muscle will have an eosinophilic hue, will demonstrate cytoplasmic striation, and will lack the homogeneous, glassy appearance of amyloid.

RADIATION ATYPIA OF NONNEOPLASTIC BREAST TISSUE

With the increasing popularity of breast-conserving treatment for breast carcinoma employing limited surgery and primary high-dosage radiotherapy, we can expect that FNA biopsy will be performed following irradiation treatment in some of these patients. The histologic changes of irradiated nonneoplastic breast tissue include epithelial atypia in the terminal duct lobular unit and larger ducts along with stromal and vascular changes.[39] Bondeson reported the cytologic FNA biopsy findings of severe atypia in disassociated epithelial cells of normal breast tissue following irradiation.[40] Knowledge of prior radiotherapy is crucial to avoiding a potential false-positive diagnosis of malignancy in patients who are actually presenting with new benign breast masses.[40,41,42] In the reported cases, FNA cytologic specimens were generally hypocellular, although scattered markedly atypical cells were present. Peterse reported the cytologic findings in 41 patients who underwent breast-

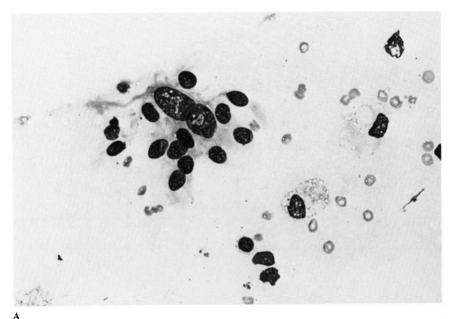

A

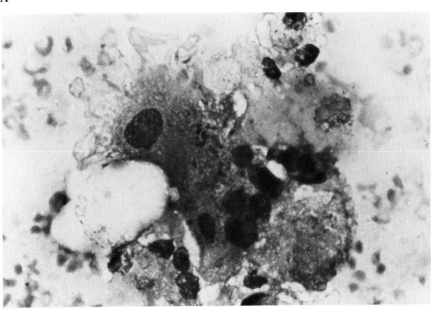

B

Fig. 7.17. A. FNA of breast demonstrating radiation atypia characterized by a few groups of cells showing considerable anisonucleosis with unremarkable nuclear:cytoplasmic ratio (Diff-Quik stain; × 200). **B.** Cluster of atypical but benign ductal cells following irradiation of breast (Diff-Quik stain; × 400). (Courtesy of Dr. Jack Frable, Medical College of Virginia, Richmond, VA).

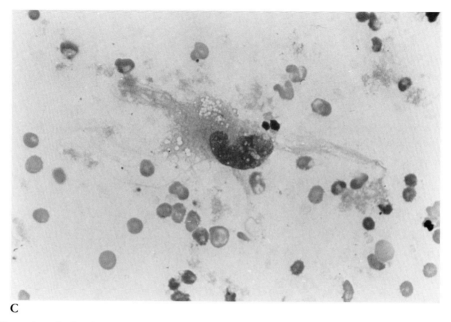

C

Fig. 7.17. C. Single atypical degenerating cell demonstrating radiation effect (Diff-Quik stain; ×400). (Courtesy of Dr. Jack Frable, Medical College of Virginia, Richmond, VA).

conserving treatment and irradiation therapy and then developed a new palpable breast lesion.[43] FNA biopsies demonstrated a recurrent breast carcinoma in 6 of the 41 patients. In the remaining 37 patients, three patterns of the nonneoplastic lesions were demonstrated: epithelial atypia in 14 cases, fat necrosis in 10 cases, and poorly cellular smears without evidence of epithelial atypia or fat necrosis in the remaining 13 cases.[43] The authors noted that the radiation-induced atypia may include the presence of considerable anisocytosis and anisonucleosis, but the nuclear:cytoplasmic ratio of the atypical cells remained within normal limits (Fig. 7.17). The epithelial cells also may possess prominent nucleoli with irregular cytoplasmic vacuolization. However, prominent cellular dissociation and necrotic debris, which are often seen in aspirates from breast carcinoma, were not encountered in the FNA smears of the irradiated nonneoplastic breast. In addition, aspirates from irradiated nonneoplastic breast tissue contained a background of bipolar nuclei, a helpful benign diagnostic feature. With a prior history of radiotherapy to the breast, a conservative approach is recommended whenever cytologic atypia is found.[39-43]

REFERENCES

1. Weiss RL, Matsen JM: Group B streptococcal breast abscess. *Arch Pathol Lab Med* 111:74–75, 1987.

2. Azzopardi JG: Problems in Breast Pathology, Vol 11. Major Problems in Pathology. Bennington L, Ed. London, WB Saunders, 1979, vol 11, pp 42–55, 346–378.

3. Haagensen CD: Diseases of the Breast. Philadelphia, WB Saunders, 1986.

4. Waldvogel FA: *Staphylococcus aureus* (including toxic shock syndrome), *In:* Mandell GL, Douglas RG Jr, Bennett JE, Eds. Principles and Practice of Infectious Diseases, ed 2. New York, John Wiley & Sons 156:1092–1117, 1985.

5. Petrek J: Postmenopausal breast abscess. *South Med J* 75:1198–1199, 1982.

6. Eckland DA, Zeigler MG: Abscess in the nonlactating breast. *Arch Surg* 107:398–401, 1973.

7. Habif DV, Perzin KH, Lipton R, et al: Subareolar abscess associated with squamous metaplasia of lactiferous ducts. *Am J Surg* 119:523–526, 1970.

8. Frable WJ: Major Problems in Pathology, Vol 14. Thin Needle Aspiration Biopsy. Philadelphia, WB Saunders, 1983.

9. Klemi PH, Joensuu H: Comparison of DNA ploidy in routine fine needle aspiration biopsy samples and paraffin-embedded tissue samples. *Anal Quant Cytol Histol* 10:195–199, 1988.

10. Kline TS: Handbook of Fine Needle Aspiration Biopsy Cytology. St. Louis, Mosby, 1988.

11. Kline TS: Masquerades of malignancy: a review of 4,241 aspirations from the breast. *Acta Cytol* 25:263–266, 1981.

12. Silverman JF, Lannin DR, Unverferth M, et al: Fine needle aspiration cytology of subareolar abscess of the breast: spectrum of cytomorphologic findings and potential diagnostic pitfalls. *Acta Cytol* 30:413–419, 1986.

13. Koss LG, Woyke J, Olszewski W: Aspiration biopsy: cytologic interpretation and histologic bases. New York, Igaku-Shoin, 1984, pp 53–104.

14. Hashimoto CH, Cobb CJ: Cytodiagnosis of hibernoma: a case report. *Diagn Cytopathol* 3:326–329, 1987.

15. DeMay RM, Kay S: Granular cell tumor of the breast. *Pathol Annu* 19:121–148, 1984.

16. Ingram DL, Mossler JA, Snowhite J, et al: Granular cell tumors of the breast. Steroid receptor analysis and localization of carcinoembryonic antigen, myoglobin, and S1OO protein. *Arch Pathol Lab Med* 108:897–901, 1984.

17. Lowhagen T, Rubio C: The cytology of the granular cell myoblastoma of the breast. *Acta Cytol* 21:314–345, 1977.

18. Feldman PS, Covell JL: Breast and lung. *In:* Fine Needle Aspiration Cytology and Its Clinical Application. Chicago, American Society of Clinical Pathologists Press, 1985, pp 27–43.

19. Galblum LI, Oertel YC: Subareolar abscess of the breast diagnosed by fine needle aspiration. *Am J Clin Pathol* 80:496–499, 1983.

20. Zuska JJ, Crile G Jr, Ayres WW: Fistulas of laciferous ducts. *Am J Surg* 81:312–317, 1951.

21. Silverman JF, Lannin DR, Meelheim D, et al: Subaveolar abscess of the breast: the role of fine needle biopsy in the diagnosis and management. *Contemp Surg* 28:45–48, 1986.

22. Oertel YC, Galblum LI: Fine needle aspiration of the breast: diagnostic criteria. *Pathol Annu* 1:375–407, 1983.

23. Carney M, Unverferth M, Silverman JF: Fine needle aspiration cytology of subareolar abscess. *Cytotechnol Bull* 22:60–64, 1985.

24. Kline TS, Joshi LP, Neal HS: Fine needle aspiration of the breast: diagnoses and pitfalls: a review of 3,545 cases. *Cancer* 44:1458–1464, 1979.

25. Oberman HA: Invasive carcinoma of the breast with granulomatous response. *Am J Clin Pathol* 88:718–721, 1987.

26. Gansler TS, Wheeler JE: Mammary sarcoidosis. Two cases and literature review. *Arch Pathol Lab Med* 108:673–675, 1984.

27. Doria MI, Tani EM, Skoog, L: Sarcoidosis presenting initially as a breast mass: detection by fine-needle aspiration biopsy. *Acta Cytol* 31:378–379, 1987.

28. Jayaram G: Cytomorphology of tuberculous mastitis: a report of nine cases with fine-needle aspiration cytology. *Acta Cytol* 29:974–978, 1985.

29. Nayar M, Saxema HMK: Tuberculosis of the breast. A cytomorphologic study of needle aspirates and nipple discharges. *Acta Cytol* 28:325–328, 1984.

30. Macansh S, Greenberg M, Barraclough B, et al: Fine needle aspiration cytology of granulomatous mastitis: report of a case and review of the literature. *Acta Cytol* 34:38–42, 1990.

31. Tabatowski K, Elson CE, Johnston WW: Silicone lymphadenopathy in a patient with a mammary prosthesis: fine needle aspiration cytology, histology and analytical electron microscopy. *Acta Cytol* 34:10–14, 1990.

32. Silverman JF, Dabbs DJ, Norris HT, et al: Localized primary (AL) amyloid tumor of the breast: cytologic, histologic, immunocytochemical and ultrastructural observations. *Am J Surg Pathol* 10:539–545, 1986.

33. Lew W, Seymour A: Primary amyloid tumor of the breast, case report and literature review. *Acta Cytol* 29:7–11, 1985.

34. Fernandez BB, Hernandez FJ: Amyloid tumor of the breast. *Arch Pathol* 95:102–105, 1973.

35. Kyle RA, Bayrd ED: Amyloidosis: review of 236 cases. *Medicine* 54:271–299, 1975.

36. Kyle RA, Greipp PR: Amyloidosis (AL). Clinical and laboratory features in 229 cases. *Mayo Clin Proc* 58:665–683, 1983.

37. Libbey CA, Skinner M, Cohen AS: The abdominal fat aspirate for the diagnosis of systemic amyloid. *Arch Intern Med* 143:1549–1552, 1983.

38. Westermark P, Stenkvist B: A new method for the diagnosis of systemic amyloidosis. *Arch Intern Med* 132:522–523, 1973.

39. Schnitt SJ, Connolly JL, Harris JR, et al: Radiation-induced changes in the breast. *Hum Pathol* 16:545–550, 1984.

40. Bondeson L: Aspiration cytology of radiation-induced changes of normal breast epithelium. *Acta Cytol* 31:309–310, 1987.

41. Gupta RK: Radiation-induced cellular changes in the breast: a potential diagnostic pitfall in fine needle aspiration cytology. *Acta Cytol* 33:141–142, 1989.

42. Pedio G, Landolt U, Zobeli L: Irradiated benign cells of the breast: a potential diagnostic pitfall in fine needle aspiration cytology. *Acta Cytol* 32:127–128, 1988.

43. Peterse JL, Thunnissen FBJM, van Heerde P: Fine needle aspiration cytology of radiation-induced changes in nonneoplastic breast lesions. Possible pitfalls in cytodiagnosis. *Acta Cytol* 33:176–180, 1989.

8

Head and Neck
Including Thyroid

SALIVARY GLAND

Diffuse enlargement or nodularity of the salivary gland may be caused by neoplasia, cystic lesions, or inflammation.[1] Inflammatory lesions (sialadenitis) may be of viral, bacterial, or autoimmune origin. It is not uncommon to encounter salivary gland masses or swellings suspicious for neoplasia that prove on needle aspiration to be benign cysts or inflammatory lesions.[2] In addition, intraparotid lymph nodes can enlarge and simulate a primary or secondary salivary gland neoplasm (especially one of the parotid gland). Therefore, FNA biopsy of salivary gland lesions is useful in diagnosing inflammatory lesions and confirming or excluding a neoplastic process. Types of nonneoplastic encountered on ABC of benign salivary lesions are presented in Table 8.1.

Inflammatory lesions of the salivary gland may be related to any of a number of causes but most often are associated with sialolithiasis. Calculi especially form in Wharton's duct of the submaxillary (submandibular) gland and cause obstruction with secondary infection (Fig. 8.1). Salivary duct stones form by deposition of calcium salts around a central nidus which may contain desquamated epithelial cells, bacteria, and products of bacterial decomposition serving as a foreign body (Fig. 8.2). Acute bacterial infections are most often present in association with obstruction of the duct due to calculi or trauma. Poor oral hygiene with dehydration and altered immune defense status are also associated with acute bacterial infections of the salivary glands. Occasionally, elderly patients with a recent history of major surgery develop sialadenitis, presumably on the basis of dehydration associated with decreased secretory function and secondary bacterial invasion. The parotid gland is most commonly involved, although the submandibular gland can also be affected. *Streptococcus viridans* and *Staphylococcus aureus* cause most cases of acute bacterial sialadenitis; pneumococcal and gram-negative bacteria are less common organisms. Mumps virus is the commonest viral cause of parotid gland swelling.[3] Coxsackie A

169

TABLE 8.1. Nonneoplastic Salivary Gland Lesions

Acute sialadenitis
Chronic sialadenitis, including postirradiation sialadenitis
Sialolithiasis
Granulomatous sialadenitis: TB, fungal, cat scratch, foreign body, sarcoid
Benign lymphoepithelial lesion including Sjögren's syndrome, Mikulicz's disease
Lymphoepithelial cysts

virus, ECHO virus, and the virus of lymphocytic choriomeningitis can also involve the parotid gland.[2] Mumps often occurs in children in the 4- to 5-year age group but may involve older children and adults.

Cytomorphologic findings of acute sialadenitis consist of sheets of neutrophils with scattered histiocytes and debris. Fragments of calculi may be present; these are refractile and stain only at the periphery with the Diff-Quik stain. Small clusters of acinar cells may be present including occasional groups showing features of inflammatory atypia (Fig. 8.3).

Chronic sialadenitis is usually secondary to sialolithiasis or as a sequela to postsurgical scarring. It is most commonly seen involving the submandibular salivary gland. Chronic recurrent sialadenitis, a poorly understood lesion, frequently affects the parotid gland.[3] Chronic sialadenitis is also seen following radiation therapy. Although FNA biopsy may not be needed in the usual case, it is quite helpful in excluding malignancy in patients with a prior history of head and neck cancer. Cytomorphologic findings include the presence of numerous chronic inflammatory

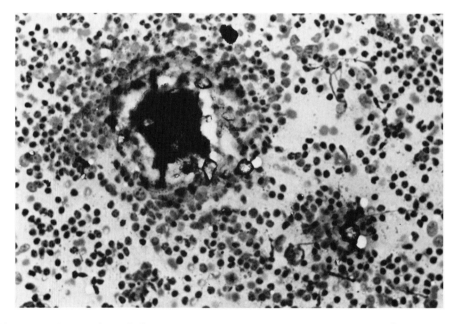

Fig. 8.1. Clumps of calcified material with surrounding extensive chronic inflammation in aspirate of sialolithiasis (Diff-Quik stain; ×100).

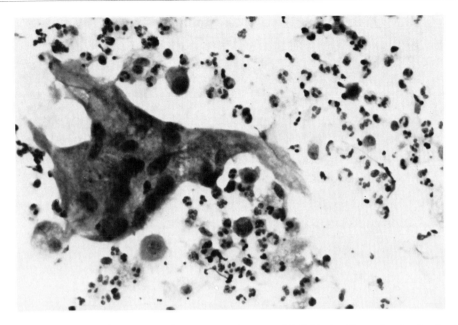

Fig. 8.2. Aspirate of acute sialadenitis secondary to sialolithiasis. Note the foreign-body type reaction to calculus material (Diff-Quik stain; × 400).

cells associated with some histiocytes and a few scattered fibroblastic cells. Potential pitfalls for a false-positive diagnosis of malignancy in postirradiation chronic sialadenitis include radiation atypia and atypical squamous metaplasia. Aspirates of chronic sialadenitis generally tend to be less cellular than those of acute sialadenitis. The differential diagnosis of salivary gland aspirates containing increased numbers of chronic inflammatory cells includes FNA biopsies of intraparenchymal lymph nodes, benign lymphoepithelial lesion, Warthin's tumor (adenolymphoma), and lymphoma. The cytologic features of these entities is discussed below.

Granulomatous Sialadenitis

The salivary glands can be involved in granulomatous processes related to tuberculosis, sarcoidosis, cat scratch disease, fungal infections, and foreign body reactions. The granulomatous inflammation can represent either a primary process or secondary involvement due to direct extension of the granulomatous inflammation from nearby lymph nodes or the oral cavity or as part of a systemic process.[2] Most commonly, an enlarged intraparotid or periparotid lymph node, or both, is involved, which can simulate a localized neoplasm.

Sarcoidosis is a multisystem granulomatous disorder of unknown etiology, most frequently involving the lymph nodes, lungs, skin, or eyes,[4] although salivary gland involvement can occasionally be present.[5-8] Parotid, sublingual, and submaxillary glands often demonstrate asymptomatic enlargement.[4] Heerfordt's syndrome (uveoparotid fever) is a form of sarcoidosis causing parotid gland enlargement, uveitis, and facial paralysis. Cytologic features as reported by Mair and associates,

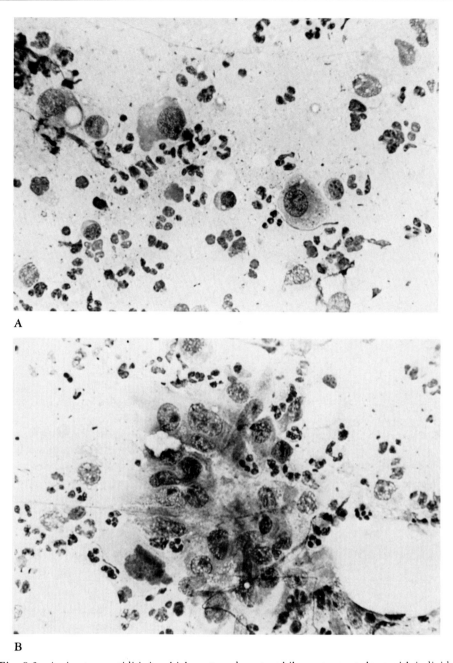

A

B

Fig. 8.3. A. Acute parotiditis in which scattered neutrophils are present along with individually scattered acinar cells showing atypical features of nuclear enlargement and mild hyperchromasia (Diff-Quik stain; ×200). **B.** Cluster of atypical acinar cells demonstrating inflammatory atypia. Note extensive acute inflammation in the background and also within the group of acinar epithelium (Diff-Quik stain; ×200).

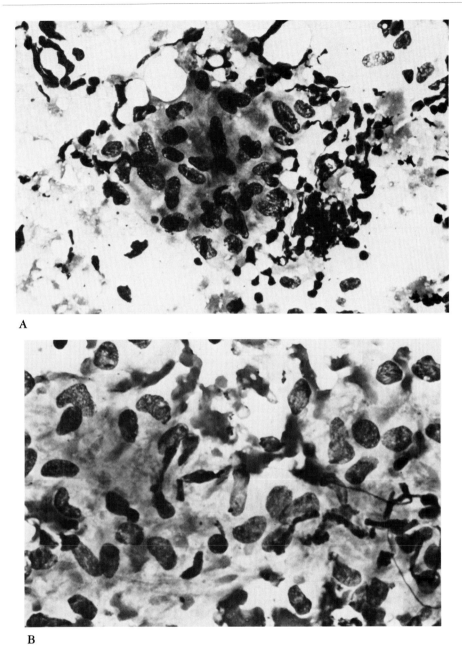

A

B

Fig. 8.4. **A.** FNA of sarcoid of parotid gland showing fragment of granulomatous inflammation in which epithelioid cells are arranged in a loose cluster (Diff-Quik stain; ×400). **B.** High-power view of epithelioid histiocytes having oval to spindle-shaped nuclei including some having a boomerang configuration (Diff-Quik stain; ×630).

Aggarwal and associates, and Qizilbash[1,2,4,9] include noncaseating epithelioid cell granulomas associated with multinucleated giant cells and associated benign-appearing salivary gland acini and ductal tissue (Fig. 8.4). The differential diagnosis includes tuberculous, fungal infections, and foreign body reaction to calcific material.[4] Therefore, appropriate special stains for organisms should be performed along with culture of the aspirated material. In aspirates of sarcoid, background necrosis is usually absent in the smears. Tuberculous infection of the salivary gland most often involves the parotid gland. Cytologic evidence of necrotizing granulomas will be seen. Special stains for mycobacteria and culture are needed for a definitive diagnosis.

Inflammation and Atypias in Benign Lymphoepithelial Lesion and Salivary Gland Neoplasms

Benign lymphoepithelial lesion is believed to be an autoimmune process that can cause unilateral or bilateral enlargement of salivary or lacrimal glands.[2,10] The term Mikulicz's disease is now used synonymously when a benign lymphoepithelial lesion causes enlargement of the salivary and lacrimal gland. The term Sjögren's syndrome is used when keratoconjunctivitis sicca, xerostomia, and a connective tissue disorder such as rheumatoid arthritis are also present. The cytologic findings consist of numerous lymphoid cells including small and large reactive lymphocytes along with plasma cells and histiocytes. Some elongated histiocytic-appearing cells may be present. Usually, ductal cells are quite sparse and acinar cells are not present. The ductal cells are arranged in small cohesive groups or sheets surrounded by a chronic inflammatory cell process. Recently, Weidner and associates reported five cases of benign lymphoepithelial cysts of the parotid gland in which some of the patients underwent aspiration biopsy. Cytologic findings included a cellular lymphoid background consisting principally of small mature lymphocytes admixed with small, flat, tightly cohesive epithelial groupings. Some of the epithelial cells had foamy and slightly granular cytoplasm containing mucin, while other cells resembled squamous metaplastic cells. In three of the cases, extracellular mucinous material was present, and in one case the lesion was virtually acellular except for the presence of amorphous masses of mucin.[11] Elliot and Oertel recently reported the fine-needle aspiration cytologic features of five cases of lymphoepithelial cyst of the salivary gland in a series of 14 surgically excised cases.[12] In the Diff-Quik-stained smears, proteinaceous background material was present along with a mixed population of lymphocytes, histiocytes, plasma cells, and metaplastic type squamous cells. Benign lymphoepithelial cysts have not been associated with Sjögren's syndrome or Mikulicz's disease. Lymphoepithelial cysts have been associated, however, with positive serology for human immunodeficiency virus (HIV).[12]

The cytologic differential diagnosis includes Warthin's tumor, although oncocytic cells are not present in benign lymphoepithelial cysts[11] (see Fig. 8.5). However, occasional cases of Warthin's tumor may only demonstrate inflammatory cells, mucoid material, and metaplastic squamous and mucin-producing cells which would be indistinguishable from benign lymphoepithelial cysts. Occasionally, squamous metaplasia may be prominent in Warthin's tumor. Aspirates from such cases can contain atypical squamous cells, which could be a potential pitfall for a false-positive

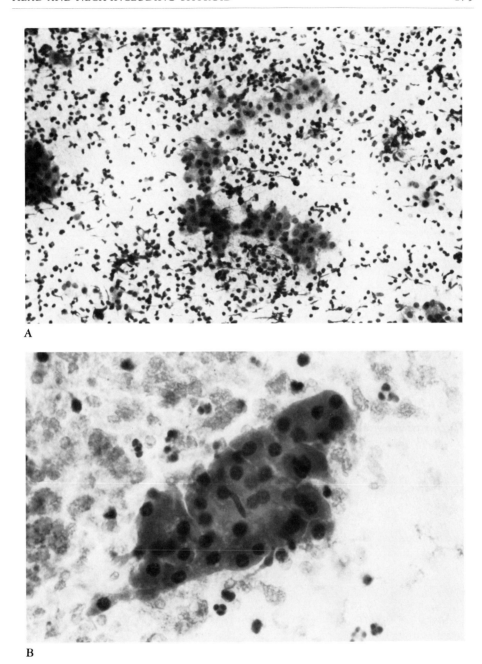

A

B

Fig. 8.5. A. Low-power view of Warthin's tumor showing a few scattered groups of onco-cytic cells along with numerous chronic inflammatory cells in the background (Papanicolaou stain; × 100). **B.** High power view of oncocytic cells having a cuboidal shape with abundant granular eosinophilic cytoplasm (Papanicolaou stain; × 400).

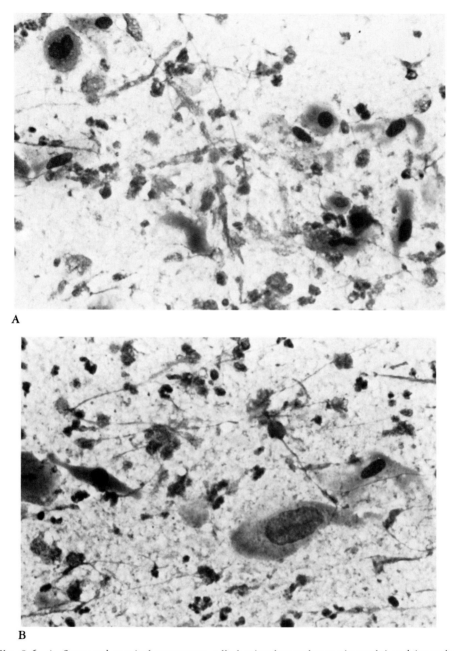

A

B

Fig. 8.6. A. Scattered atypical squamous cells having hyperchromatic nuclei and irregular shapes in an aspirate of Warthin's tumor undergoing squamous metaplasia (Diff-Quik stain; ×200). **B.** Scattered markedly atypical squamous cells in aspirate of Warthin's tumor (Diff-Quik stain; ×400).

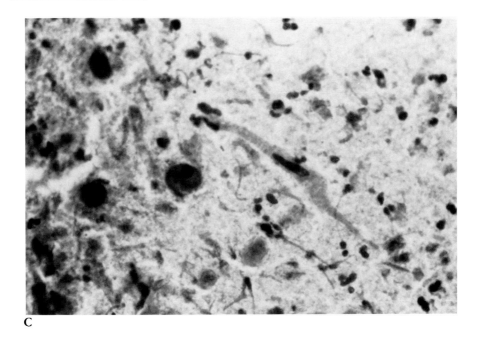

C

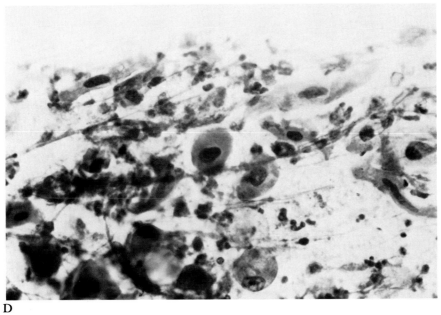

D

Fig. 8.6. C. and **D.** Scattered atypical squamous cells along with neutrophils and necrotic material in the background from an aspirate of Warthin's tumor (Papanicolaou stain; ×400).

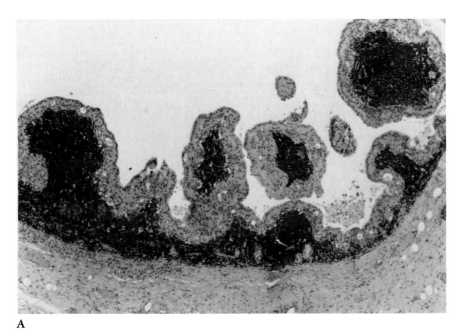

A

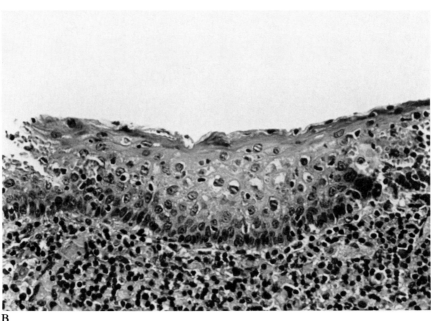

B

Fig. 8.7. A. Resected Warthin's tumor showing characteristic histologic findings of cystic spaces lined by oncocytic cells with underlying nodules of lymphocytes (H&E stain; × 100). **B.** Portion of the cyst lining shows extensive squamous metaplasia with some acute inflammation (H&E stain; × 400).

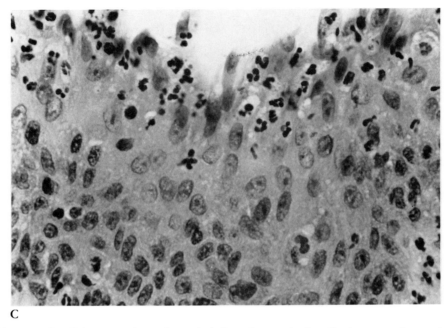

C

Fig. 8.7. C. High-power view of acutely inflamed metaplastic cells demonstrating nuclear enlargement and irregularity with prominent nucleoli. These cells were the source of the atypical squamous cells seen in the FNA biopsy (H&E stain; ×630).

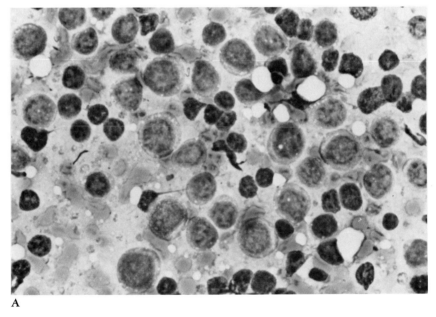

A

Fig. 8.8. A. Aspirate of large non-cleaved lymphoma involving the submaxillary gland. Note numerous atypical lymphoid cells having enlarged nuclei with no evidence of nuclear irregularity. A few smaller lymphoid cells are present (Diff-Quik stain; ×400).

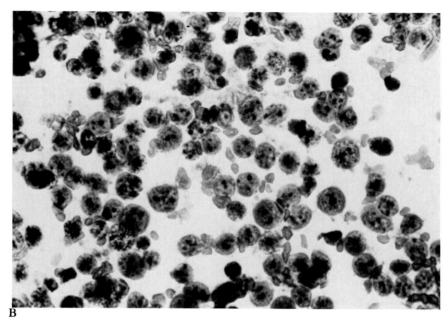

B

Fig. 8.8. B. Monomorphic population of atypical lymphoid cells consistent with large non-cleaved lymphoma of submaxillary gland (Papanicolaou stain; × 400).

diagnosis of metastatic squamous cell carcinoma involving a periparotid lymph node (Fig. 8.6). Inflamed branchial cleft cyst also enters into the differential diagnosis. Although the squamous cells may show cytologic atypia, definite malignant features will not be present. A conservative approach is warranted in this setting, especially in a patient without a previous history of a head and neck squamous cell carcinoma. Tissue confirmation may be needed before definitive treatment (Fig. 8.7). For a definitive diagnosis of Warthin's tumor, oncocytic cells arranged in cohesive sheets should be present along with lymphoid cells. Specimens of Warthin's tumor that are cystic, contain abundant background debris, and oncocytic cells may be cytologically confused with benign lymphoepithelial cysts and benign lymphoepithelial lesions. Aspirates from malignant lymphomas consist of a uniform monomorphic population of atypical lymphoid cells and therefore should not be confused with usual cases of benign lymphoepithelial lesions or chronic sialadenitis (Fig. 8.8).

BRANCHIAL CLEFT CYST

Branchial cleft cyst is lateral cervical lesion that usually occurs behind the angle of the mandible, in the anterior triangle of the neck, or at the junction of the upper third and lower two thirds of the sternocleidomastoid muscle. It may, however, occur in other cervical neck locations. Although these lesions occur in a wide age range, the majority of the patients are young adults. Characteristically, these lesions present as slowly growing lesions and are relatively asymptomatic, circumscribed,

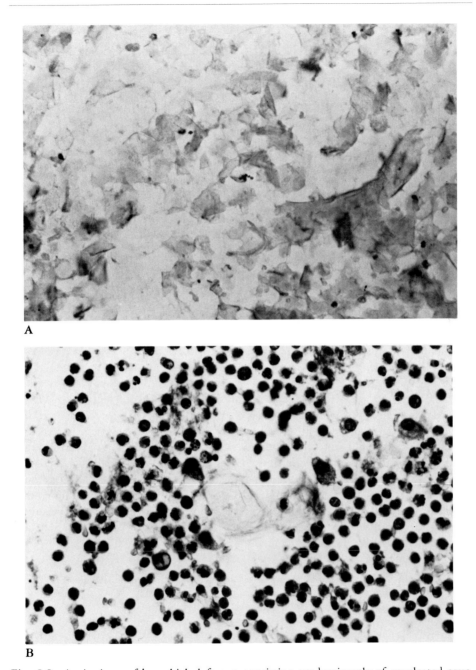

Fig. 8.9. A. Aspirate of branchial cleft cyst consisting predominantly of anucleated squamous cells (Papanicolaou stain; × 100). **B.** Inflamed branchial cleft cyst showing no significant atypia of the squamous cells although some cases have been reported in which inflammatory atypia can be confused with a metastatic squamous cell carcinoma (Papanicolaou stain; × 100).

TABLE 8.2. Salivary Gland Lesions That Are Potential Pitfalls for False-Positive Diagnosis of Malignancy

Lesion	Potential False-Positive Diagnosis
Postirradiation chronic sialadenitis	Radiation atypia mistaken for recurrent carcinoma
Warthin's tumor with squamous metaplasia	Squamous atypias mistaken for squamous cell carcinoma
Inflamed branchial cleft cyst	Squamous atypia mistaken for squamous cell carcinoma
Mucus retention cyst	Squamous metaplasia and mucinous cells mistaken for mucoepidermoid

and movable. Histologically, the cyst wall contains lymphoid tissue and the cyst is lined by stratified squamous epithelium, although some pseudostratified columnar epithelium may be present. FNA cytologic findings generally reveal benign squamous cells associated with granular debris and lymphoid cells (Fig. 8.9). Koss believes that the presence of even slight nuclear atypia in an aspirate of a neck mass clinically considered to be a branchial cleft cyst most often represents a metastasis from a well differentiated squamous cell carcinoma to a cervical lymph node.[13] Warson and associates recently reported the cytologic findings of an inflamed branchial cleft cyst in which elongated, spindle-shape keratinized cells having atypical, hyperchromatic nuclei were present[14] (Fig. 8.8). The lesion was considered to be highly suspicious for well differentiated squamous cell carcinoma. Resection of the mass revealed an acutely inflamed branchial cleft cyst. The authors caution that an inflamed branchial cleft cyst could be a potential pitfall for a false-positive diagnosis of metastatic squamous cell carcinoma. Another lesion that can have similar cytologic findings is a Warthin's tumor with squamous metaplasia. We believe that any lateral cervical mass containing atypical keratinized squamous cells should be resected for definitive diagnosis. Benign aspirated lesions that are potential pitfalls for a false-positive diagnosis of malignancy are presented in Table 8.2.

ORBIT

Most FNA biopsies of the orbit have been performed for the diagnosis of neoplastic conditions. Recently there have been two reports of aspergillosis of the orbit diagnosed by ABC.[15,16] Most reported cases of orbital aspergilloma have been in previously healthy individuals, although patients may have received systemic corticosteroids.[15] In contrast, rhinocerebral phycomycosis usually occurs in severely debilitated patients and carries a very poor prognosis. At times it may be difficult to differentiate aspergillosis from phycomycosis cytologically. The use of immunocytochemical stains for aspergillosis may prove to be a useful technique in making a diagnosis of a specific fungus, especially when a limited amount of diagnostic material is available.[15]

CERVICOFACIAL ACTINOMYCOSIS

Actinomycosis commonly involves the cervicofacial, ileocecal, and pulmonary regions, in that order of frequency.[17] Cervicofacial actinomycosis usually presents as a firm, indurated, minimally painful swelling of the submandibular region.[18] Other sites of involvement include the lacrimal gland, orbit, tongue, hypopharynx, larynx, maxilla, and parotid gland.[19] Occasional patients are symptomatic with high fever and weight loss. *Actinomyces* is an anaerobic, gram-positive bacterium of the order Actinomycetales. Cultures of the lesion often are negative.[18] The average duration from clinical presentation to diagnosis can average 3 months.[18] Pollock and associates suggest that because of the variable clinical presentation, relative infrequency of the lesion, and poor culture results, aspiration cytology may be an effective means of recognizing the organisms and obtaining material for microbiologic examination.[18] Cytologic findings will include the presence of sulfur granules consisting of clumps of branching, thin, pleomorphic rods. Other organisms that enter into the differential diagnosis include streptomyces and *Nocardia*. In contrast to actinomyces, *Nocardia* is positive with modified acid-fast stains.[18]

THYROID GLAND

The term thyroiditis is used to describe not only specific thyroid diseases but any disorder of the thyroid that has prominent inflammation or fibrosis. Thyroiditis has been classified according to etiology, duration, or morphology of the process, although the cause of many of these disorders often is in doubt.[20,21] Most often, thyroiditis is classified on the basis of the duration of the clinical course as being acute, subacute, or chronic. Although most patients with thyroiditis are euthyroid, transient episodes of hyperfunction and hypofunction are not uncommon, and permanent hypothyroidism can sometimes be present secondary to extensive parenchymal destruction.[20,22] Since thyroiditis can present either with diffuse enlargement or a prominent nodule, it can be mistaken for a neoplasm.[21] We believe that FNA biopsy of the thyroid is the most cost-effective and accurate method of evaluating patients with thyroid nodules and thereby eliminates unnecessary surgery.[23]

Thyroid nodules are common; they are identified in approximately 4% of the U.S. population.[24-28] Although thyroiditis is the most common disease affecting the thyroid, the vast majority of the nodules are caused by benign nodular goiter, followed by thyroiditis (Table 8.3). Therefore, recognition of the cytopathologic features of thyroiditis is important for accurate diagnosis and for avoiding false-negative and false-positive diagnoses of malignancy.

Acute Thyroiditis

Acute thyroiditis is an uncommon inflammatory disease of the thyroid caused by bacterial, fungal, and very rarely parasitic infections.[20] In a recent literature review, 224 cases of acute thyroiditis was reported including 153 bacterial, 33 fungal, and 11 parasitic infections.[29] Acute bacterial thyroiditis occurs in a wide age range and

TABLE 8.3. Nonneoplastic Thyroid Lesions

Acute thyroiditis
Subacute (granulomatous) thyroiditis
Riedel's struma
Hashimoto's thyroiditis
Amyloid goiter
Granulomatous inflammation; infectious and foreign body (Teflon and suture
    granulomas)

is slightly more common in women than in men. Preceding infections such as upper
respiratory tract infection or pharyngitis are often noted before acute thyroiditis
becomes apparent.[30] The typical signs and symptoms are anterior neck pain, tenderness, fever, dysphagia, dermal erythema, or dysphonia with concurrent pharyngitis
or pharyngeal pain.[29] The majority of patients with acute bacterial thyroiditis have
leukocytosis of more than 10,000 per ml with normal total serum thyroxine and
radioactive iodine uptake. Thyroid autoantibodies are not present. Since acute suppurative thyroiditis resolves with appropriate antibiotic treatment, it is seldom aspirated. However, FNA biopsy can be used to confirm the clinical diagnosis and to
provide a specimen for culture.[20] The most common bacterial organisms responsible
for acute suppurative thyroiditis are *Staphylococcus aureus, Streptococcus pyogenes,
Streptococcus pneumoniae,* and *Enterobacter.*[20] Cytomorphologic findings include the
presence of numerous inflammatory cells consisting predominantly of neutrophils,
necrotic debris, and bacteria which are best appreciated in the Diff-Quik stain.[31]
Recently, a case of disseminated cryptococcosis presenting as thyroiditis was diagnosed by FNA biopsy.[32]

Subacute (Granulomatous) Thyroiditis

Subacute (granulomatous) thyroiditis is a self-limited, spontaneously remitting inflammatory disease of the thyroid that most likely has a viral etiology.[20] Synonyms
for subacute thyroiditis include deQuervain's disease, giant cell thyroiditis, viral
thyroiditis, nonsuppurative thyroiditis, and struma granulomatosa.[20,21] Subacute
thyroiditis is reported to be most common in women from their teens to their 40's
and is rarely seen in children. The clinical presentation of subacute thyroiditis
ranges from an abrupt onset of chills, fever, and pain in the thyroid region to some
patients complaining only of a low grade fever and vague tenderness of the anterior
neck. Often patients have malaise, fatigue, myalgia, and mild fever. The thyroid
gland characteristically is only slightly to moderately enlarged with the affected lobe
or lobes firm to hard and quite tender to palpation. Most often the clinical course
lasts for 2 to 5 months, although approximately 20% of the patients have a more
chronic relapsing course. If the disease is severe or prolonged, hypothyroidism may
persist for weeks to months, but less than 5% of the patients have permanent
hypothyroidism. Pertinent laboratory findings include an elevated erythrocyte sedimentation rate with a normal white blood cell count. Thyroid function test findings
have varying patterns depending on the stage of the disease. Complete restoration
of normal thyroid function usually occurs within a few months.

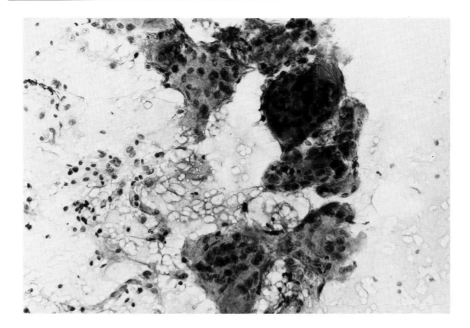

Fig. 8.10. Numerous multinucleated foreign-body type giant cells in aspirate of subacute thyroiditis (Papanicolaou stain; × 100).

Fine-needle aspiration biopsy can be useful in confirming a diagnosis of subacute thyroiditis, but it is seldom used since most patients respond well to medical management. This generally includes treatment with salicylates, although corticosteroids may be prescribed in severe cases.[20] Sanders and associates reported a case of painless giant cell thyroiditis diagnosed by FNA biopsy.[33] Our experience with subacute thyroiditis is similar to the cytologic results reported by Kini.[21] The spectrum of cytomorphologic features of subacute thyroiditis reflects the characteristic microscopic findings of destruction of the thyroid parenchyma. The findings include a foreign-body type giant cell reaction around inspissated colloid along with a mixed inflammatory cell infiltrate consisting predominantly of lymphocytes, plasma cells, and neutrophils (Fig. 8.10). Multinucleated foreign body type giant cells can be seen near colloid and/or follicular epithelium (Fig. 8.11). Other findings include epithelioid histiocytes, stromal fragments, and fibroblasts. The cytologic differential diagnosis should include other thyroid entities associated with giant cells such as Hashimoto's thyroiditis and papillary carcinoma.

Two related types of subacute thyroiditis are subacute lymphocytic (painless) thyroiditis and postpartum subacute lymphocytic thyroiditis, both of which may undergo aspiration.[20] Subacute lymphocytic thyroiditis is a poorly understood condition that appears to be a common type of thyroiditis in U.S. adults.[20] Presenting signs and symptoms include evidence of hyperthyroidism and variable thyroid enlargement. Patients without clinical hyperthyroidism and only slight enlargement of the gland may be unrecognized because of the self-limited nature of the process and the lack of clinical sequelae. Although there are histologic similarities with classic subacute granulomatous thyroiditis, most patients with subacute lymphocytic

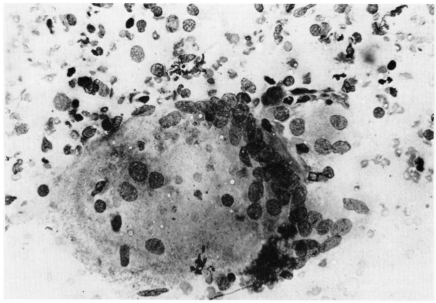

A

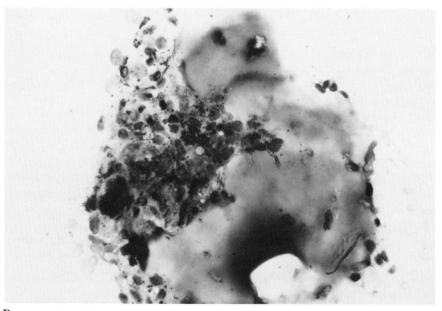

B

Fig. 8.11. A. Scattered multinucleated giant cells in aspirate of subacute thyroiditis (Diff-Quik stain; ×400). **B.** Multinucleated histiocytes surrounding clump of colloid material (Diff-Quik stain; ×200).

thyroiditis demonstrate greater numbers of lymphoid cells, fewer plasma cells, and no neutrophils or giant cells in the tissue.[20]

Invasive Fibrous Thyroiditis (Riedel's Struma)

The most uncommon type of thyroiditis is invasive fibrous thyroiditis (chronic sclerosing thyroiditis, Riedel's struma), which primarily affects women and leads to complete destruction of the thyroid gland by fibrosclerosis. Patients classically present with a stony hard or woody mass, fixed to surrounding neck structures via extension of the fibrosclerotic process beyond the capsule of the thyroid. Although the disease is rare, it is important to recognize, since it may readily be clinically confused with malignancy. Unfortunately, FNA biopsy will yield little cellular material, necessitating histologic confirmation by wedge resection or lobectomy.[20,21] The differential diagnoses include the fibrous variant of Hashimoto's thyroiditis and granulomatous thyroiditis. When cytologic material is present in an aspirate of invasive fibrous thyroiditis, it usually consists of a few scattered lymphocytes, neutrophils, histiocytes, and fibroblasts.[34,35]

Chronic Lymphocytic Thyroiditis (Hashimoto's Thyroiditis)

Hashimoto's thyroiditis was first reported in 1912 as a chronic disorder of the thyroid ("struma lymphomatosa"). Although chronic lymphocytic thyroiditis most commonly occurs in women between 30 and 50 years of age, it can be seen in any age group including children. In fact, Hashimoto's thyroiditis is the most common thyroid disease of children in the United States. Chronic lymphocytic thyroiditis usually begins as a diffuse enlargement of the thyroid gland with or without nodularity. Most patients have painless enlargement of the thyroid, although a few report mild neck pain or tenderness as initial symptoms. Since the gland is diffusely irregular with some variation in symmetry, the patient can present with a thyroid nodule. Solitary 1- to 3-cm thyroid nodules were reported as the presenting sign in the majority of patients undergoing FNA biopsy in one series.[35]

Although at one time thought to be uncommon, Hashimoto's thyroiditis is being increasingly recognized in the U.S. population. At the Mayo Clinic more than 500 new cases of Hashimoto's thyroiditis are identified each year, and evidence of Hashimoto's thyroiditis is found in approximately 2% of women at autopsy.[20] It is believed that the greater utilization of FNA biopsy and serologic tests for autoantibodies has led to a more frequent recognition of this chronic inflammatory disorder of the thyroid, although Hashimoto's thyroiditis may also be increasing in frequency. Speculation exists that the increased iodine content of the North American diet has possibly led to an alteration in the thyroglobulin molecule, which then elicits an autoimmune response.[20,36] Approximately 80 and 97% of patients with Hashimoto's thyroiditis, respectively, have serum antibodies to thyroglobulin or microsomal antigen. Although many patients do not require treatment, if thyroid enlargement causes local pressure symptoms, thyroid hormone therapy is instituted which often reduces the size of the goiter. If hypothyroidism is present, thyroid replacement is needed. During the early phases of the disease, mild thyrotoxicosis

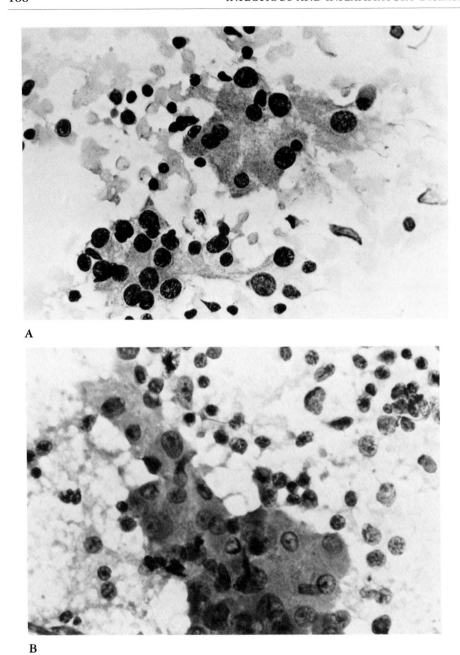

Fig. 8.12. A. Aspirate of Hashimoto's thyroiditis consisting of clusters of oxyphilic cells and scattered lymphocytes. Note the anisonucleosis of the Hurthle cells (Papanicolaou stain; ×400). **B.** High-power view of Hurthle cells showing some variation in nuclear size with the presence of small nucleoli. Note numerous chronic inflammatory cells in the background (Papanicolaou stain; ×630).

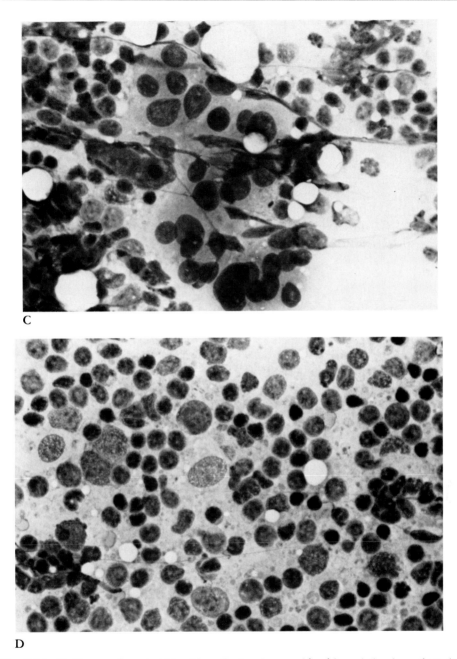

C

D

Fig. 8.12. C. Cluster of atypical Hurthle cells showing considerable variation in nuclear size and shape along with associated chronic inflammatory cells (Diff-Quik stain; ×400). D. Aspirate of Hashimoto's thyroiditis in which some fields show predominantly lymphoid cells with very few Hurthle or follicular cells. Benign features include polymorphic population of small mature to larger reactive lymphoid cells along with histiocytes (Diff-Quik stain; ×630).

may be present, and occasionally hypothyroidism occurs late in the disease. It has been increasingly appreciated that patients with Hashimoto's thyroiditis have an increased risk for development of malignancy, particularly primary malignant lymphoma of the thyroid.[37]

Cytomorphologic features of Hashimoto's thyroiditis include a polymorphic inflammatory cell reaction including many mature lymphocytes, plasma cells and transformed lymphoid cells, and histiocytes including some containing cytoplasmic phagocytized debris (Fig. 8.12). Multinucleated foreign-body type giant cells can be present but are an infrequent component. Oncocytic epithelial cells (Hurthle cells) arranged in small microtissue fragments or clusters along with reactive-appearing follicular cells are present.[21,38] In general, the epithelial cells are quite cohesive with good cell orientation, and considerable nuclear pleomorphism can be present. Hurthle cells are generally larger than follicular cells and have characteristic acidophilic granular cytoplasm in the Papanicolaou-stained smears. Anisonucleosis is characteristically present and nucleoli may also be seen, but macronucleoli, a feature of Hurthle cell neoplasms, are not a common finding.[39] Colloid is often scant in amount, and a ropelike detritus can be present.[40]

The cytologic differential diagnosis of Hashimoto's thyroiditis includes a number of entities such as granulomatous thyroiditis, Hurthle cell nodules and neoplasms, follicular neoplasms, papillary carcinoma, and malignant lymphoma. A potential false-positive diagnosis of epithelial neoplasm can be made in aspirates of Hashimoto's thyroiditis. Since atypical and pleomorphic Hurthle cells occur in Hashimoto's thyroiditis, a false-positive diagnosis of Hurthle cell neoplasm can occur. In Hashimoto's thyroiditis, however, atypical follicular and Hurthle cells occur mostly in cohesive groups and clusters, in contrast to the loosely cohesive or isolated arrangement of uniform-appearing oxyphilic cells of Hurthle cell neoplasia. In addition, Hurthle cell tumors have oncocytic cells with prominent cherry red macronucleoli and well defined cytoplasm (Fig. 8.13). The presence of increased numbers of lymphoid cells both surrounding and infiltrating the Hurthle cells in Hashimoto's thyroiditis is an important and helpful diagnostic feature.[39,41,42] Since many patients are medically managed with no confirmatory tissue biopsy, it is difficult to evaluate the accuracy of aspiration cytology for the diagnosis of Hashimoto's thyroiditis.[39,41]

Hurthle cell nodules arising in Hashimoto's thyroiditis can pose an especially difficult diagnostic problem, since this lesion can be cytologically confused with Hurthle cell neoplasm. Hurthle cell nodules are nonencapsulated proliferations of Hurthle cells in Hashimoto's thyroiditis which cytologically can demonstrate features mimicking neoplasia such as the presence of three-dimensional clusters, anisonucleosis, and prominence of nucleoli (Fig. 8.14). Both Guarda and Kini report that a very helpful diagnostic clue in arriving at a correct diagnosis of Hurthle cell nodule is the appreciation of lymphocytes infiltrating the oncocytic cell groups.[21,39,42]

Follicular cells can be reactive and atypical in appearance in Hashimoto's thyroiditis and lack a follicular pattern. All of these features can potentially cause a false-positive diagnosis of follicular neoplasm. However, follicular neoplasms will demonstrate cells having uniformly enlarged nuclei and arranged in a syncytial tissue fragment, in contrast to the cohesive groups of follicular cells in Hashimoto's thyroiditis. The presence of increased numbers of lymphocytes and plasma cells should also help in suggesting the correct diagnosis of Hashimoto's thyroiditis. Papillary

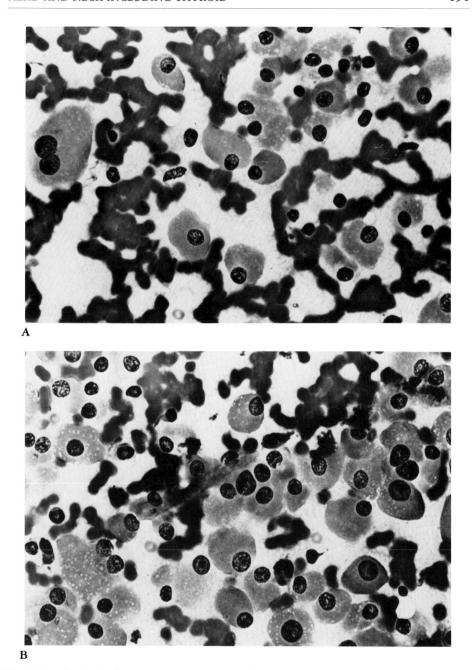

A

B

Fig. 8.13. A. FNA of Hurthle cell neoplasm of thyroid consisting of individually scattered Hurthle cells showing some variation in nuclear size with the presence of small nucleoli. A few binucleated cells are present (Diff-Quik stain; ×200). **B.** Another example of Hurthle cell neoplasm consisting of individually scattered cells having enlarged nuclei with prominent cherry red macronucleoli (Diff-Quik stain; ×200).

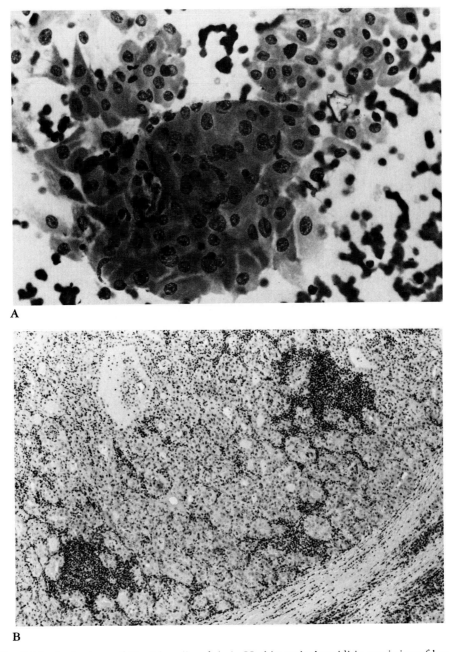

Fig. 8.14. A. Aspirate of Hurthle cell nodule in Hashimoto's thyroiditis consisting of loose cluster of Hurthle cells including some having small nucleoli. A helpful diagnostic feature of Hurthle cell nodule is the presence of some lymphocytes within the groups of cells (Diff-Quik stain; ×200). **B.** Resected lesion demonstrating Hurthle cell nodule in Hashimoto's thyroiditis. Note nonencapsulated proliferation of Hurthle cells (H&E stain; ×100).

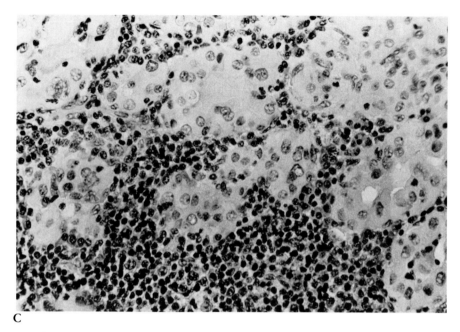

C

Fig. 8.14. C. High-power view of Hurthle cell nodule showing groups of Hurthle cells in which there are surrounding lymphocytes along with lymphocytes infiltrating the clusters (H&E stain; ×400).

hyperplasia of the follicular epithelium can also occur in Hashimoto's thyroiditis and thereby lead to a false-positive diagnosis of papillary carcinoma. However, in papillary carcinoma the nuclei are enlarged and have a powdery chromatin pattern.[21] Although intranuclear inclusions can be encountered in Hashimoto's thyroiditis in rare instances, they are a much more common feature of papillary carcinoma. Syncytial tissue fragments with or without a follicular pattern, papillary and/or monolayer groupings, and psammoma bodies are additional cytologic findings found in papillary carcinoma. However, it must be realized that papillary carcinoma can occur in the setting of Hashimoto's thyroiditis.[21] In those cases, a spectrum of cytologic findings shared by papillary carcinoma and Hashimoto's thyroiditis will be appreciated.[21,38] In addition, focal lymphocytic thyroiditis can coexist with nodular hyperplasia or be adjacent to a neoplasm.[40] Surgical exploration in those cases of lymphocytic thyroiditis diagnosed by FNA with repeatedly negative serology antibody titers may be needed to exclude a neoplasm.[40]

Lastly, malignant lymphoma will consist of a monomorphic population of atypical lymphoid cells in contrast to the polymorphic population of inflammatory cells seen in Hashimoto's thyroiditis[42,43] (Fig. 8.15). However, malignant lymphoma arising in Hashimoto's thyroiditis can be a difficult diagnostic problem when cytologic evidence of both processes is present in the smears. Kini and associates was able to identify 17 of 24 patients as having lymphoma coexisting with thyroiditis.[39,44,45]

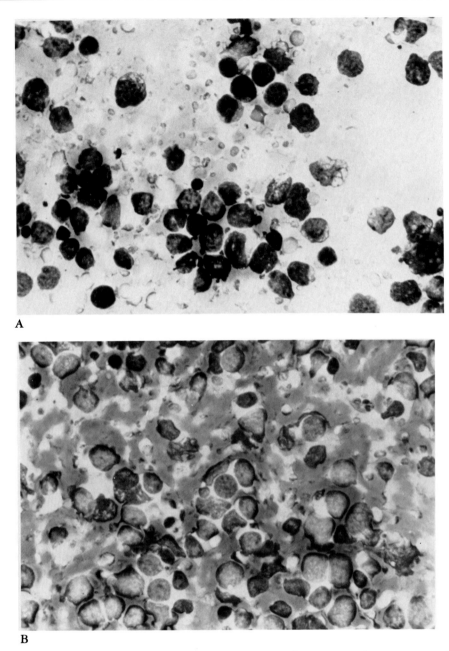

Fig. 8.15. A. FNA of large cell lymphoma of the thyroid consisting of numerous atypical cells demonstrating nuclear cleavage (Diff-Quik stain; ×400). **B.** Another example of primary thyroid lymphoma in which large atypical lymphoid cells are present (Diff-Quik stain; ×400).

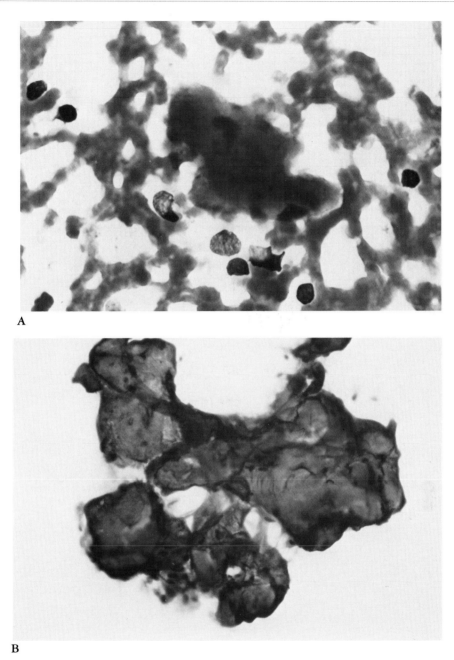

A

B

Fig. 8.16. **A.** Aspirate of medullary carcinoma of the thyroid in which numerous clumps of amorphous, acellular amyloid are present (Diff-Quik stain; ×400). **B.** Clump of amyloid in aspirate of medullary carcinoma (Papanicolaou stain; ×400).

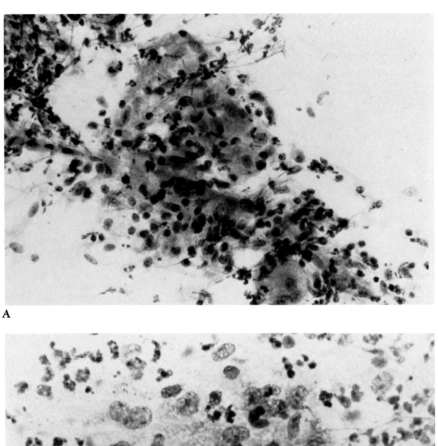

A

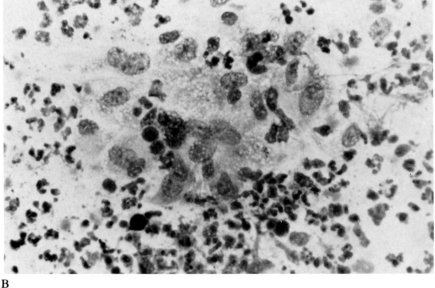

B

Fig. 8.17. A. FNA biopsy of soft tissue in the region of the thyroid in a patient having a history of thyroid surgery. Cytologic findings reveal features consistent with a suture granuloma characterized by loose fragments of epithelioid histiocytes associated with inflammatory cells (Diff-Quik stain; ×100). **B.** Loose cluster of granulomatous inflammation (Diff-Quik stain; ×400).

Other Unusual Thyroid Nodules

FNA biopsy of the thyroid has been used to diagnose amyloid goiter, a rare condition that induces a progressive enlargement of the thyroid gland.[46,47] The differential diagnosis includes medullary carcinoma of the thyroid, which also contains amyloid (Fig. 8.16). Lucas and associates reported the presence of irregular clumps of amorphous acellular material in a cell block from a thyroid aspirate which also showed the typical apple-green birefringence of the Congo red–stained amyloid following polarization.[46] Wilson and Gartner reported the FNA cytologic findings of an unusual Teflon granuloma mimicking a thyroid tumor following clinical injection of Teflon material into the left posterior vocal cord for impaired phonation.[49] Of particular interest was the misinterpretation of atypical histiocytic cells, both individually arranged and in cluster, as malignant cells. This case again illustrates the potential false-positive diagnosis of malignancy in aspirates of granulomatous inflammation.[48] We have performed FNA biopsies of suture granulomas in patients having previous thyroid surgery (Fig. 8.17).

REFERENCES

1. Qizilbash AH, Sianos J, Young JEM, et al: Fine needle aspiration biopsy cytology of major salivary glands. *Acta Cytol* 29:503–512, 1985.

2. Qizilbash AH, Young JEM: Guides to Clinical Aspiration Biopsy: Head and Neck. New York, Igaku-Shoin, 1988, p 16.

3. Batsakis JG: Tumors of the Head and Neck. Clinical and Pathological Considerations, ed. 2. Baltimore, Williams & Wilkins, 1979, pp. 100–120.

4. Mair S, Leiman G, Levinsohn D: Fine needle aspiration cytology of parotid sarcoidosis. *Acta Cytol* 33:169–172, 1989.

5. O'Dwyer P, Farrar WB, James AG, et al: Needle aspiration biopsy of major salivary gland tumours. *Cancer* 57:554–557, 1986.

6. Hammer JE, Scofield HH: Cervical lymphadenopathy and parotid gland swelling in sarcoidosis: a study of 31 cases. *J Am Dent Assoc* 74:1224–1230, 1967.

7. Miglets AW, Viall JH, Kataria YP: Sarcoidosis of the head and neck. *Laryngoscope* 87:2038–2048, 1977.

8. Tarpley TM Jr, Anderson L, Lightbody P, et al: Minor salivary gland involvement in sarcoidosis. *Oral Surg* 33:755–762, 1972.

9. Aggarwal AP, Jayaram G, Mandal AK: Sarcoidosis diagnosed on fine-needle aspiration cytology of salivary glands: a report of three cases. *Diagn Cytopathol* 5:289–292, 1989.

10. Godwin JT: Benign lymphoepithelial lesion of the parotid gland. *Cancer* 5:1089–1103, 1952.

11. Weidner N, Geisinger KR, Sterling RT, et al: Benign lymphoepithelial cysts of the parotid gland. *Am J Clin Pathol* 85:395–401, 1986.

12. Elliott JN, Oertel YC: Lymphoepithelial cysts of the salivary glands. Histologic and cytologic features. *Am J Clin Pathol* 93:39–43, 1990.

13. Koss LG: Diagnostic Cytology and Its Histopathologic Bases. ed. 3. Philadelphia, JB Lippincott, 1979, pp 1026–1027.

14. Warson F, Blommaert D: Inflamed branchial cleft cyst: a potential pitfall in aspiration cytology. *Acta Cytol* 30:201–202, 1986.

15. Oneson RH, Feldman PS, Newman SA: Aspiration cytology and immunohistochemistry of an orbital aspergilloma. *Diagn Cytopathol* 4:59–61, 1988.

16. Austin P, Dekker A, Kennerdell JS: Orbital aspergillosis. Report of a case diagnosed by fine needle aspiration biopsy. *Acta Cytol* 27:166–169, 1983.

17. Das DK, Bhatt NC, Khan VA, et al: Cervicofacial actinomycosis: diagnosis by fine needle aspiration cytology. *Acta Cytol* 278–280, 1989.

18. Pollock PG, Koontz FP, Viner TF, et al: Cervicofacial actinomycosis: rapid diagnosis by thin-needle aspiration. *Arch Otolaryngol* 104:491–494, 1978.

19. Finegold SM: Anaerobic Bacteria in Human Disease. New York, Academic Press, 1977.

20. Hay ID: Thyroiditis: a clinical update. *Mayo Clin Proc* 60:836–843, 1985.

21. Kini SR: Guides to Clinical Aspiration Biopsy. Igaku-Shoin, New York, 1987.

22. Levine SN: Current concepts of thyroiditis. *Arch Intern Med* 143:1952–1956, 1983.

23. Silverman JF, West RL, Larking EW, et al: The role of fine-needle aspiration biopsy in the rapid diagnosis and management of thyroid neoplasm. *Cancer* 57:1164–1170, 1986.

24. Miller JM, Hamburger JI, Kini S: Diagnosis of thyroid nodules: use of fine needle aspiration and needle biopsy. *JAMA* 241:481–484, 1979.

25. Weir SD, Park HK, Larkin EW, et al: Needle biopsy in the evaluation of the thyroid nodule. *NC Med J* 43:710–712, 1982.

26. Werk EE, Vernon BM, Gonzalez JJ, et al: Cancer in thyroid nodules. *Arch Intern Med* 144:474–476, 1984.

27. Ramacciotti CE, Pretorius HT, Chu EW, et al: Diagnostic accuracy and use of aspiration biopsy in the management of thyroid nodules. *Arch Intern Med* 144:1169–1173, 1984.

28. Colacchio TA, LoGerfo P, Feind CR: Fine needle cytologic diagnosis of thyroid nodules: review and report of 300 cases. *Am J Surg* 140:568–571, 1980.

29. Berger SA, Zonszein J, Villamena P, et al: Infectious diseases of the thyroid gland. *Rev Infect Dis* 5:108–122, 1983.

30. Takai S-I, Miyauchi A, Matsuzuka F, et al: Internal fistula as a route of infection in acute suppurative thyroiditis. *Lancet* 1:751–752, 1979.

31. Persson PS: Cytodiagnosis of thyroiditis. *Acta Med Scand* 483:8–100, 1968.

32. Szporn AH, Tepper S, Watson CW: Disseminated cryptococcosis presenting as thyroiditis: fine needle aspiration and autopsy findings. *Acta Cytol* 29:440–453, 1985.

33. Sanders LR, Moreno AJ, Pittman DL: Painless giant cell thyroiditis diagnosed by fine needle aspiration and associated with intense thyroidal uptake of gallium. *Am J Med* 80:971–975, 1986.

34. Tempka T, Aleksandrowicz J, Till M: Le thyroidogramme. *Sangre* 19:336–340, 1948.

35. Friedman M, Shimaoka K, Rao U, et al: Diagnosis of chronic lymphocytic thyroiditis (nodular presentation) by needle aspiration. *Acta Cytol* 25:513–522, 1981.

36. Bagchi N, Brown TR, Urdaniva E, et al: Induction of autoimmune thyroiditis in chickens by dietary iodine. *Science* 230:325–327, 1985.

37. Holm L-E, Blomgren H, Lowhagen T: Cancer risks in patients with chronic lymphocytic thyroiditis. *N Engl J Med* 312:601–604, 1985.

38. Ravinsky E, Safneck JR: Differentiation of Hashimoto's thyroiditis from thyroid neoplasms in fine needle aspirates. *Acta Cytol* 32:854–861, 1988.

39. Kini SR, Miller JM, Hamburger JI: Cytopathology of Hurthle cell lesions of the thyroid gland by fine needle aspiration. *Acta Cytol* 25:647–652, 1981.

40. Tseleni-Balafouta S, Kyroudi-Voulgari A, Paizi-Biza P, et al: Lymphocytic thyroiditis in fine-needle aspirates: differential diagnostic aspects. *Diagn Cytopathol* 5:362–365, 1989.

41. Kline TS: Handbook of Fine Needle Aspiration Biopsy Cytology, ed. 2. New York, Churchill Livingstone, 1988.

42. Guarda LA, Baskin HJ: Inflammatory and lymphoid lesions of the thyroid gland. Cytopathology by fine-needle aspiration. *Am J Clin Pathol* 87:14–22, 1987.

43. Matsuda M, Sone H, Koyama H, et al: Fine-needle aspiration cytology of malignant lymphoma of the thyroid. *Diagn Cytopathol* 3:244–249, 1987.

44. Hamburger JI, Miller JM, Kini SR: Clinical-Pathological Evaluation of Thyroid Nodules: Handbook and Atlas. Southfield, MI, 1979. Private publication.

45. Kini SR, Miller JM, Hamburger JI: Problems in the cytologic diagnosis of the "cold" thyroid nodule in patients with lymphocytic thyroiditis. *Acta Cytol* 25:506–512, 1981.

46. Lucas A, Sanmarti A, Salinas I, et al: Amyloid goiter. Diagnosis by fine-needle aspiration biopsy of the thyroid. *J Endocrinol Invest* 12:43–46, 1989.

47. Gharib H, Goellner JR: Diagnosis by amyloidosis by fine-needle aspiration biopsy of the thyroid. *N Engl J Med* 305:586, 1981.

48. Wilson RA, Gartner WS: Teflon granuloma mimicking a thyroid tumor. *Diagn Cytopathol* 3:156–158, 1987.

9

Thoracic Lesions

Although fine-needle aspiration (FNA) cytology of the lung is used most often to diagnose suspected pulmonary malignancies, it has also been shown to be a valuable procedure in the diagnosis of infectious and inflammatory diseases.[1-15] The procedure was first employed in 1883 by Leyden for the diagnosis of pneumonia.[1] Since that initial report, others have performed aspiration biopsies of pneumonic processes to obtain material for culture.[5,8,9,14-20] Bacterial, fungal, viral, and parasitic infectious diseases can be diagnosed by aspiration biopsy.

Granulomatous lesions are the most common type of inflammatory process involving the lung to be diagnosed by FNA cytology.[1] Lalli and associates reported five cases of tuberculosis, five cases of aspergillosis, and one case of cryptococcosis diagnosed by FNA biopsy in a series of 1,223 patients.[12] Schwinn and associates reported the biopsy results of 290 patients, 60 of whom had nonneoplastic diseases.[10] Of the 60 patients, 44 had a specific diagnosis established by a combination of cytology, cell block, culture, and clinical correlation. Fifteen granulomatous lesions were identified, including six cases of tuberculosis, three cases of nonspecific granulomatous disease, and two cases of histoplasmosis, coccidioidomycosis, and sarcoidosis. Schwinn and associates believed that the cell block was the most contributory diagnostic component of the aspirate in these 15 cases.[10] In another series, Zavala and Schoell reported 25 cases of infectious and inflammatory pulmonary processes among 50 consecutive patients examined by FNA cytology.[8] The authors reported one case of tuberculosis, one case of histoplasmosis, and two cases of cryptococcosis diagnosed by combined smear, culture, and cytologic examination. Zavala and Schoell advocated a combination of procedures, with emphasis on culture, permitting a specific diagnosis to be rendered in 60% of the cases, with a sensitivity of 83% and a specificity of 100%. Bhatt and associates reported the value of aspiration cytology in the evaluation of opportunistic infections in the immunocompromised patient. Three infections were diagnosed by identifying organisms in the cytology smears.[7] *Pneumocystis carinii* was confirmed with the Gomori methenamine silver (GMS) stain in a patient clinically suspected of having that infection. In the other two cases, the hyphae of *Mucor* and *Aspergillus* were identified in the Papanicolaou-stained smears, along with special stain confirmation. The

TABLE 9.1. Nonneoplastic Pulmonary Lesions that Might Be Sampled by FNA Biopsy

> Abscess
> Granulomatous processes: sarcoid, fungi, TB, etc.
> *Pneumocystis carinii* (pneumocystoma)
> Irradiation and/or chemotherapy—related abnormalities
> Viral infections
> Other parasites, eg, *Dirofilaria*
> Pulmonary infarction
> Pseudolymphoma and other inflammatory pseudotumors
> Amyloid
> Pneumoconiosis
> Aspiration pneumonia
> Wegener's granulomatosis

accompanying cellular reactions were not described in this report. Bonfiglio is one of the few authors to stress the cytologic features of granulomatous disease in making a specific diagnosis. He noted that granulomas should be suspected when variable amounts of necrotic debris associated with lymphocytes, histiocytes, and multinucleated Langhans'-type giant cells are present. If these cytologic features are identified, special stains for fungi and tuberculosis on the smears are recommended.[21] A listing of nonneoplastic pulmonary lesions examined by ABC is presented in Table 9.1, and specific infections are discussed below.

TUBERCULOSIS

Dahlgren and Ekstrom described the aspiration cytology of pulmonary tuberculosis and stressed the cytomorphologic findings as a clue in making a specific diagnosis.[22] The cytologic features of tuberculosis included the presence of finely grained, necrotic material in the background associated with epithelioid cells, multinucleated Langhans' type giant cells, and occasional small calcified fragments. In their series, 42 of the 57 patients had the cytologic diagnosis confirmed by culture. However, in Robicheaux and associates' series of aspiration biopsy cytology of pulmonary tuberculosis, only the culture was diagnostic (positive in 9 of 12 cases).[23] This experience is more in keeping with the relatively unsuccessful identification of mycobacteria in exfoliative cytologic specimens as noted by Johnston and Frable.[24] These authors commented that the cytologic diagnosis of granulomas in bronchial washings and sputum cytology is infrequent, since one rarely identifies epithelioid-type histiocytes, caseation-type debris, or tissue fragments of necrotic material.[24] Dahlgren and Lind, in a series of FNA biopsies of the lung, reported the superiority of FNA biopsy in diagnosing tuberculosis when compared with routine sputum cytology.[25] Bailey and associates reported that combined examination of FNA smears and bacteriologic culture is the most effective way of diagnosing tuberculosis.[26] In a large series of FNA biopsy of tuberculosis, Rajwanshi and associates noted that acid-fast bacilli could be identified in nearly 41% of the cases.[27] In those cases having an associated cellular reaction and necrosis, acid-fast bacilli positivity was 50%, whereas it was nearly 67% positive in cases having only acellular necrotic material in the smears. This is similar to the experience of Bailey and associates, who obtained a higher positivity rate in cases without typical granulomas (47.4%) than in those cases with granulomas (26.6%).[26] However, Rajwanshi cautions that the absence of acid-fast bacilli in smears showing an otherwise typical cytologic appearance of tuberculosis should not deter from suggesting the possibility of tuberculosis.[27] It is well known that 10,000 to 100,000 acid-fast bacilli per ml need to be present before the mycobacterium can be recognized microscopically.[28] Therefore, any specimen showing either the characteristic appearance of granulomatous inflammation or acellular necrotic material with or without inflammation should be submitted for culture[26,27] (Fig. 9.1). Although the presence of epithelioid cells, Langhans' type giant cells, epithelioid granulomas, inflammation, and necrosis may suggest the diagnosis of tuberculosis, other granulomatous processes can involve the lung.[1]

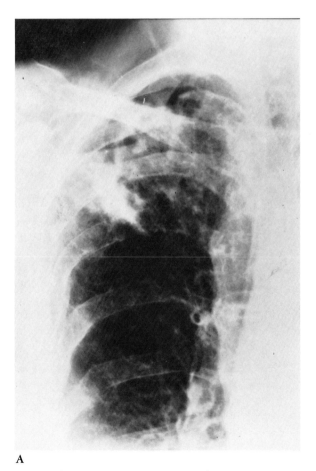

A

Fig. 9.1. A. Radiograph demonstrating stellate-shaped lesion in right upper lobe of lung, radiologically thought to be malignant.

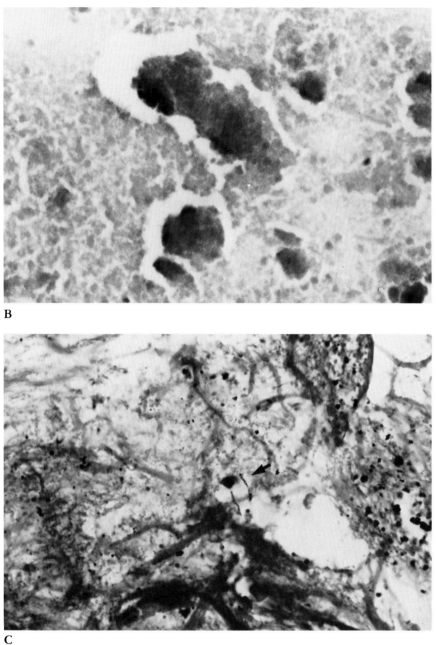

Fig. 9.1. B. The aspirated material consists entirely of amorphous clumps of granular material (Diff-Quik stain; ×100). **C.** Cell block from aspirate containing abundant debris and scattered beaded acid-fast bacilli (*arrow*) (AFB stain; ×200).

FUNGAL INFECTIONS

The cytomorphologic features of many fungal infections have been discussed and illustrated in Chapter 4. The morphologic identification of fungi as well as culture are extremely important in making a specific diagnosis.[29,30] Moreover, the diagnosis should be suspected whenever granulomatous inflammation is seen in the smears from a pulmonary aspirate.[1,31]

Cryptococcosis

Cryptococcosis is a fungal infection of worldwide distribution caused by the ubiquitous yeast *Cryptococcus neoformans*.[32] The respiratory tract is the primary portal of entry with dissemination and spread to the central nervous system especially common in susceptible individuals.[33] The pulmonary infection is asymptomatic in up to one third of the cases.[33] In clinically symptomatic cases, the patient can present with cough, chest pain, mucoid sputum, weight loss, and low grade fever.[33]

The radiologic findings are variable and nonspecific in pulmonary cryptococcosis, ranging from a single mass to a diffuse pneumonic infiltrate.[34,35] The diagnosis of pulmonary cryptococcosis can at times be challenging, since the disease can present with a variety of radiologic, clinical, and histologic patterns.[31,32,33,36] In cryptococcosis, the histologic reaction will vary with the stage of disease. Initial lesions may be gelatinous, whereas older lesions are granulomatous.[34] The early lesions consist of gelatinous masses of fungi with little inflammation, fibrosis, or granuloma formation.[32,37] Therefore it is not surprising that earlier aspiration biopsy cytology reports stressed mainly the presence of organisms rather than the associated cytomorphologic findings.[38,39,40]

Cryptococci have been cytologically identified in sputum,[35,41] bronchial washings,[24] and FNA biopsy specimens.[37,38,40,42] The fungi measure from 5 to 20 microns in diameter and can show a single narrow teardrop-shaped bud with surrounding gelatinous capsule, which can vary in thickness[24,33] (Fig. 9.2). Special stains demonstrating the mucinous capsule are often helpful in making a relatively specific diagnosis.[41] In older lesions, granulomatous inflammation can be recognized in fine-needle aspirates and may be the only clue to the infectious etiology of the nodule[1,31] (Fig. 9.3).

Histoplasmosis

Histoplasmosis is found throughout North America in soil contaminated by bird and bat excreta and is endemic to parts of the United States, particularly the Ohio–Mississippi Valley.[1,43] It is estimated that approximately 40% of Americans have been infected by *H. capsulatum,* with up to 80% of adult populations in some midwestern states having a positive skin test.[43] Therefore, the skin test has little value in those endemic areas, having a high positivity rate. The disease has an incubation time of 10 to 14 days, with most infections being subclinical or asymptomatic. A self-limited, flulike syndrome or pneumonia can occur, however. A more aggressive course has been noted in infants, and in elderly and immunosuppressed patients.[43]

The radiologic appearance is variable, with some cases having radiologic evidence

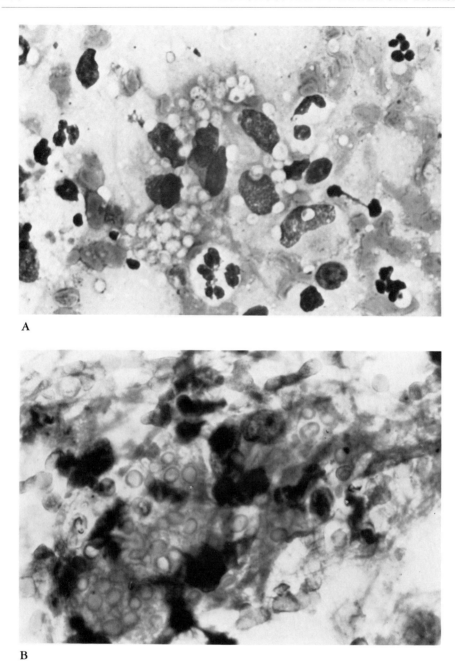

Fig. 9.2. A. Loose cluster of epithelioid histiocytes containing numerous cryptococci. Note prominent gelatinous capsule around the organisms (Diff-Quik stain; ×400). **B.** Numerous intracytoplasmic organisms having pink mucinous capsules. (Mucicarmine; ×600).

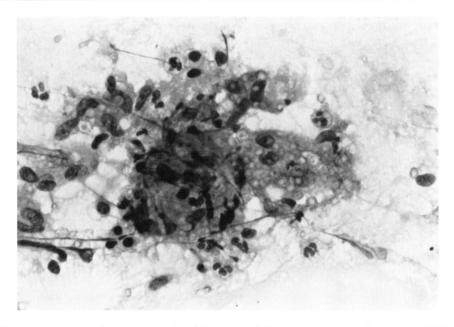

Fig. 9.3. Aspirate of cryptococcosis of lung containing granulomatous fragments. Within some of the epithelioid histiocytes, numerous cryptococci are present (Papanicolaou stain; ×400).

of a small pulmonary nodule whereas others present with a pneumonic infiltrate. Associated hilar adenopathy may be present along with plural effusions. Some nodules may calcify, while others undergo cavitation.[43] The calcified nodules may be radiologically confused with tuberculosis, whereas the noncalcified may be confused with primary or metastatic carcinoma. Older lesions show a greater tendency toward extensive calcification.[12,32] In yeast phase, *H. capsulatum* measure 2 to 4 microns in diameter and have a rigid cell wall.

In our experience, in contrast to other fungi which may be readily appreciated in Papanicolaou-stained smears, the yeast of *H. capsulatum* are most often seen with special stains[1,24] (Fig. 9.4). The Gomori methenamine silver (GMS) stain is preferred since it clearly separates the organisms from calcified debris in the background. In one prior reported case of histoplasmosis diagnosed by FNA cytology, the organism was identified in smears stained with GMS.[1]

Aspergillus Infections

Pulmonary *Aspergillus* infections may be invasive or noninvasive and occur in both immunocompetent and immunocompromised patients.[7,14,44,45] Characteristic septate, acute angle–branching hyphae are suggestive for aspergillosis (Fig. 9.5). Correct morphologic identification is important because microbiologic isolation and identification may take up to several weeks.[46] The hyphae of *Aspergillus* can be confused with other fungi, such as *Pseudallescheria, Fusarium, Trichosporon,* dematiacious Hyphomycetes, *Candida,* and Zygomycetes. Phillips and Weiner advocate the use of immunohistochemical stains to make a specific diagnosis of aspergillosis.[46]

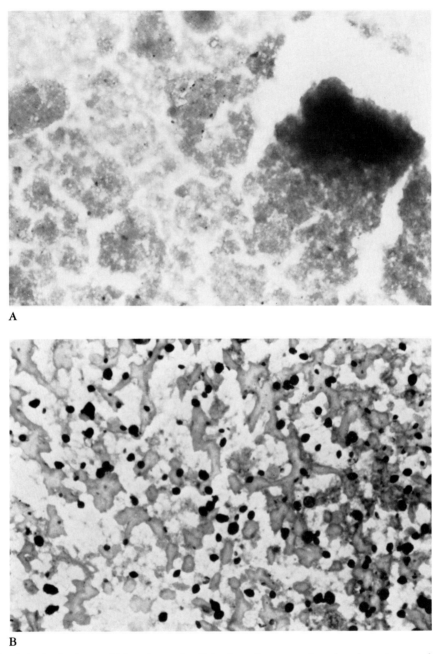

A

B

Fig. 9.4. A. Aspirate of histoplasmosis of the lung demonstrating abundant clumps of necrotic material consistent with caseation-type necrosis (Diff-Quik stain; ×400). **B.** Numerous yeast of histoplasmosis capsulatum measuring 2–4 microns in diameter (GMS stain; ×400).

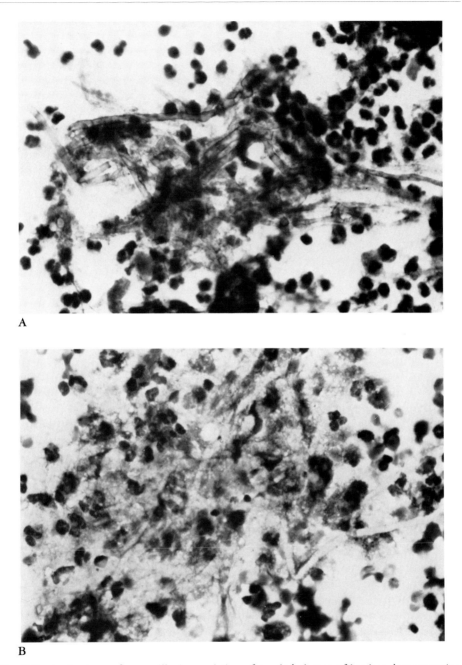

A

B

Fig. 9.5. A. Aspirate of aspergillosis consisting of tangled cluster of hyphae demonstrating acute-angle branching and septation (Papanicolaou stain; ×400). **B.** Similar group of aspergillosis not as well demonstrated in the Diff-Quik stained material (Diff-Quik stain; ×400).

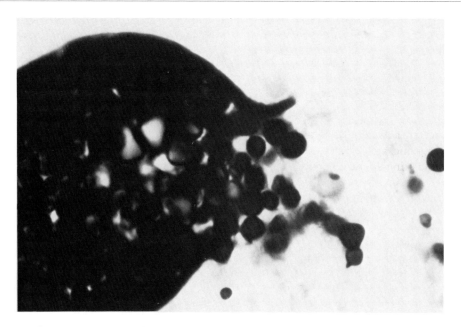

Fig. 9.6. Large spherule of coccidioidomycosis with released endospores (GMS stain; ×400).

This technique can readily be applied to cytology smears. A possible aid in diagnosing *aspergillosis* infection is the finding of calcium oxalate crystals in the cytology smears.[47,48,49] Farley believes that the presence of birefringent needlelike, wheat sheaf–shaped crystals is a helpful marker for an associated aspergillous infection.[48]

Coccidioidomycosis

Coccidioidomycosis is a fungal infection that is endemic to the southwestern part of the United States and therefore is important in the differential diagnosis of solitary pulmonary nodules in individuals living in or traveling through that region. The infection is acquired by inhaling airborne arthrospores. Many individuals are asymptomatic or have mild flulike symptoms and therefore are unaware that they have acquired pulmonary coccidioidomycosis.[50,51] Since the chest x-ray finding of a solitary coin lesion can be indistinguishable from malignancy, FNA biopsy can be a useful procedure in making a correct diagnosis. In immunocompromised patients from endemic regions, coccidioidomycosis is the most common fungal infection.[50,51]

The morphologic features of coccidioidomycosis have been well described.[50] With the Papanicolaou stain, the spherules of *Coccidiodes* are orange to reddish-purple. Mature spherules are round with double walls and contain endospores, which range in size from 2 to 5 microns (Fig. 9.6). Immature sporangia range in size from 4 to 40 microns and do not contain endospores. With the Diff-Quik stain, the spherules do not stain but appear as colorless, highly refractile structures. Older, nonviable spherules can have a folded, fractured, or collapsed structure. These types of spherules are more commonly observed in chronic cavitary pulmonary disease. Mycelial elements can also be present and appear as branched septate hyphae, approximately 2 microns in thickness and having spaced barrel-shaped arthroconidia, which range from 2 to 4 microns in width and 3 to 6 microns in length. Mycelial forms are believed to form when the organism is exposed to sufficiently aerobic conditions.[50]

Other confirmatory tests that have been used to diagnose coccidioidomycosis include complement fixation serology and culture. However, the serologic tests results are variable, and unless dissemination is present the titers may not be elevated. In addition, as with histoplasmosis, a positive skin test is quite common in endemic areas.[50,52,53] Culture may not be positive, especially in patients with longstanding solitary nodules.[50,51] Forseth and associates reported the presence of spherules in 49 of 96 patients with coccidioidomycosis. However, only 3 of 35 cultures from biopsy-proved coccidioidal lesions were positive (8.6% yield).[51]

Other fungi and related organisms identified in FNA biopsy include *Blastomyces*[54] and *Actinomyces*[55] (Fig. 9.7). The morphologic appearance of these organisms has been discussed in Chapter 4. Entering into the differential diagnosis of fungal infection is pulmonary sarcoidosis, which has also been diagnosed by FNA biopsy.[11]

VIRAL INFECTIONS

Cytomegalovirus and herpes simplex are members of the herpes family of viruses that can cause pulmonary infections, especially in immunocompromised patients[56] (Fig. 9.8). Although the diagnosis can be made in routine exfoliative cytologic specimens,[21,24] there have been only a few ABC reports of viral infections.[56] The morphologic features of different viral infections are outlined in Chapter 4. Immunoperoxidase and DNA studies may also prove helpful in confirming the cytologic impression of viral infection.[57,58] The differential diagnosis of viral infection includes reactive alveolar cells, drug reactions, repair, or malignancy.[24]

PNEUMOCYSTIS

Pneumocystis carinii pneumonitis is the commonest life-threatening opportunistic infection in AIDS patients, occurring in up to 85% of this patient population and carrying up to a 50% mortality.[58] This protozoan is universally acquired as a clinically inapparent infection in early childhood.[59] Histologic examination of lung tissue from patients with *Pneumocystis* pneumonia reveals the alveolar spaces to contain an eosinophilic honeycomb-type exudate when the hematoxylin and eosin stain is employed. The interstitial septae may have a mild diffuse infiltration of lymphocytes, and some cases will also show increased numbers of plasma cells. In occasional chronic infection, septal fibrosis may be present.

Respiratory specimens used to document the presence of *Pneumocystis carinii* in AIDS and other immunocompromised patients include random and induced sputum samples, bronchoscopic washing, bronchoalveolar lavage, fine-needle aspiration, and transbronchial and open lung biopsies. As demonstrated in a number of studies, bronchoalveolar lavage has emerged as the procedure of choice with the

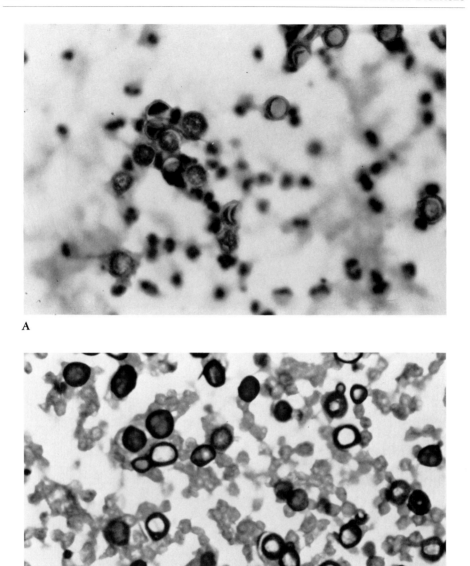

A

B

Fig. 9.7. A. Aspirate of blastomycosis consisting of numerous fungal yeasts having internal structure with well defined cell wall (Papanicolaou stain; ×600). **B.** Blastomycosis in cell block of lung aspirate. Note broad base budding (GMS stain; ×600).

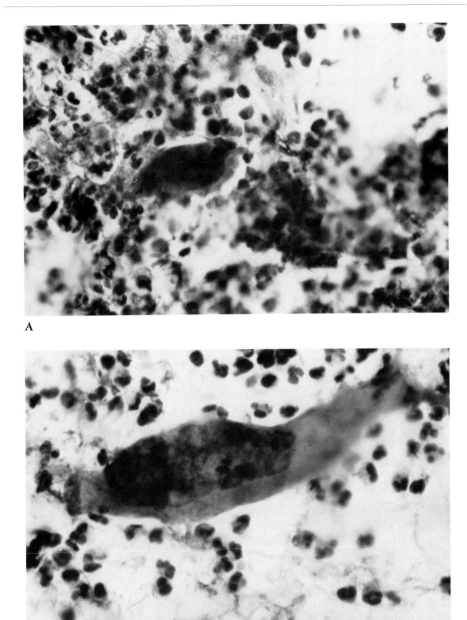

Fig. 9.8. A. Scattered atypical multinucleated cells showing considerable degenerative changes in a patient with prior history of squamous cell carcinoma. Note the associated extensive acute inflammation (Papanicolaou stain; ×400). **B.** High-power view of one of the atypical bizarrely shaped cells showing multinucleation with considerable nuclear degeneration. Although recurrent squamous cell carcinoma was considered, the morphologic appearance suggested a herpetic infection (Papanicolaou stain; ×600).

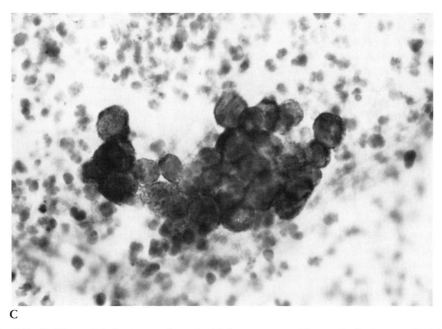

C

Fig. 9.8. C. Herpetic infection confirmed with immunoperoxidase stain for herpes. Positive cytoplasm staining of numerous atypical cells (Immunoperoxidase stain; ×400).

greatest sensitivity in the diagnosis of *Pneumocystis* pneumonia when compared with bronchial washing, brushing, and sputum cytology.[60] Diagnostic results in the range of 80% or better have been reported for bronchoalveolar lavage, which is similar to the results reported with transbronchial biopsies. Bedrossian recently reviewed the variety of useful respiratory techniques for the bronchoscopic diagnosis of *Pneumocystis*, with transbronchial biopsy having a diagnostic yield of 83%, bronchoalveolar lavage 82%, and washing and brushing cytology 53%.[60] In reported sputum series, diagnostic yields in the range of 15 to 78% have been described.[61-73] *Pneumocystis carinii* detection is enhanced in induced sputum specimens, especially when combined with immunoperoxidase or indirect fluorescent antibody stains on the smears.[61,62,63] However, other authors, such as del Rio, believe that although *Pneumocystis carinii* can be identified in expectorated sputum from patients with AIDS, the sensitivity of the test is still quite low.[67] Although bronchoalveolar lavage currently is the primary procedure used for diagnosing pneumonitis in patients with AIDS, percutaneous FNA biopsy has been employed in selected cases.[9,74-77] FNA biopsy is usually performed in those occasional patients having atypical radiologic presentations such as cavitary or nodular lesions of *Pneumocystis* pneumonia[78] (Fig. 9.9). One major disadvantage of FNA biopsy in the evaluation of lung nodules in AIDS is the possible increased pneumothorax complication rate in patients already having significant respiratory compromise.[74]

A number of different stains have been used on cytologic material to demonstrate *Pneumocystis carinii*.[60,79,80,81] Cyst wall stains include GMS, Gram–Weigert, Grocott, PAS, and toluidine blue.[60] Intracystic bodies and trophozoites can be demonstrated by crystal violet, Diff-Quik, Giemsa, May–Grunwald–Giemsa (MGG), PAS, and Wright–Giemsa.[60] Recently, immunofluorescence or immunoperoxidase stains or hybridization probes have been used to diagnose *Pneumocystis* pneumo-

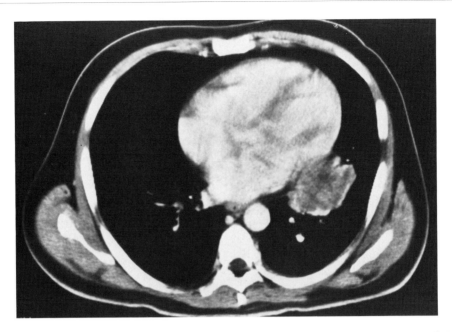

Fig. 9.9. Computed tomographic (CT) scan of pneumocystoma characterized by a nodular lesion of *Pneumocystis carinii.*

nia.[60,61,63,68,71,79,82] These routine and special stains can be readily applied to the aspirated smears. For rapid identification of *Pneumocystis carinii,* Diff-Quik stain on the smears from the aspirate or cytospin preparations from the bronchoalveolar lavage can be routinely employed. In Diff-Quik stained material, up to eight intracystic trophozoites within the nonstaining cyst can be demonstrated. The Papanicolaou-stained smears will show the honeycomb cast of *Pneumocystis* (Fig. 9.10). Rapid GMS stain, which can be accomplished within 1 to 5 minutes, can be used for confirmation.[83] In many laboratories, the GMS stain is the standard stain to confirm *Pneumocystis carinii.*

LUNG ABSCESS

Lung abscesses are usually caused by bacteria such as staphylococci or *Klebsiella* and are often secondary to bronchial obstruction. The aspirated material generally consists of tannish-yellow or green semisolid, purulent material. The smears demonstrate sheets of neutrophils, many of which are undergoing liquefactive necrosis, along with necrotic cells, cell debris, fibrin, and histiocytes. In some cases, bacteria can be readily identified in the Diff-Quik stain, both in the background and within the cytoplasm of neutrophils and especially histiocytes (Fig. 9.11).

The cytologic smears should be carefully evaluated to exclude the possibility of an associated carcinoma. The extensive inflammation associated with some carcinomas potentially could lead to a false-negative diagnosis of malignancy in some aspirates. This most often occurs with squamous cell carcinoma of the lung, although other types of carcinoma may undergo extensive necrosis and inflammation and therefore simulate a lung abscess.[84] Wallace and associates reported that between 8 and 17% of patients who have radiologic evidence of a cavitary pulmonary infiltration or lung

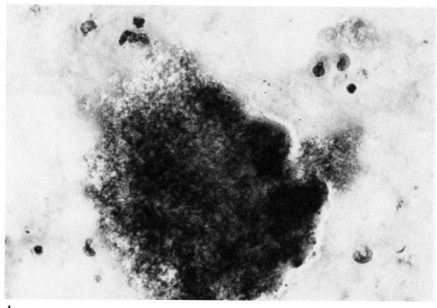

A

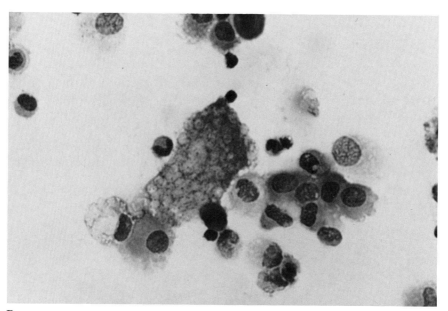

B

Fig. 9.10. **A.** Aspirate of this nodule demonstrating numerous clumps of honeycomb material consistent with *Pneumocystis carinii* (Papanicolaou stain; ×400). **B.** Diff-Quik stain of
Pneumocystis carinii (×200).

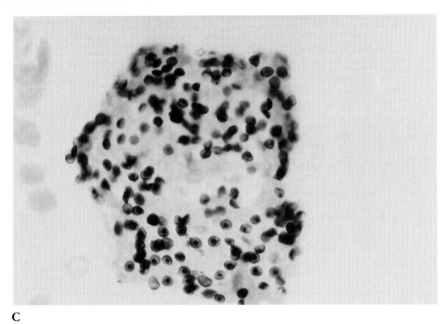

C

Fig. 9.10. C. GMS stain of *Pneumocystis carinii* (×400).

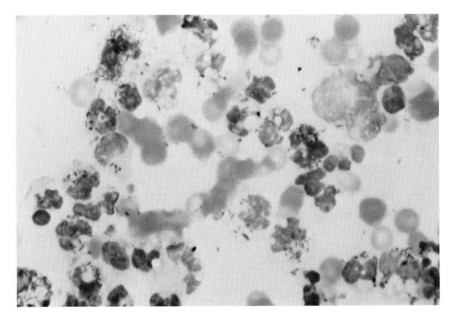

Fig. 9.11. Aspirate of lung abscess consisting of numerous neutrophils including many containing intracytoplasmic bacteria (Diff-Quik stain; ×400).

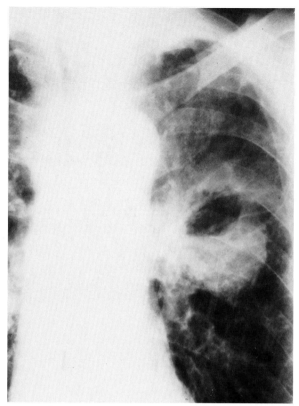

Fig. 9.12. Radiograph of squamous cell carcinoma of the lung demonstrating prominent cavitation which can be confused with a lung abscess.

abscess had been found to have an underlying bronchogenic carcinoma[85] (Fig. 9.12). This incidence rises with age: patients older than 45 years have associated carcinoma in up to one third the cases of lung abscess.[85,86]

"Carcinomatous" lung abscess can be frequently difficult to differentiate radiologically from simple abscesses.[85,87] Wallace and associates reported that combined bronchoscopic and sputum cytology allowed a specific diagnosis of carcinoma to be made in 22 of 25 patients (88%).[85] The abscess may form because of an obstructing carcinoma of the lung (postobstruction pneumonia) or as a reaction to tumor. In addition to an intense acute inflammatory cell exudate, a foreign body reaction to keratinous debris is present in some cases of squamous cell carcinoma of the lung. Subtle cytologic clues such as the presence of keratinous fragments or ghost cells may be appreciated along with only rare dysplastic or malignant cells[84] (Fig. 9.13). Therefore, a conservative approach is necessary since inflammation, degeneration, and inflammatory atypia may also lend to a false-positive diagnosis of malignancy. No false-positive cytologic diagnosis occurred in the nonmalignant group studied by Wallace and associates, even though cellular atypia in the setting of inflammation and infection was frequently reported.[85]

Inflammatory atypia of epithelial cells, fibroblasts, and histiocytes has been reported as a potential cause for a false-positive diagnosis of malignancy in tuberculosis, aspergillosis, and actinomycosis.[21,24,88-91] An unequivocal diagnosis of malig-

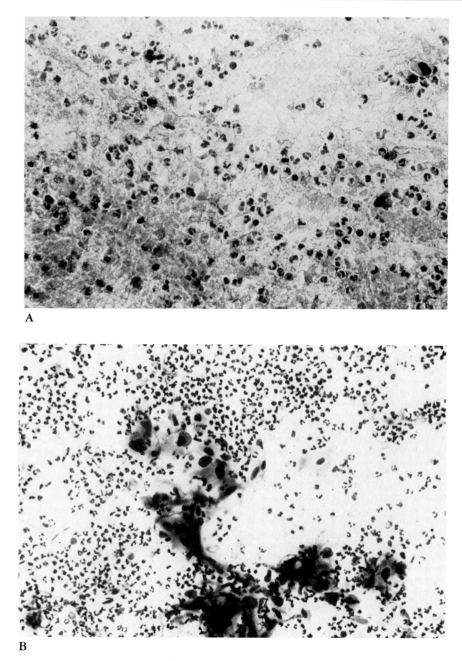

A

B

Fig. 9.13. A. Low-power view of squamous cell carcinoma in which extensive acute inflammation and a few scattered dysplastic keratinized cells are present (Diff-Quik stain; × 100). **B.** Another case of squamous cell carcinoma associated with extensive acute inflammation. In this field, a loose cluster of malignant keratinized cells is present (Diff-Quik stain; × 100).

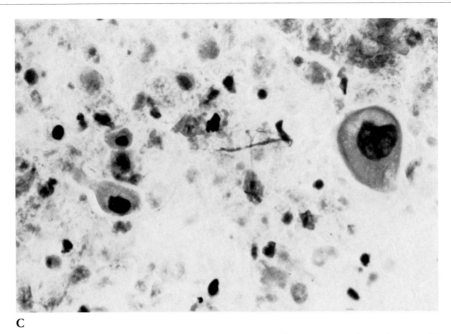

C

Fig. 9.13. C. Examination of other fields in aspirate of squamous cell carcinoma of lung showing extensive acute inflammation and necrosis along with diagnostic malignant keratinized cells (Papanicolaou stain; ×400).

nancy should not be made if there are limited numbers of atypical epithelial cells. In addition, a diagnosis of malignancy should not be made if only degenerating or poorly preserved atypical cells are present. Metaplastic cells can be mistaken for malignant squamous cells, especially when there is nuclear irregularity, clumped chromatin, and the presence of large nucleoli.[17] In general, however, metaplastic cells have a low nuclear:cytoplasmic ratio and the cells are few in number. Degenerating histiocytes with hyperchromatic nuclei and nucleoli may be mistaken for adenocarcinoma because of the vacuolated or foamy nature of the cytoplasm.[17] However, macrophages and histiocytes have eccentric, reniform-shaped nuclei with lower nuclear:cytoplasmic ratio. The most common malignancy confused with atypical histiocytes is bronchoalveolar cell carcinoma.

A potential for a false-positive diagnosis of malignancy can also occur in lung aspirates from patients who have received chemotherapy or irradiation. The atypical cells may be of pulmonary epithelial origin or from the mesothelium. Reactive fibroblasts may also have an atypical appearance (Fig. 9.14). Helpful features to suggest the correct diagnosis of chemotherapeutic or irradiation changes include the repairlike arrangement of the cells (Fig. 9.15). Some of the atypical cells will also demonstrate cytoplasmic vacuolization and a degenerative quality to the nuclei (Fig. 9.16). The cytologic features of repair and chemotherapy/irradiation effect are detailed in Tables 9.2 and 9.3. A listing of pitfalls for false-positive diagnosis of malignancy in respiratory specimens and the types of benign elements mistaken for specific carcinomas are presented in Tables 9.4 and 9.5.

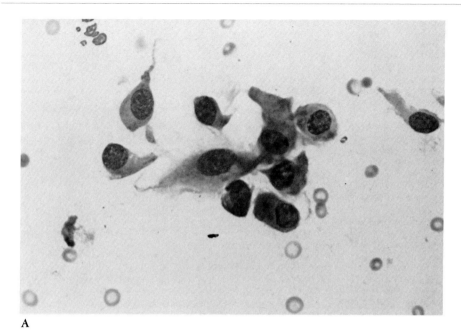

A

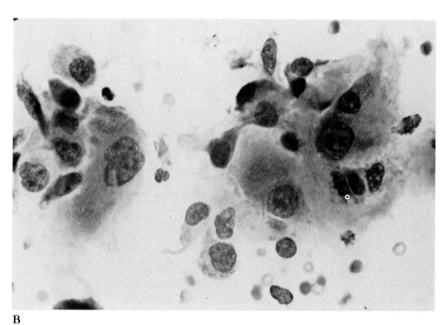

B

Fig. 9.14. A. Scattered single elongated to spindle-shaped cells having slightly enlarged and irregular nuclei consistent with mesenchymal repair (Diff-Quik stain; ×200). **B.** Loose cluster of cells demonstrating mesenchymal repair in lung aspirate (Diff-Quik stain; ×400).

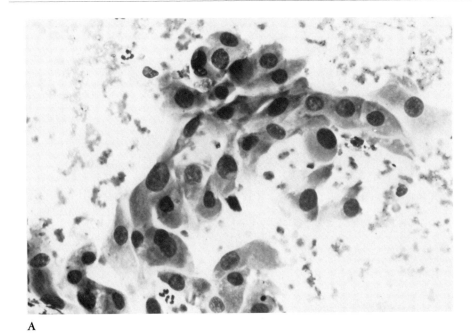

A

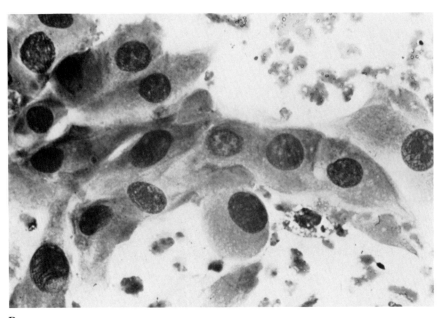

B

Fig. 9.15. A. Aspirate in renal transplant patient having a lung lesion showing features of epithelial repair characterized by a loose, sheetlike grouping of cells (Diff-Quik stain; × 200). **B.** High-power view of a group of cells showing epithelial repair characterized by sheetlike arrangement of cells having enlarged hyperchromatic to vesicular nuclei with one or more prominent nucleoli. However, note no loss of polarity or significant atypia (Diff-Quik stain; × 600).

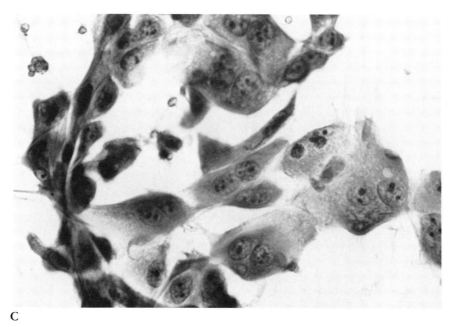

C

Fig. 9.15. C. Aspirate of lung showing epithelial repair demonstrating a slightly greater degree of atypicality. Note the enlarged vesicular nuclei, prominent nucleoli, and mitotic figures (Papanicolaou stain; ×600).

PULMONARY INFARCT

Pulmonary embolism and pulmonary infarct are extremely common causes of morbidity and mortality and may escape detection, since the majority of the lesions are asymptomatic or mimic other lung lesions.[92,93] Only 10 to 13% of the cases are diagnosed antemortem.[92] Clinically and radiologically, a solitary pulmonary infarct can simulate a peripheral lung neoplasm.[92] We previously reported the cytologic findings of a pulmonary infarction diagnosed by FNA cytology in a 54-year-old white man with a prior history of renal transplant surgery[94] (Fig. 9.17). Although the diagnosis of pulmonary embolus was unsuspected, the cytologic findings suggested the correct diagnosis which was confirmed by subsequent radiologic studies. Cytomorphologic findings included the presence of numerous histiocytes containing refractile intracytoplasmic coarse pigment consistent with hemosiderin, which was confirmed with the Gomori iron stain (Fig. 9.18). Some groups of squamous metaplastic cells and possibly mesothelial cells were also present. Although not a problem in our case, the cytologic features of pulmonary infarct can be a potential source for a false-positive diagnosis of malignancy[95,96] (Fig. 9.19).

A number of authors have stressed that atypical bronchoalveolar cells can be present in different types of pulmonary specimens including sputum, bronchial-washing, and bronchial-brushing samples following pulmonary infarction.[24,92,95,96,97] Bewtra and associates reported that atypical bronchoalveolar glandular cells arranged in three-dimensional clusters and having enlarged nuclei with macronucleoli

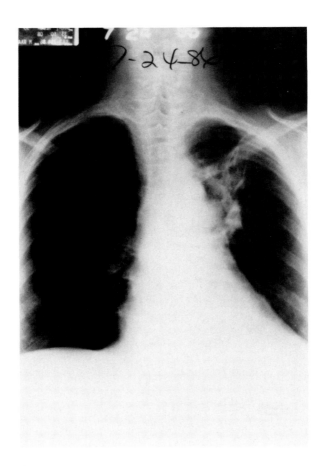

A

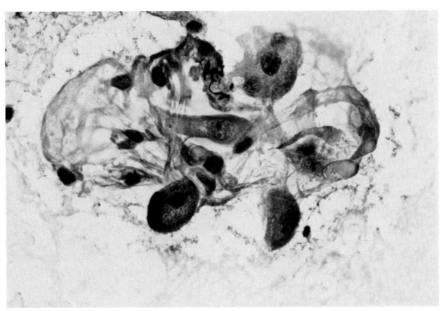

B

224

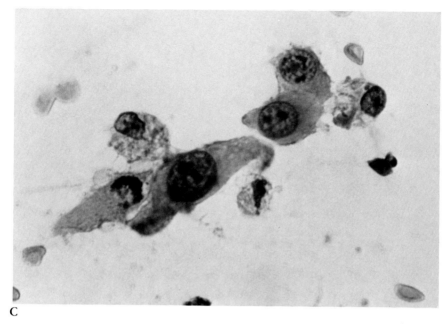

C

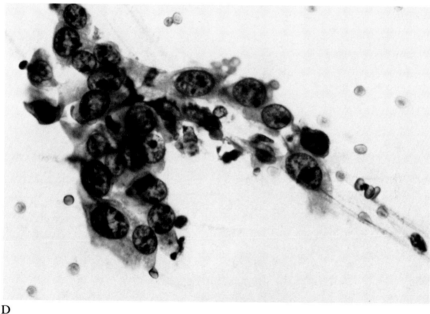

D

Fig. 9.16. **A.** Chest X-ray of patient who received irradiation therapy for squamous cell carcinoma and now presents with an ill-defined lesion of the left upper lobe. **B.** Aspirate of lesion demonstrating loose cluster of atypical cells in which the nuclei are irregular with prominent nucleoli. Features favoring atypical repair include degenerative quality of nuclei and bichromasia of cytoplasm (Papanicolaou stain; ×400). **C.** Another case demonstrating atypical repair in a lung aspirate. Note individual cells having a greater degree of hyperchromasia and irregularity of nucleoli. However, overall cellularity was limited and more diagnostic repairlike groupings were seen elsewhere in the smears (Papanicolaou stain; ×400). **D.** Atypical repair grouping in lung aspirate demonstrating considerable hyperchromasia and irregularity of nucleoli with overlapping of nuclei. However, overall configuration of the group favors the diagnosis of repair reaction (Papanicolaou stain; ×400).

225

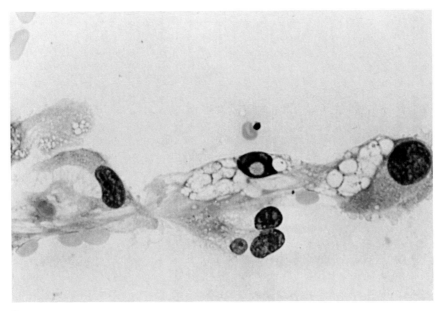

E

Fig. 9.16. E. Aspirate of lung in patient who had received irradiation. Note irradiation effect including nuclear and cytoplasmic enlargement with maintenance of unremarkable nuclear:cytoplasmic ratio. Prominent cytoplasmic and nuclear vacuolization are also present (Diff-Quik stain; × 400).

TABLE 9.2. Cytomorphologic Differential Diagnostic Features of Epithelial Repair Versus Malignancy

Epithelial Repair	*Pulmonary Malignancy*
Groups of cells	Groups of cells
Few single cells	Many single cells
Flat metaplastic sheets	Syncytial arrangement
Distinct cell borders	Variable cytoplasmic borders
Cellular polarity maintained	Loss of polarity
Enlarged nuclei	Enlarged nuclei
Round or oval nuclei with smooth nuclear membrane	Irregular nuclear borders
Uniform nuclei	Variable nuclei
Vesicular, hypochromatic nuclei with even chromatin distribution	Opaque to hyperchromatic nuclei with irregular chromatin distribution
Nucleoli	Nucleoli
Normal mitotic figures	Abnormal mitotic figures
No diathesis	Clean background or diathesis

TABLE 9.3. Radiation Changes

Nuclear and cytoplasmic enlargement
Nuclear and/or cytoplasmic vacuolization
Bi- and multinucleation
Anisonucleosis
Karyorrhexis, karyolysis
Macronucleoli, multiple
Amphophilia, pale staining
Cytophagocytosis
Loss of sharp cytoplasmic border

TABLE 9.4. Pitfalls for False-Positive Diagnosis of Malignancy in Respiratory Cytology

Reserve cell hyperplasia
Irritation form of bronchial cells ("Creola bodies")
Atypical squamous metaplasia
Atypical bronchoalveolar cell hyperplasia
Regeneration and repair
Radiation/chemotherapy effect
Viral cytopathic changes
Megakaryocytes
Vegetable cells
Degenerating macrophages

TABLE 9.5. Pitfalls in Respiratory Cytology

Benign	Malignancy (False-Positive Diagnosis)
Repair	Squamous cell carcinoma
Squamous metaplasia	Squamous cell carcinoma
Irritated (hyperplastic) bronchial cells, "Creola bodies"	Adenocarcinoma
Reserve cells	Small cell carcinoma
Pneumocytes	Bronchoalveolar cell carcinoma

could be confused with malignant cells in cases of pulmonary infarction. The authors believed that these adenomatous-type groups of atypical cells and clusters of bronchioloalveolar cells were the most specific cytologic feature of pulmonary infarct.[92] Other cytologic findings in exfoliative respiratory specimens following pulmonary infarction include the presence of squamous metaplastic cells and Creola bodies. Frable and Johnston[24] have further noted that abnormally enlarged cells arranged in sheetlike groups and clusters with some depth of focus can be present in pulmonary infarcts.[97] The sheetlike arrangement of cells can be confused with squamous cell carcinoma, whereas the groups showing some depth of focus can be misdiagnosed

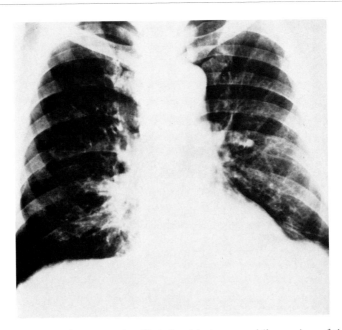

Fig. 9.17. Chest X-ray demonstrating ill-defined lesion near hilar region of the right lung.

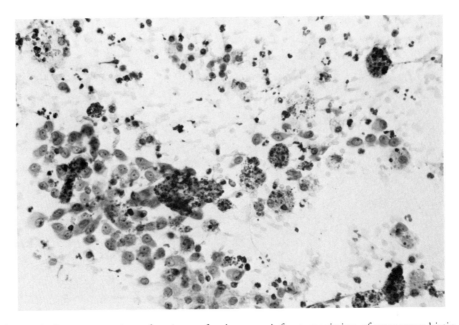

Fig. 9.18. Low-power view of aspirate of pulmonary infarct consisting of numerous histio-cytes containing refractile hemosiderin-type pigment. A few scattered respiratory cells are seen along with loose, sheetlike groupings of mesothelial cell (Papanicolaou stain; × 100). (From Silverman JF, Weaver MD, Show R, et al: Fine needle aspiration cytology of pulmo-nary infarct. *Acta Cytol* 29:162–166, 1985. With permission.)

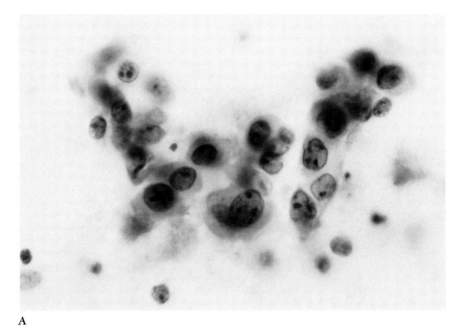

A

B

Fig. 9.19. A. Atypical alveolar lining cells in aspirate of pulmonary infarct. Note aniso-nucleosis and nuclear irregularity with presence of one or more prominent nucleoli. However, the grouping does retain the features of epithelial repair (Papanicolaou stain; ×400). **B.** Resected lesion showing histologic features of a pulmonary infarct (H&E stain; ×100).

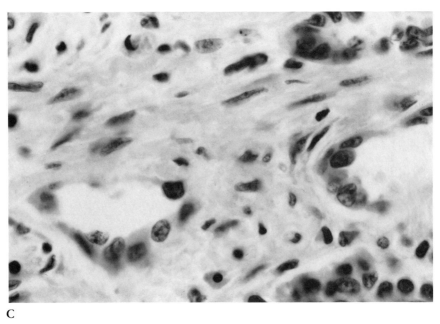

C

Fig. 9.19. C. At the periphery of the infarct, prominent regeneration and repair of alveolar lining cells are seen. Cells such as these probably accounted for the atypical epithelial cells noted in the aspirated specimen (H&E stain; ×400).

as adenocarcinoma. Although the atypical cells can be seen in different types of pulmonary material, bronchial brushings were thought to be the most difficult and problematic to interpret, since the better preserved cells could cytologically simulate malignancy.[97] Frable suggested that the marked variation in cell size and shape, poor nuclear detail and reactive appearance, along with a common cell border and tight clustering of the atypical cells are helpful features for a correct diagnosis of pulmonary infarction.

Infarction of the lung parenchyma is also a sequela of pulmonary dirofilariasis.[17,98] The diagnostic cytologic finding is the presence of a worm showing features of *Dirofilaria immitis* in the aspirated material[17,98] (Fig. 9.20). Other pulmonary lesions to be considered when the aspirate demonstrates extensive necrosis include caseation necrosis, tumor necrosis (Fig. 9.21), and Wegener's granulomatosis (Fig. 9.22).

PNEUMOCONIOSIS

Roggli and associates have reported the presence of asbestos bodies in FNA biopsies of the lung in two patients, one of whom had considerable occupational exposure to asbestos particles[99] (Fig. 9.23). One of the cases was associated with an *Aspergillus* infection, whereas the other patient had an adenocarcinoma of the lung. Tao and associates reported the cytologic diagnosis of intravenous talc granulomatosis by FNA biopsy in a 44-year-old former drug addict.[100] Cytomorphologic features

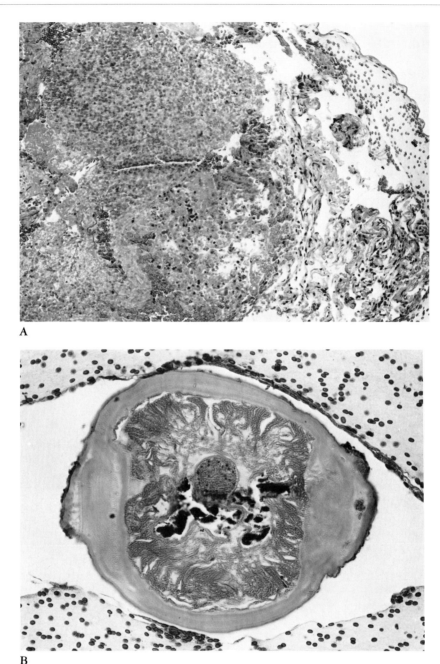

A

B

Fig. 9.20. A. Cell block of lung aspirate consisting of hemorrhagic and infarcted tissue (H&E stain; ×120). **B.** Cross-section of worm (*Dirofilaria immitis*) (H&E stain; ×275). Both photomicrographs courtesy of Dr. J-G. Hsiu, DePaul Hospital, Norfolk, VA. (From Hawkins AG, Hsiu J-G, Smith RM, et al: Pulmonary dirofilariasis diagnosed by fine needle aspiration biopsy: a case report. *Acta Cytol* 29:19–22, 1985. With permission.)

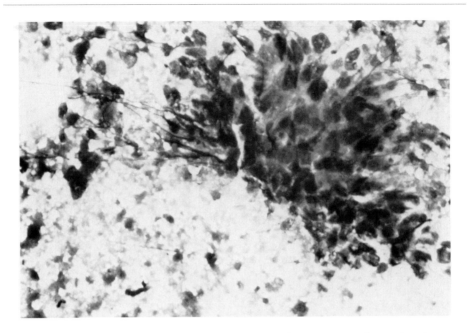

Fig. 9.21. Extensive tumor necrosis in lung aspirate; after a prolonged search only a rare group of malignant cells were found in the smears (Diff-Quik stain; ×400).

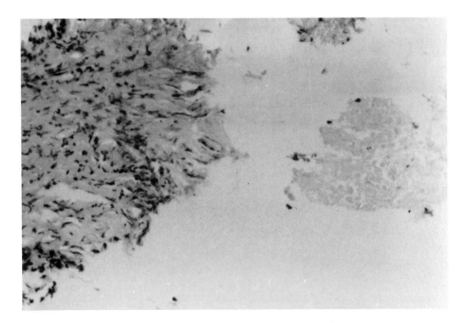

Fig. 9.22. Aspirate of Wegener's granulomatosis showing no diagnostic features for that entity except for a clump of necrotic material along with a nearby fragment of inflamed lung parenchyma in cell block (H&E; ×400) (Courtesy of Dr. G. F. Worsham, Roper Hospital, Charleston, SC).

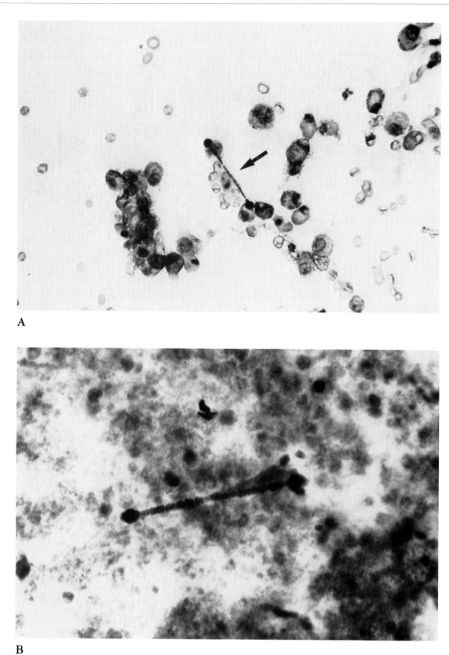

A

B

Fig. 9.23. A. Ferruginous body in middle of field of a lung aspirate from a patient with-
asbestosis (*arrow*) (Papanicolaou stain; ×200). B. High-power view of ferruginous body
having dumbbell-shaped configuration. Extensive necrosis in background (Papanicolaou stain;
×400).

included the presence of numerous mononuclear to multinucleated macrophages containing aggregates of silicate crystals which were best seen by polarization of the smears. The background of the slides contained fibroblasts, lymphocytes, and foreign-body type giant cells, some of which had intracytoplasmic birefringent platelike crystals.[101]

ASPIRATION PNEUMONIA

Covell and Feldman reported a case of aspiration pneumonia (phytopneumonitis) diagnosed by FNA cytology.[102] Cytologic findings included the presence of a chronic inflammatory cell exudate and abundant foreign material consistent with vegetable matter. This material was variably sized and had angulated shapes with thick refractile cell walls and numerous basophilic round bodies about 4 to 7 microns in diameter in the cytoplasm. The angulated structure and the cell wall were diagnostic of cells of plant origin, and the basophilic bodies represented storage vacuoles. This case is especially important since the radiologic appearance of aspiration pneumonia can mimic lung cancer. In addition there is a potential to misdiagnose the vegetable material as representing either fungi or malignant cells.

OTHER NONNEOPLASTIC PULMONARY LESIONS

Inflammatory pseudotumors can clinically and radiologically mimic a neoplastic process.[103] Pulmonary inflammatory pseudotumors have been traditionally diagnosed by open lung biopsy. Histologically, a polymorphic population of cells are present including fibroblasts admixed with plasma cells, lymphocytes, and histiocytes.[104-107] Machicao and associates recently reported a series of four patients with inflammatory pseudotumors diagnosed by FNA biopsy.[103] Cytologic findings included uniform spindle-shaped fibroblasts arranged in small clusters and large groups, along with uniform sheets of pneumocytes. A potential for a false-positive diagnosis of malignancy existed, since isolated atypical cells having features of histiocytes and fibroblasts were present (Fig. 9.24). These cells were larger than the usual histiocytes and fibroblasts and had abundant vacuolated cytoplasm and large nuclei, with a finely granular chromatin pattern. Some of the cells possessed macronucleoli. Although the cytologic findings of inflammatory pseudotumor are nonspecific, recognition of the other benign cytologic features of the lesion should avert a misdiagnosis of malignancy.

Frable has illustrated an FNA case of *Wegener's granulomatosis* in a 53-year-old male presenting with a 5-cm pulmonary mass.[108] The cytomorphologic features were nonspecific and consisted of fibrin, inflammatory cells, and large pale histiocytic-appearing cells. Histologic examination demonstrated an inflammatory and granulomatous process of the lung associated with a prominent vasculitis consistent with Wegener's granulomatosis. In a small series of FNA biopsies of Wegener's granulomatosis, Fekete and associates reported the presence of neutrophils en-

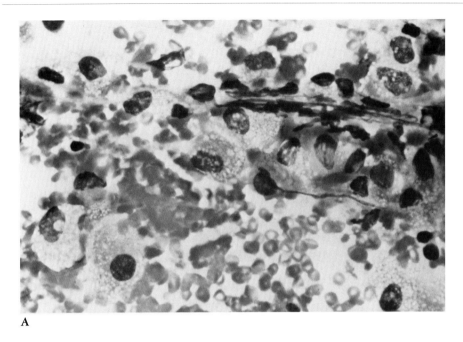

A

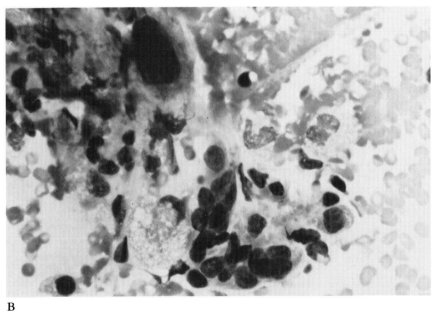

B

Fig. 9.24. A. Aspirate of inflammatory pseudotumor consisting of numerous vacuolated cells having slightly enlarged and irregular hyperchromatic nuclei. Potentially, these reactive histiocytes could be confused with a clear cell carcinoma (Diff-Quik stain; ×400). **B.** Aspirate of inflammatory pseudotumor of the lung in which scattered histiocytes demonstrate considerable nuclear enlargement and hyperchromasia (Diff-Quik stain; ×400).

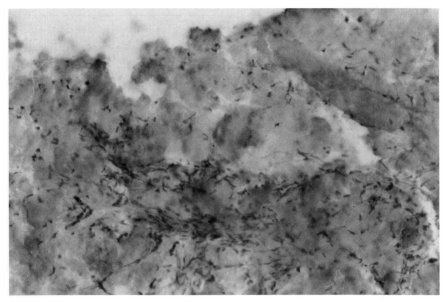

A

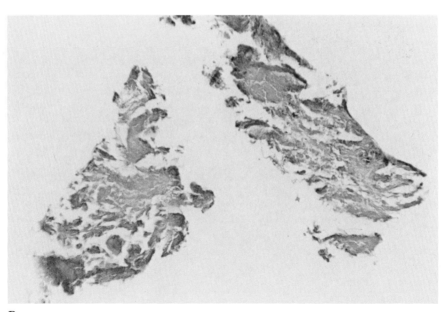

B

Fig. 9.25. A. FNA of amyloid tumor of lung demonstrating amorphous clumps of amyloid with scattered interspersed stromal cells (Papanicolaou stain; ×400) (Courtesy of Dr. G. Fred Worsham, Roper Hospital, Charleston, SC). **B.** Cell block from FNA of lung revealing clumps of Congo red–positive material (Congo red stain; ×200) (Courtesy of Dr. G. Fred Worsham).

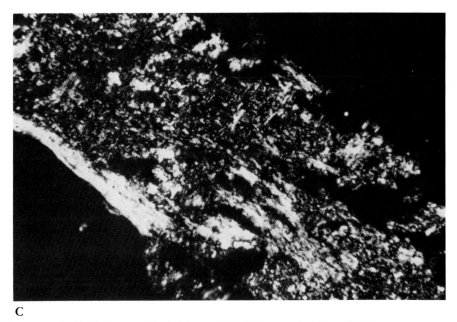

C

Fig. 9.25. C. Birefringent, polarizable amyloid (Congo red stain; × 400).

trapped within necrotic debris and benign multinucleated giant cells often having nuclei arranged in rings or horseshoes.[109] These relatively nonspecific findings should alert the cytologist to the possibility of Wegener's granulomatosis, especially when the classic clinical findings are present.[110] Unfortunately, respiratory involvement usually precedes generalized, renal, and other limited forms of pulmonary Wegener's granulomatosis. Therefore, the reader is cautioned not to make a definitive diagnosis, since open lung biopsy will most likely be necessary for a specific diagnosis of Wegener's granulomatosis.

Other unusual nonneoplastic pulmonary masses examined by FNA biopsy include extramedullary hematopoiesis[111] and lipid pneumonia.[112]

Amyloidosis involving the thoracic region has been diagnosed by FNA biopsy.[113,114] The cytologic findings include the presence of clumps of large waxy amorphous material measuring up to 500 microns and staining metachromatically with the Diff-Quik and other Romanovsky stains. Amyloid is Congo red positive and demonstrates characteristic apple-green birefringence with polarization (Fig. 9.25). Other secondary changes can be present, including a foreign body reaction to the amyloid material.[115]

REFERENCES

1. Silverman JF, Marrow HG: Fine needle aspiration cytology of granulomatous diseases of the lung, including nontuberculous *Mycobacterium* infection. *Acta Cytol* 29:535–541, 1985.

2. Perlmutt LM, Johnston WW, Dunnick NR: Percutaneous transthoracic needle aspiration: a review. *AJR* 152:451–455, 1989.

3. Alonzo P, Sanchez S, Ramirez E, et al: Transthoracic needle biopsy in neoplastic and nonneoplastic pathology: experience in a general hospital. *Diagn Cytopathol* 2:284–289, 1986.

4. Klein JO: Diagnostic lung puncture in the pneumonias of infants and children. *Pediatrics* 44:486–492, 1969.

5. Garcia de Olarte D, Trujillo H, Uribe A, et al: Lung puncture-aspiration as a bacteriologic diagnostic procedure in acute pneumonias of infants and children. *Clin Pediatr* 10:346–350, 1971.

6. Arroyo J, Gordan V, Postic B: Transthoracic needle aspiration in the management of pulmonary infections. *J SC Med Assoc* 77:427–432, 1981.

7. Bhatt ON, Miller R, Le Riche J, et al: Aspiration biopsy in pulmonary opportunistic infections. *Acta Cytol* 21:206–209, 1977.

8. Zavala DC, Schoell JE: Ultrathin needle aspiration of the lung in infectious and malignant disease. *AM Rev Respir Dis* 123:125–131, 1981.

9. Bandt PD, Blank N, Castellino RA: Needle diagnosis of pneumonitis. Value in high-risk patients. *JAMA* 220:1578–1580, 1972.

10. Schwinn CP, Sargent EN, Turner AF, et al: Cytopathology of percutaneous pulmonary needle aspiration biopsy. In: *Compendium on Diagnostic Cytology,* Eds. Wied GL, Koss LG, Reagan JW. Chicago, Tutorials of Cytology, 1983, pp 325–341.

11. Vernon SE: Nodular pulmonary sarcoidosis. Diagnosis with fine needle aspiration biopsy. *Acta Cytol* 29:473–479, 1985.

12. Lalli AF, McCormack LJ, Zelch M, et al: Aspiration biopsies of chest lesions. *Radiology* 127:35–40, 1978.

13. Diefenthal HC, Tashjian J: The role of plain films, CT, tomography, ultrasound, and percutaneous needle aspiration in the diagnosis of inflammatory lung disease. *Semin Respir Infect* 3:83–105, 1988.

14. de Vivo F, Pond GD, Rhenman B, et al: Transtracheal aspiration and fine needle aspiration biopsy for the diagnosis of pulmonary infection in heart transplant patients. *J Thorac Cardiovasc Surg* 96:696–699, 1988.

15. Lyon AB: Bacteriologic studies of 165 cases of pneumonia and postpneumonic empyema in infants and children. *Am J Dis Child* 23:72–87, 1922.

16. Netter A: L'epidemie d'influenza de 1918. *Bull Acad Med* 80:275–286, 1918.

17. Kline TS: *Handbook of Fine Needle Aspiration Biopsy Cytology,* ed 2. New York, Churchill Livingstone, 1988.

18. Finland M: Diagnostic lung puncture. *Pediatrics* 44:471–473, 1969.

19. Gibney RTN, Man GCW, King EG, et al: Aspiration biopsy in the diagnosis of pulmonary disease. *Chest* 80:300–303, 1981.

20. Johnston WW: Percutaneous fine needle aspiration biopsy of the lung: a study of 1,015 patients. *Acta Cytol* 28:218–232, 1984.

21. Bonfiglio TA: Fine needle aspiration biopsy of the lung. *Pathol Annu* 16:159–180, 1981.

22. Dahlgren SE, Ekstrom P: Aspiration cytology in the diagnosis of pulmonary tuberculosis. *Scand J Resp Dis* 53:196–201, 1972.

23. Robicheaux G, Moinuddin SM, Lee LH: The role of aspiration biopsy cytology in the diagnosis of pulmonary tuberculosis. *Am J Clin Pathol* 83:719–722, 1985.

24. Johnston WW, Frable WJ: *Diagnostic Respiratory Cytology.* In: *Masson Monographs in Cytopathology,* Ed. WW Johnston. Vol I. New York, Masson Publishing USA, 1979, pp 96–117.

25. Dahlgren SE, Lind B: Comparison between diagnostic results obtained by transthoracic needle biopsy and by sputum cytology. *Acta Cytol* 16:53–58, 1972.

26. Bailey TM, Akhtar M, Ali MA: Fine needle aspiration biopsy in the diagnosis of tuberculosis. *Acta Cytol* 29:732–736, 1985.

27. Rajwanshi A, Bhambhani S, Das DK: Fine-needle aspiration cytology diagnosis of tuberculosis. *Diagn Cytopathol* 3:13–16, 1987.

28. Pagel W, Simmonds FAH, Macdonald J, et al: Pulmonary tuberculosis, ed. 4. London, Oxford University Press, 1964:245.

29. Johnston WW, Schlein B, Amatulli J: Cytopathologic diagnosis of fungus infections. I. A method for the preparation of simulated cytopathologic material for the teaching of fungus morphologic in cytology specimens. II. The presence of fungus in clinical material. *Acta Cytol* 13:488–495, 1969.

30. Johnston WW: The cytopathology of mycotic infections. *Laboratory Medicine* 2:34–40, 1971.

31. Silverman JF, Johnsrude IS: Fine needle aspiration cytology of granulomatous crypto-coccosis of the lung. *Acta Cytol* 29:157–161, 1985.

32. Binford CH, Dooley JR: Diseases caused by fungi and actinomycetes. In: *Pathology of Tropical and Extraordinary Diseases,* Eds. CH Binford, DH Connor. Vol 2. Washington, DC, Armed Forces Institute of Pathology, 1976, pp 551–559.

33. Littman ML, Walter JE: Cryptococcosis: current status. *Am J Med* 45:922–933, 1968.

34. Gordonson J, Birnbaum W, Jacobson G, et al: Pulmonary crytococcosis. *Radiology* 112:557–561, 1974.

35. Rosen SE, Koprowska I: Cytologic diagnosis of a case of pulmonary cryptococcosis. *Acta Cytol* 26:499–502, 1982.

36. Hatcher CR Jr, Sehdeva J, Waters WD, et al: Primary pulmonary cryptococcosis. *J Thorac Cardiovasc Surg* 61:39–49, 1971.

37. Walts AE: Localized pulmonary cryptococcosis: diagnosis by fine needle aspiration. *Acta Cytol* 27:457–459, 1983.

38. Dormer BA, Scher P: Tumor of lung due to *Cryptococcus histolyticus. Clin Proc* 6:269–273, 1947.

39. Roger V, Nasiell M, Nasiell K, et al: Cytologic findings indicating pulmonary tubercu-losis: II. The occurrence in sputum of epithelioid cells and multinucleated giant cells in pulmonary tuberculosis, chronic non-tuberculous inflammatory lung disease and bronchogenic carcinoma. *Acta Cytol* 16:538–542, 1972.

40. Whitaker D, Sterrett GF: Cryptococcus neoformans diagnosed by fine needle aspiration cytology of the lung. *Acta Cytol* 20:105–107, 1976.

41. Prolla J: The detection of *Cryptococcus neoformans* in sputum cytology. *Acta Cytol* 14:87–91, 1970.

42. Lalli AF, McCormack LJ, Zelch M, et al: Aspiration biopsies of chest lesions. *Radiology* 127:35–40, 1978.

43. Sinner WN: Needle biopsy of histoplasmosis. *Fortschr Rontgenstr* 133:590–593, 1980.

44. Colby TV, Weiss RL: Current concepts in the surgical pathology of pulmonary infec-tions. *Am J Surg Pathol* 11:25–37, 1987.

45. McCalmont TH, Geisinger KR, Silverman JF: Fine-needle aspiration cytology of asper-gillosis in cardiac transplant patients. *Arch Surg* 126:394–396, 1991.

46. Phillips P, Weiner MH: Invasive aspergillosis diagnosed by immunohistochemistry with monoclonal and polyclonal reagents. *Hum Pathol* 18:1015–1024, 1987.

47. Reyes CV, Kathuria S, MacGlashan A: Diagnostic value of calcium oxalate crystals in respiratory and pleural fluid cytology. A case report. *Acta Cytol* 23:65–68, 1979.

48. Farley ML, Mabry L, Munoz LA, et al: Crystals occurring in pulmonary cytology specimens. Association with *Aspergillus* infection. *Acta Cytol* 29:737–744, 1985.

49. Lee SH, Barnes WG, Schaetzel WP: Pulmonary aspergillosis and the importance of oxalate crystal recognition in cytology specimens. *Arch Pathol Lab Med* 110:1176–1179, 1986.

50. Freeman SI, Ang EP, Haley RS: Identification of coccidioidomycosis of the lung by fine needle aspiration biopsy. *Acta Cytol* 30:420–424, 1986.

51. Foreth J, Rohwedder JJ, Levine BE, et al: Experience with needle biopsy for coccidioidal lung nodules. *Arch Intern Med* 146:319–320, 1986.

52. Cunningham RT, Einstein H: Pulmonary cavities due to coccidioidomycosis with spontaneous rupture. In: *Proceedings of the Twenty-Fifth Annual Coccidioidomycosis Study Group Meeting,* Sacramento, CA, April 11, 1980, p 6.

53. Stevens DA, Levine HB, Deresinski SC, et al: Epidemiological and clinical skin testing studies with spherulin: Coccidioidomycosis. New York, Stratton Intercontinental Medical Book Corporation, 1977, pp 107–114.

54. Trumbull ML, Chesney TM: The cytological diagnosis of pulmonary blastomycosis. *JAMA* 245:836–838, 1981.

55. Valicenti JF, Daniell C, Gobien RP: Thin needle aspiration cytology of benign intrathoracic lesions. *Acta Cytol* 25:659–664, 1981.

56. Buchanan AJ, Gupta RK: Cytomegalovirus infection of the lung: Cytomorphologic diagnosis by fine-needle aspiration cytology. *Diagn Cytopathol* 2:341–342, 1986.

57. Bedrossian UK, Lozano de Arce EA, et al: Immunoperoxidase method to detect herpes simplex virus in cytologic specimens. *Lab Med* 15:673–676, 1984.

58. Fauci AS, Masur H, Gelmann EP, et al: NIH conference. The acquired immunodeficiency syndrome: an update. *Ann Intern Med* 102:800–813, 1985.

59. Linder J, Rennard S: *Bronchoalveolar Lavage.* Chicago, ASCP Press, 1988, pp 67–69.

60. Bedrossian CWM, Mason MR, Gupta PK: Rapid cytologic diagnosis of *Pneumocystis:* A comparison of effective techniques. *Semin Diagn Pathol* 6:245–261, 1989.

61. Baughman RP, Strohofer SS, Clinton BA, et al: The use of an indirect fluorescent antibody test for detecting *Pneumocystis carinii. Arch Pathol Lab Med* 113:1062–1065, 1989.

62. Ng VL, Gartner I, Weymouth LA, et al: The use of mucolysed induced sputum for the identification of pulmonary pathogens associated with human immunodeficiency virus infection. *Arch Pathol Lab Med* 113:488–493, 1989.

63. Blumenfeld W, Kovacs JA: Use of a monoclonal antibody to detect *Pneumocystis carinii* in induced sputum and bronchoalveolar lavage fluid by immunoperoxidase staining. *Arch Pathol Lab Med* 112:1233–1236, 1988.

64. Ghali VS, Garcia RL, Skolom J: Fluorescence of *Pneumocystis carinii* in Papanicolaou smears. *Hum Pathol* 15:907–909, 1984.

65. Leigh TR, Parsons P, Hume C, et al: Sputum induction for diagnosis of *Pneumocystis carinii* pneumonia. *Lancet* 2:205–206, 1989.

66. O'Brien RJ, Quinn JL, Miyahara BT, et al: Diagnosis of *Pneumocystis carinii* pneumonia by induced sputum in a city with moderate incidence of AIDS. *Chest* 95:136–138, 1989.

67. del Rio C, Guarner J, Honig EG, et al: Sputum examination in the diagnosis of *Pneumocystis carinii* pneumonia in the acquired immunodeficiency syndrome. *Arch Pathol Lab Med* 112:1229–1232, 1988.

68. Elvin KM, Bjorkman A, Linder et al: *Pneumocystis carinii* pneumonia: detection of parasites in sputum and bronchoalveolar lavage fluid by monoclonal antibodies. *Br Med J* 297:381–384, 1988.

69. Blumenfeld W, Griffiss JM: *Pneumocystis carinii* in sputum. Comparable efficacy of screening stains and determination of cyst density. *Arch Pathol Lab Med* 112:816–820, 1988.

70. Zaman MK, Wooten OJ, Suprahmanya B, et al: Rapid noninvasive diagnosis of *Pneumocystis carinii* from induced liquefied sputum. *Ann Intern Med* 109:7–10, 1988.

71. Kovacs JA, Ng VL, Masur H, et al: Diagnosis of *Pneumocystis carinii* pneumonia: Improved detection in sputum with use of monoclonal antibodies. *N Engl J Med* 318:589–593, 1988.

72. Bigby TD, Margolskee D, Curtis JL, et al: The usefulness of induced sputum in the diagnosis of *Pneumocystis carinii* pneumonia in patients with the acquired immunodeficiency syndrome. *Am Rev Respir Dis* 133:515–518, 1986.

73. Pitchenik AE, Ganjei P, Torres A, et al: Sputum examination for the diagnosis of *Pneumocystis carinii* pneumonia in the acquired immunodeficiency syndrome. *Am Rev Respir Dis* 133:226–229, 1986.

74. Wallace JM, Batra P, Gong H Jr, et al: Percutaneous needle lung aspiration for diagnosing pneumonitis in the patient with acquired immunodeficiency syndrome (AIDS). *Am Rev Respir Dis* 131:389–391, 1985.

75. Batra P, Wallace JM, Ovenfors C-O: Efficacy and complications of transthoracic needle biopsy of lung in patients with *Pneumocystis carinii* pneumonia and AIDS. *J Thorac Imaging* 2:79–80, 1987.

76. Jacobs JB, Vogel C, Powell RD, et al: Needle biopsy in *Pneumocystis carinii* pneumonia. *Radiology* 93:525–530, 1989.

77. Castellino RA: Percutaneous pulmonary needle diagnosis *Pneumocystis carinii* pneumonitis. *Natl Cancer Inst Monogr* 43:137–140, 1976.

78. Saldana MJ, Mones JM: Cavitation and other atypical manifestations of *Pneumocystis carinii* pneumonia. *Semin Diagn Pathol* 6:273–286, 1989.

79. Strigle SM, Gal AA: A review of pulmonary cytopathology in the acquired immunodeficiency syndrome. *Diagn Cytopathol* 5:44–54, 1989.

80. Moas CM, Evans DA, Stein-Streilein J, et al: Cresyl violet: A rapid, simple, easily interpretable stain for detecting *Pneumocystis carinii* in sputum. *South Med J* 82:957–959, 1989.

81. Chandra P, Delaney MD, Tuazon CU: Role of special stains in the diagnosis of *Pneumocystis carinii* infection from bronchial washing specimens in patients with the acquired immune deficiency syndrome. *Acta Cytol* 32:105–108, 1988.

82. Gal AA, Klat EC, Koss MK, et al: The effectiveness of bronchoscopy in the diagnosis of *Pneumocystis carinii* and cytomegalovirus pulmonary infections in the acquired immunodeficiency syndrome. *Arch Pathol Lab Med* 111:238–241, 1987.

83. Shimono LH, Hartman B: A simple and reliable methenamine silver stain for *Pneumocystis carinii* and fungi. *Arch Pathol Lab Med* 110:855–856, 1986.

84. Koss LG, Woyke S, Olszewski W: *Aspiration Biopsy. Cytologic Interpretation and Histologic Bases.* New York, Igaku-Shoin, 1984, pp 293–295.

85. Wallace RJ Jr, Cohen A, Awe RJ, et al: Carcinomatous lung abscess. Diagnosis by bronchoscopy and cytopathology. *JAMA* 242:521–522, 1979.

86. Brock RC: *Lung Abscess.* Springfield, IL, CC Thomas, 1952, p 130.

87. Bernhard WF, Wylie RH, Malcolm JA: The carcinomatous abscess. A clinical paradox. *N Engl J Med* 266:914–919, 1962.

88. Flower CDR, Verney GI: Percutaneous needle biopsy of thoracic lesions: an evaluation of 300 biopsies. *Clin Radiol* 30:215–218, 1979.

89. Khouri NF, Stitik FP, Erozan YS, et al: Transthoracic needle aspiration biopsy of benign and malignant lung lesions. *AJR* 144:281–288, 1985.

90. Sinner WN: Pulmonary neoplasms diagnosed with transthoracic needle biopsy. *Cancer* 43:1533–1540, 1979.

91. Johnson RD, Gobien RP, Valicenti JF Jr: Current status of radiologically directed pulmonary thin needle aspiration biopsy: An analysis of 200 consecutive biopsies and review of the literature. *Ann Clin Lab Sci* 13:225–239, 1983.

92. Bewtra C, Dewan N, O'Donahue WJC: Exfoliative sputum cytology in pulmonary embolism. *Acta Cytol* 27:489–496, 1983.

93. Silverman JF, Weaver MD, Shaw R, et al: Fine needle aspiration cytology of pulmonary infarct. *Acta Cytol* 29:162–166, 1985.

94. Sasahara AA, Sharma GVRK, Barsamian EM, et al: Pulmonary thromboembolism. *JAMA* 249:2945–2950, 1983.

95. Johnston WW, Frable WJ: The cytopathology of the respiratory tract. *Am J Pathol* 84:372–424, 1976.

96. Scoggins WG, Smith RH, Frable WJ, et al: False positive cytologic diagnosis of lung carcinoma in patient with pulmonary infarct. *Ann Thoracic Surg* 24:474–480, 1977.

97. Frable WJ: Pulmonary infarcts. Check Sample Program. Cytopathology: No. C-17. ASCP Commission on Continuing Education. Chicago, American Society of Clinical Pathology, 1974.

98. Hawkins AG, Hsiu J-G, Smith RM, et al: Pulmonary dirofiliariasis diagnosed by fine needle aspiration biopsy: a case report. *Acta Cytol* 29:19–22, 1985.

99. Roggli VL, Johnston WW, Kaminsky DB: Asbestos bodies in fine needle aspirates of the lung. *Acta Cytol* 28:493–498, 1984.

100. Tao L-C, Morgan RC, Donat EE: Cytologic diagnosis of intravenous talc granulomatosis by fine needle aspiration biopsy. A case report. *Acta Cytol* 28:737–739, 1984.

101. Kung ITM, Johnson FB, So S-Y, et al: Blue bodies in cytology specimens in a case of pulmonary talcosis. *Am J Clin Pathol* 81:675–678, 1984.

102. Covell JL, Feldman PS: Fine needle aspiration diagnosis of aspiration pneumonia (phytopneumonitis). *Acta Cytol* 38:77–80, 1984.

103. Machicao CN, Sorensen K, Abdul-Karim FW, et al: Transthoracic needle aspiration biopsy in inflammatory pseudotumors of the lung. *Diagn Cytopathol* 5:400–403, 1989.

104. Tchertkoff V, Bok YL, Wagner BM: Plasma cell granuloma of lung. *Dis Chest* 44:440–443, 1963.

105. Bahadori M, Liebow AA: Plasma cell granulomas of the lung. *Cancer* 31:191–208, 1973.

106. Carter D, Eggleston J: Facile on tumors of the lower respiratory tract. Washington, DC: Armed Forces Institute of Pathology, 1974:300–307.

107. Berardi RS, Chen HP, Stines GJ: Inflammatory pseudotumors of the lung. *Surg Gynecol Obstet* 156:89–96, 1983.

108. Frable WJ: *Thin-Needle Aspiration Biopsy. Major Problems in Pathology,* vol 14. Philadelphia, WB Saunders, 1983.

109. Fekete PS, Campbell WJ Jr, Bernardino ME: Transthoracic needle aspiration biopsy in Wegener's granulomatosis. Morphologic findings in five cases. *Acta Cytol* 34:155–160, 1990.

110. Fauci, AS, Wolff SM: Wegener's granulomatosis: studies in eighteen patients and a review of the literature. *Medicine* 52:535–561, 1973.

111. Walker AN, Feldman PS, Walker GK: Fine needle aspiration of thoracic extramedullary hematopoiesis. *Acta Cytol* 27:170–172, 1983.

112. Nathanson L, Frenkel D, Jacobi M: Diagnosis of lipoid pneumonia by aspiration biopsy. *Arch Intern Med* 72:627–634, 1943.

113. Hsiu J-G, Stitik FP, D'Amato NA, et al: Primary amyloidosis presenting as a unilateral hilar mass: report of a case diagnosed by fine needle aspiration biopsy. *Acta Cytol* 30:55–58, 1986.

114. Tomashefski JF, Cramer SF, Abramowsky C, et al: Needle biopsy diagnosis of solitary amyloid nodule of the lung. *Acta Cytol* 24:224–227, 1980.

115. Silverman JF, Dabbs DJ, Norris HT, et al: Localized primary (AL) amyloid tumor of the breast. Cytologic, histologic, immunocytochemical and ultrastructural observations. *Am J Surg Pathol* 10:539–545, 1986.

10
Abdomen and Retroperitoneum

A variety of infections and inflammatory processes can involve the abdomen and retroperitoneum (Table 10.1). Correlation with clinical signs and symptoms and the radiologic location and appearance of the lesion is critical for making a correct diagnosis. A discussion of infectious and inflammatory lesions involving the liver, pancreas, kidney, adrenal gland, and other abdominal retroperitoneal structures is presented.

LIVER

Abscess

Most liver abscesses are bacterial in origin. Pyogenic abscesses of the liver are usually secondary to acute cholangitis, pylephlebitis, septicemia, subphrenic abscess, or trauma.[1] Radiographically, single or multiple lesions can be present, which may mimic primary or metastatic malignancies of the liver. Aspiration cytology of a pyogenic abscess will demonstrate sheets of neutrophils along with considerable background debris. In the Diff-Quik stain, bacterial organisms are often readily identified, although Gram stain can better classify the bacterial population (Fig. 10.1). Whenever a liver abscess is encountered, material should be submitted for microbiologic examination.

Although amoebic liver abscesses are believed to be an unusual complication of amoebic enterocolitis, approximately 40% of cases of amoebic colitis are associated with solitary or multiple liver abscesses.[1,2] Usually a solitary, large, irregular encapsulated lesion is present in the right hepatic lobe. The abscess cavity is filled with a chocolate pasty material, often having the consistency of anchovy paste. There have been only a few FNA reports of extracolonic amebiasis.[3,4] The diagnosis is based on finding trophozoites of *Entamoeba histolytica* measuring from 12 to 60

TABLE 10.1. Nonneoplastic Abdominal and Retroperitoneal Lesions

> Abscess: Bacterial, fungal, parasitic
> Cysts: Congenital, parasitic (eg, hydatid)
> Granulomas: TB, fungal, foreign body
> Xanthogranuloma: Liver, kidney, gallbladder, etc.
> Malacoplakia: Genital, urinary, GI, etc.
> Fat necrosis
> Foreign body reaction
> Infarct: Renal, etc.

microns and having a single round nucleus with chromatin beading along the nuclear membrane, and surrounding granular cytoplasm containing diagnostic red blood cells. The viable trophozoites are usually present in the advancing wall of the abscess, while degenerating and necrotic organisms are present in the center of the lesion.[5] The diagnosis can be confirmed with the highly sensitive indirect hemagglutination test.[1,3]

Other parasites that can be appreciated in hepatic FNA specimens include the trematode *Schistosoma mansoni,* which has ova with a characteristic lateral spine.[5] Frias-Hidvegi has also illustrated an example of *Giardia lamblia* appreciated in a percutaneous fine-needle aspiration biopsy of the biliary tree[5] (Fig. 10.2). The organisms were more readily identified in the Giemsa-stained material than by the traditional Papanicolaou method. Tao has illustrated an example of FNA cytology of clonorchiasis of the liver.[1] The cytologic diagnosis was based on finding ova of the liver fluke *Clonorchis sinensis* associated with large numbers of eosinophils and Charcot-Leyden crystals in the smears.

Although hepatic involvement with actinomycosis is quite unusual, Shurbaji and associates recently reported the FNA cytologic findings of hepatic actinomycosis in a 43-year-old woman with a long-term history of using an intrauterine contraceptive device (IUD). Cytologic examination of the liver aspirate showed clumps of *Actinomyces* organisms present in a necrotic background. The Brown and Brenn stain demonstrated gram-positive filaments, showing variation in size and acute-angle branching (Fig. 10.3). Immunoperoxidase staining with species-specific antiserum performed on the smears identified the organisms as *Actinomyces israelii.*

Cysts

Solitary or multiple cysts of the liver can be congenital, neoplastic, or parasitic in origin. Hydatid disease caused by the hydatid tapeworm, *Echinococcus granulosus,* is most prevalent in sheep-raising countries and occurs infrequently in the United States. The tapeworm's definitive hosts are dogs and wolves, who expel ova in feces. When ova are swallowed by the human host, six-hook embryos develop in the duodenum.[1,5] The embryos then enter the bloodstream which is filtered by the liver. In the liver, the hydatid cyst develops a multilayered wall that contains an inner germinal layer from which brood capsules develop (Fig. 10.4). From these capsules numerous scoleces develop which contain suckers and two rows of hooklets (Fig. 10.5). FNA cytology of a hydatid cyst of the liver will demonstrate scoleces that have many hooklets, some of which may be arranged in a ringlike pattern.[1,6]

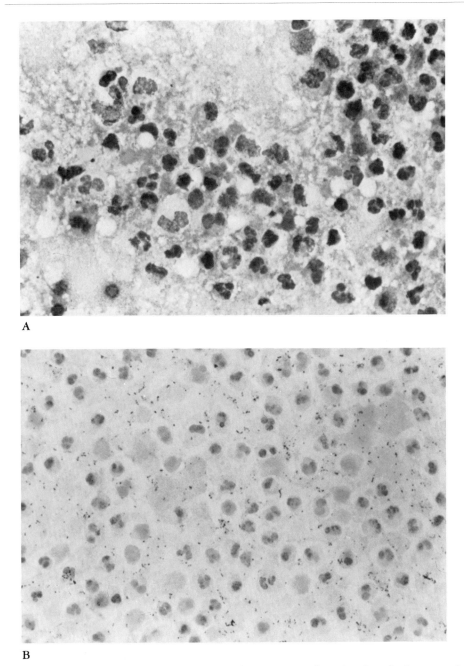

A

B

Fig. 10.1. **A.** Sheets of neutrophils, some of which are undergoing liquefactive necrosis, along with considerable debris in the background (Diff-Quik stain; ×200). **B.** Gram stain demonstrating numerous gram-positive organisms in the background (Gram stain; ×200).

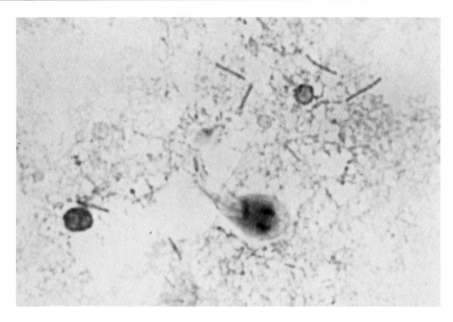

Fig. 10.2. High-power view of *Giardia lamblia* trophozoites in FNA biopsy of biliary tree. Note the pear-shaped configuration of the organism which contains two nuclei and four pairs of flagella (Papanicolaou stain; ×1300) (Courtesy of Dr. Denise Frias-Hidvegi, Northwestern University, Chicago, IL). (From Frias-Hidvegi D: *Guide to Clinical Aspiration Biopsy, Liver and Pancreas.* Igaku-Shoin, New York.)

The cyst fluid is usually clear and contains few inflammatory cells. In older cysts, scoleces may be difficult to find, but the presence of hooklets is diagnostic of hydatid disease.[1] Because of the possibility of anaphylactic shock developing following rupture of the cyst,[7] FNA biopsy should not be performed when echinococcosis is suspected.[2,8]

Granulomas

The liver is commonly involved by granulomatous disease. It is estimated that one third of the granulomas are due to sarcoid, since approximately two thirds of sarcoid patients have liver involvement. Other causes of granulomatous liver disease include infectious agents such as mycobacterium, fungi, or parasites; drug reaction; association with neoplasm; foreign body reaction; and certain liver diseases such as primary biliary cirrhosis. Clinical information, microbiologic examination, and the cytologic pattern of the granulomatous inflammation and associated host response may suggest the correct diagnosis.[9] Aspirates from tuberculous lesions demonstrate loose granulomas associated with a background of caseous necrosis. Organisms can sometimes be demonstrated with special stains, although culture is often necessary for confirmation. In contrast, sarcoidosis usually has minimal necrosis or no necrosis (Fig. 10.6). Fungi can generally be appreciated with special stains performed on the smears, although culture is often helpful and complementary. Tao and associates reported the cytologic findings of intravenous talc granulomatosis in a drug addict,

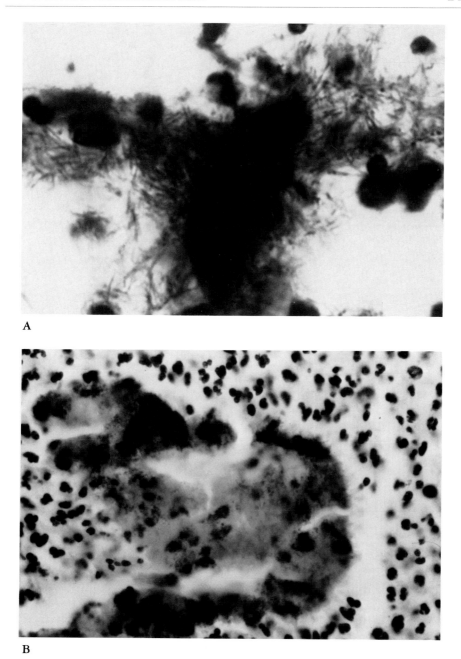

A

B

Fig. 10.3. **A.** Clumps of *Actinomyces* with considerable branching (Papanicolaou stain; ×400). **B.** Cell block demonstrating sulfur granule (Gram stain; ×400).

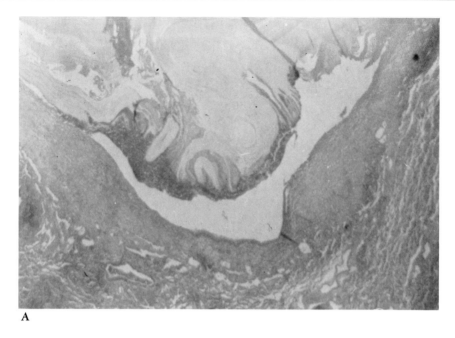

A

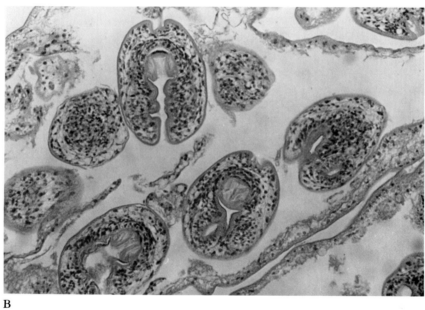

B

Fig. 10.4. **A.** Low power view of hydatid cyst (H&E stain; ×100). **B.** Inner germinal layer and brood capsules of hydatid cyst of liver (H&E stain; ×400).

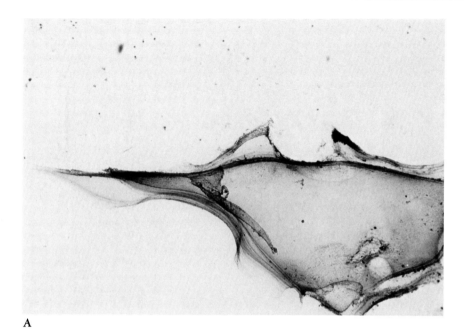

A

B

Fig. 10.5. A. FNA of hydatid cyst of soft tissue in which fragments of the chitinous membrane are present (Papanicolaou stain; ×25) (Courtesy of Dr. Valeria Ascoli, Universita "La Sapienza," Rome, Italy). **B.** Scoleces of *E. granulosus* (Papanicolaou stain; ×400).

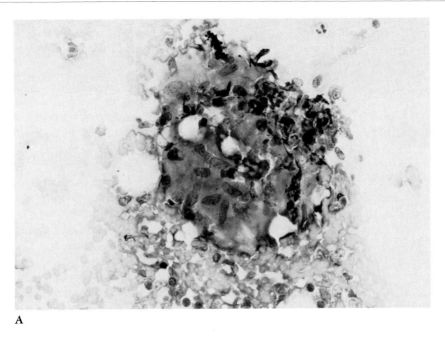

A

B

Fig. 10.6. A. Sarcoidal-type granuloma consisting of cluster of epithelioid histiocytes (Diff-Quik stain; ×400). **B.** Granulomatous inflammation consisting of loose clusters of epithelioid histiocytes and Langhans' type giant cells along with admixed chronic inflammatory cells (H&E stain; ×400).

diagnosed by FNA biopsy. When the smears were examined following polarization, strongly birefringent platelike crystals measuring from 2 to 100 microns were identified.[10]

Viral Hepatitis

Acute hepatitis is a generic term for any diffuse inflammatory process of the liver. Acute viral hepatitis is reserved for those inflammatory diseases of the liver caused by specific hepatotropic viruses. The most common viral agents are type A, type B, and non-A, non-B, which includes type C and delta agent. Other viruses that can cause hepatitis include cytomegalovirus, Epstein-Barr virus (mononucleosis hepatitis), herpes virus, and adenovirus. Depending on the viral agent, acute viral hepatitis can either undergo resolution, become a fulminant process, or develop into chronic liver disease. The chronic forms have been divided into chronic lobular hepatitis, chronic persistent hepatitis, and chronic active hepatitis. The persistent and active forms can evolve into cirrhosis.

The classic histologic features of acute viral hepatitis include a diffuse panlobular inflammatory reaction in the hepatic parenchyma, along with acidophilic bodies and ballooning degeneration of hepatocytes. There may be a portal inflammatory cell infiltrate which may be confined to the portal tract or extend into the adjacent periportal parenchyma to suggest piecemeal necrosis. The hepatic plates are scrambled or disorganized causing lobular disarray. Other changes that may be present include confluent areas of necrosis, cholestasis, fibrosis, and bile ductular proliferation. Ceroid and iron pigment may accumulate in macrophages within portal tracts and Kupffer cells in the lobules in the latter stages of acute resolving viral hepatitis.

Type A hepatitis is a self-limited process, whereas hepatitis B and non-A, non-B including hepatitis C often develop into a chronic carrier state with possible progression to chronic hepatitis with or without cirrhosis and an increased incidence of hepatocellular carcinoma.

FNA biopsy in acute viral hepatitis may show degenerative, and/or regenerative changes of the hepatocytes and inflammation. Ballooning degeneration is characterized by enlarged hepatocytes that have swollen and granular cytoplasm with large, centrally located nuclei possessing prominent nucleoli. Acidophilic bodies are characterized by small, dense cytoplasmic structures, which may or may not also have a small centrally located pyknotic nucleus. Oval to spindle-shaped Kupffer cells having scanty cytoplasm and arranged in loose groupings may be present along with other Kupffer cells having intracytoplasmic hemosiderin or ceroid pigment. Regenerative changes of the hepatocytes include binucleation and some enlarged nuclei with prominent nucleoli. The inflammatory changes in viral hepatitis consist of increased numbers of mononuclear cells, in contrast to neutrophils of alcoholic hepatitis. Alcoholic hepatitis may also demonstrate characteristic Mallory bodies within the cytoplasm of hepatocytes and prominent fatty metamorphosis.[1,2,11,12]

Although the cytologic changes of acute viral hepatitis can be appreciated, FNA biopsy should not be used to make a specific diagnosis and classification of the hepatitis. A core tissue biopsy specimen is needed to assess the architectural changes adequately. In addition, ancillary special stains such as PAS with and without diastase, trichrome stain, and immunoperoxidase stains for hepatitis B surface antigen and core are best performed on the tissue specimen.

FNA biopsies obtained from cirrhotic livers may range from scanty specimens due to fibrosis or a relatively cellular specimen.[13] Aspirates from cirrhotic liver can be a potential diagnostic pitfall for a false-positive diagnosis of malignancy owing to the atypical cytologic changes seen in regenerating hepatocytes.[2] Hepatocytes in cirrhosis may demonstrate anisonucleosis, binucleation, and increased numbers of mitotic figures[1,2,5] (Fig. 10.7). Other findings may include groups of bile ductular cells, bile thrombi, and necrosis, but little inflammation.[2,11,14,15] Aspirates from regenerative nodules consist of numerous single cells, along with other cells arranged in sheets and clusters of variable size. Stripped nuclei may also be present.[5] In the larger clusters, it is important to identify the thin liver cords formed by one or two rows of hepatocytes. Fragments of fibroconnective tissue may also be seen.[5] Although scattered atypical hepatocytes may be present, these cells have a low nuclear:cytoplasmic ratio. The cytologic atypia found in some cases of cirrhosis can also be present in viral hepatitis, in liver cells near metastatic and hepatocellular carcinoma,[16] and in liver cells following treatment with arterial infusion of chemotherapeutic agents.[5] We concur with Hidvegi that the diagnosis of cirrhosis should not be based entirely on cytologic material. Histologic examination of a core needle biopsy or wedge biopsy is needed for definite diagnosis.

The cytologic differential diagnosis of cirrhosis includes well differentiated hepatocellular carcinoma.[5] The main cytologic features supportive for a diagnosis of hepatocellular carcinoma include the presence of thick trabeculae rimmed by endothelial cells and a greater number of atypical cells when compared to cirrhosis. In addition, the atypical cells have a higher nuclear:cytoplasmic ratio with the nuclei having a coarse chromatin pattern with irregular nucleoli (Fig. 10.8). Other patterns seen in well differentiated hepatocellular carcinoma include a solid arrangement of small cells with a high nuclear:cytoplasmic ratio and pseudoglandular structures.[5] The problem of differentiating cirrhosis from hepatoma is complicated by the fact that cirrhosis is present in nearly 90% of the U.S. cases of hepatocellular carcinoma.[17] Therefore, accurate radiologic placement of the aspirating needle is crucial in making a correct diagnosis of well differentiated hepatocellular carcinoma and differentiating these changes from cirrhosis.

Other Hepatic Lesions

Xanthogranuloma of the liver, which is also known as inflammatory pseudotumor, is a rare lesion of uncertain etiology that can present as an intrahepatic mass and thereby mimic a malignant neoplasm. Lupovich and associates reported the FNA cytologic findings of inflammatory pseudotumor of the liver which was initially misdiagnosed as malignant because of the presence of atypical hepatocytes. Cytologic examination demonstrated an acute inflammatory cell process along with numerous foamy histiocytes, some plasma cells, and lymphocytes. Histologic examination of the resected mass revealed the true benign nature of the lesion. The smears were then restained by the Gram technique, which demonstrated clusters of gram-positive cocci.[18] It is believed that this lesion may represent an unusual tissue response to an intrahepatic bacterial infection. The cytologic findings are similar to xanthogranuloma of other sites that have been sampled by FNA biopsy.[19]

Xanthogranulomatous cholecystitis is an uncommon inflammatory process of the gallbladder that may be radiologically and grossly confused with a neoplastic pro-

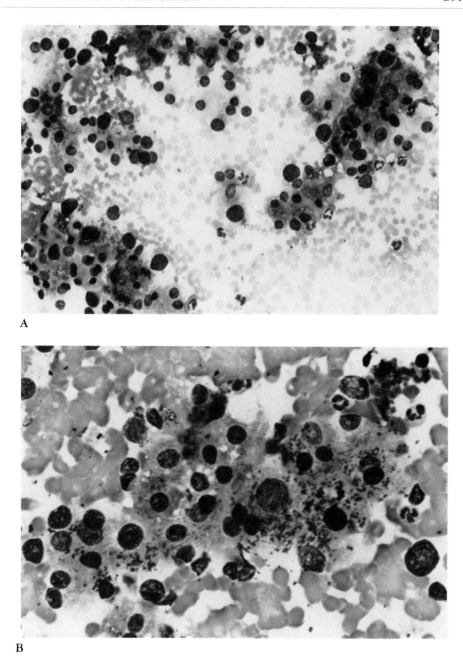

Fig. 10.7. A. Low-power view of aspirate of liver in patient with cirrhosis showing considerable anisonucleosis along with some stripped nuclei. Note bile pigment (Diff-Quik stain; ×100). **B.** Cluster of benign hepatocytes showing considerable anisonucleosis in aspirate of cirrhotic liver. Note abundant intracytoplasmic pigmentation (Diff-Quik stain; ×400).

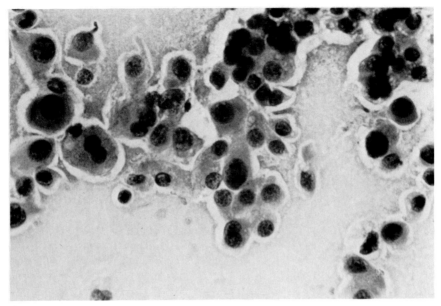

A

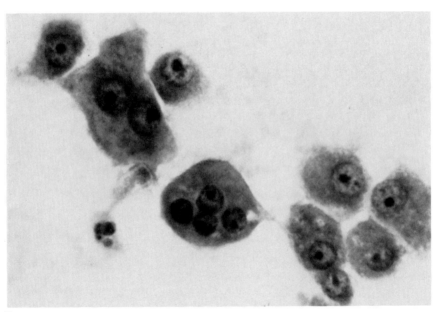

B

Fig. 10.8. A. Aspirate of well differentiated hepatocellular carcinoma showing cytologic features that can be confused with regenerating cells from cirrhosis. Note the greater degree of anisonucleosis and higher nuclear:cytoplasmic ratio which favors an hepatocellular carcinoma (Diff-Quik stain; ×200). **B.** Another example of a well differentiated hepatocellular carcinoma demonstrating malignant hepatocytes with greater degree of atypia including multinucleation and prominent nucleoli (Papanicolaou stain; ×630).

cess. Cytologic findings include the presence of abundant foamy xanthoma-type histiocytes arranged singly and in clusters associated with interspersed capillaries, multinucleated giant cells, and some columnar epithelial cells. When abdominal aspirates contain increased numbers of histiocytic-type cells, the differential diagnosis includes histiocytosis X, histiocytic lymphoma, malignant histiocytosis, malacoplakia, fat necrosis, and well differentiated renal cell carcinoma.[19]

PANCREAS

Percutaneous fine-needle aspiration biopsy is widely used in the evaluation of benign and malignant pancreatic masses.[20,21-27] Sampling by large-core cutting needle or by wedge resection has been associated with morbidity and even mortality.[28,29] In contrast, FNA cytology of the pancreas is a relatively safe and accurate intraoperative or percutaneous biopsy procedure.[2]

Pancreatitis

Pancreatitis may be secondary to alcoholism, obstruction, infection, or trauma or may be idiopathic in nature. Release of pancreatic enzymes such as amylase and lipase causes necrosis and inflammation of the pancreas and surrounding tissues. Lipolytic enzymes cause fat necrosis within the pancreas and nearby adipose tissue and at times, distant sites. The patient with pancreatitis usually presents with abdominal pain and an elevated serum amylase level.

Although FNA biopsy is not usually indicated for the diagnosis of acute pancreatitis, it is not uncommon for patients presenting with obstructing neoplastic lesions to have a secondary acute pancreatitis. Cytologic findings seen both in the primary and secondary forms of acute pancreatitis include an acute inflammatory cell reaction with extensive degeneration and necrosis of ductal and acinar cells and considerable background debris. Some of the degenerating epithelial cells can demonstrate nuclear enlargement and atypia which may be a potential pitfall for a false-positive diagnosis of malignancy (Fig. 10.9). One should be conservative when interpreting aspirates of the pancreas containing extensive acute inflammation and atypical cells, in order to avoid this pitfall.

Approximately one third of the patients with acute pancreatitis who survive progress to chronic pancreatitis.[1] Because of the increased fibrosis and atrophy of acinar cells, the aspirates from chronic pancreatitis may be paucicellular (Fig. 10.10). In our experience, however, many of the specimens show good cellularity with increased numbers of chronic inflammatory cells (predominantly lymphocytes). Some neutrophils, histiocytes, and fibroblasts may also be present. Again, atypical epithelial cells may be seen that show variation in nuclear size and shape and have nuclei with small nucleoli. Since aspirates from both pancreatitis and pancreatic carcinoma may contain inflammatory cells, there exists the distinct possibility for a false-positive or -negative diagnosis of pancreatic carcinoma and pancreatitis respectively, in aspirated material.[21]

Cytologic criteria that are helpful for the diagnosis of pancreatitis include the presence of relatively few atypical ductal cells; in contrast, to aspirates of well

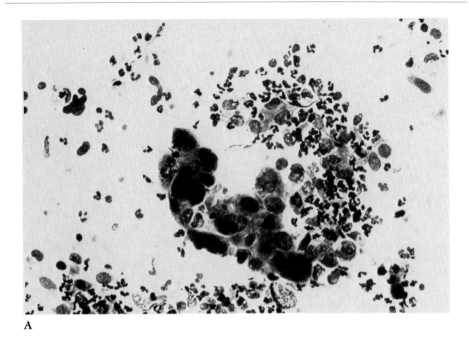

A

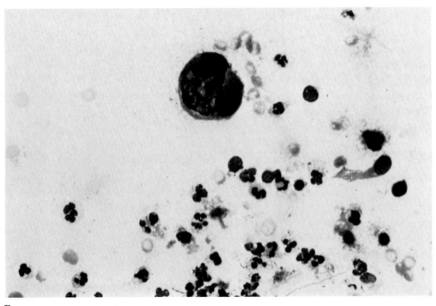

B

Fig. 10.9. A. Aspirate of acute pancreatitis showing considerable inflammatory atypia of the epithelial cells along with extensive acute inflammation (Diff-Quik stain; ×200). **B.** High-power view of single, markedly atypical degenerating cell in an aspirate of acute pancreatitis (Diff-Quik stain; ×400).

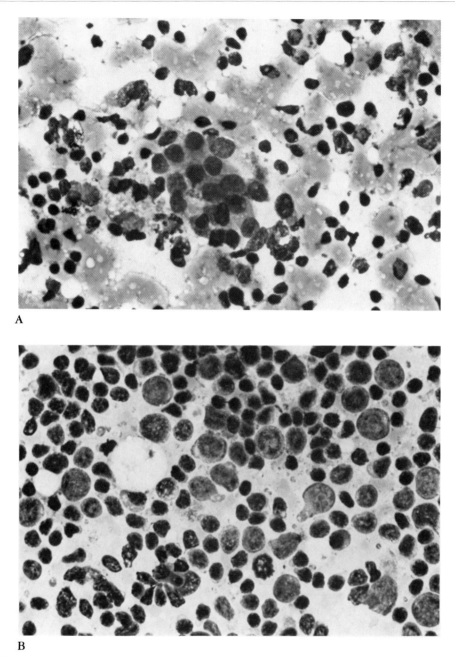

A

B

Fig. 10.10. **A.** Aspirate of chronic pancreatitis in which a small cluster of mildly atypical acinar cells is seen associated with numerous inflammatory cells (Diff-Quik stain; ×200). **B.** Aspirate of chronic pancreatitis showing considerable chronic inflammation with a paucity of epithelial cells (Diff-Quik stain; ×400).

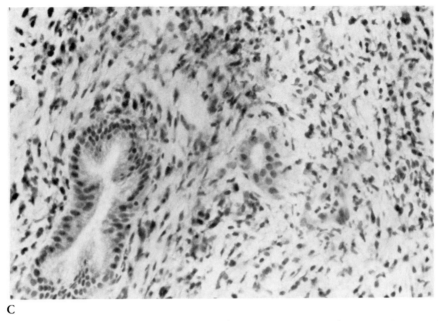

C

Fig. 10.10. C. Tissue biopsy from same case of chronic pancreatitis demonstrating atrophy of acinar cells with increased fibrosis (H&E stain; ×400).

differentiated adenocarcinoma which contain numerous atypical groups. In chronic pancreatitis, the cells generally are arranged in a regular, loose monolayer in contrast to irregular, tightly cohesive three-dimensional groups and/or syncytial clusters of atypical cells in well differentiated adenocarcinoma.[1,2] The epithelial cells in chronic pancreatitis may show a slight degree of atypia and anisonucleosis, but the cells usually have regular nuclear membranes and few or no macronucleoli (Fig. 10.11). In contrast, there is a greater degree of pleomorphism of the ductal cells in pancreatic carcinoma (Fig. 10.12).

Other potential pitfalls for a false-positive diagnosis of pancreatic carcinoma in pancreatitis include the presence of granulation tissue and mesenchymal repair. A potential exists for a false-negative diagnosis of malignancy when extensive acute or chronic pancreatitis is present in aspirates from patients with pancreatic carcinoma.[2] Mitchell and Carney reviewed 16 series of FNA biopsies of the pancreas and reported a diagnostic sensitivity of the procedure of 55 to 100%.[25] In our experience, FNA biopsy of the pancreas is an accurate procedure with a sensitivity rate of 88% and a specificity of 100%.[20] The main limitation of the procedure is the relatively high incidence of false-negative or insufficient biopsies. These instances may be related to inaccurate placement of the needle, necrosis, desmoplasia of the tumor, or underdiagnosis of a well differentiated adenocarcinoma of the pancreas.[24,25] False-negative diagnosis can especially occur when chronic pancreatitis adjacent to a pancreatic neoplasm is aspirated.[2,25]

We recently presented a series of FNA biopsies of the pancreas in which benign and malignant giant cells were encountered.[20] Giant cells of varying types were seen including multinucleated foreign-body type giant cells, most likely represent-

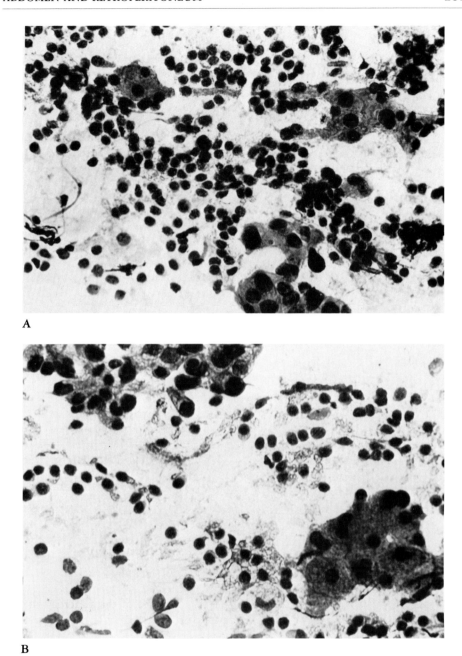

A

B

Fig. 10.11. **A.** Low-power view of aspirate of chronic pancreatitis showing some aniso-nucleosis of acinar cells along with numerous chronic inflammatory cells. (Papanicolaou stain; ×200). **B.** High power view of chronic pancreatitis demonstrating scattering of acinar cells and some lymphocytes (Diff-Quik stain; ×400).

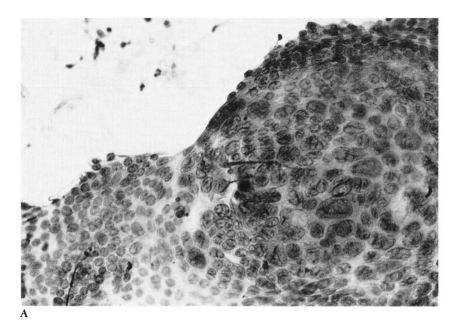

A

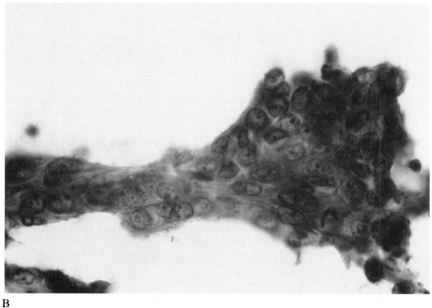

B

Fig. 10.12. A. FNA of well differentiated pancreatic carcinoma showing greater degree of nuclear atypicality including anisonucleosis and nuclear irregularity (Papanicolaou stain; ×200). **B.** High-power view of well differentiated pancreatic carcinoma demonstrating sheet of neoplastic cells showing anisonucleosis with overlapping of nuclei and some loss of polarity (Papanicolaou stain; ×200).

ing changes found in pancreatitis. The benign giant cells were noted in both benign and malignant cases (Fig. 10.13). These multinucleated-type histiocytes need to be differentiated from multinucleated tumor cells which can be found in the usual pancreatic carcinomas and in special types of poorly differentiated pancreatic malignancies, such as pleomorphic giant cell carcinoma of the pancreas and osteoclastic tumor of the pancreas.[20,22,30,31] Walts has presented a differential diagnosis of benign and malignant giant cells found in pancreatic aspirates.[32] The differential diagnosis of benign giant cells include Langhans' type giant cells, foreign-body type giant cells, and multinucleated histiocytes that can occur in the setting of pancreatic abscesses, fat necrosis, pseudocysts, and infectious and sarcoidal granulomas. Langhans'-type giant cells have peripheral bland nuclei without nucleoli. In contrast, foreign-body and multinucleated histiocytes will have haphazardly arranged nuclei or nuclei centrally clustered within the cytoplasm. Benign foreign-body type histiocytes may also contain intracytoplasmic debris. This feature, however, is not specific for benign giant cells, since cytophagocytosis can be seen in tumor giant cells of pleomorphic giant cell carcinoma of the pancreas.[22]

Malignant multinucleated giant cells include cells found in Hodgkin's disease, metastatic carcinoma, metastatic malignant melanoma, trophoblastic tumor, and sarcomas. Primary pancreatic malignancies having multinucleated tumor giant cells include pleomorphic giant cell carcinoma and osteoclastic tumor of the pancreas.[24,30-35] It is important to recognize the malignant nature of the giant cells since pleomorphic giant cell carcinoma and osteoclastic tumor of the pancreas have a worse prognosis than the usual pancreatic carcinoma[31] (Fig. 10.14).

Pancreatic Cysts

Cysts of the pancreas may be classified as congenital, retention, pseudocyst, cystic neoplasmic, or parasitic.[2,5,36] Pseudocysts may be postinflammatory, traumatic, or surgical, although some cases have an unknown etiology. A common denominator of pseudocysts of the pancreas is blockage of the pancreatic ducts with leakage of pancreatic fluid into the surrounding pancreatic tissue which results in necrosis and cyst formation. Pseudocysts lack an epithelial lining and instead have a luminal surface lined by granulation tissue with surrounding fibrosis.

FNA biopsy of a pseudocyst will reveal turbid fluid containing amorphous debris and calcified fragments with only a few inflammatory cells and histiocytes.[2,5] Some multinucleated histiocytes may be present. Fluid from pseudocysts will have an elevated amylase level,[37] in contrast to cystic carcinomas which have elevated levels of carcinoembryonic antigen (CEA) in the fluid.

KIDNEY

Although there has been an increasing number of reports of FNA biopsy of renal masses in recent years,[38,39,40] some controversy concerning its utilization for the diagnosis of renal neoplasia still exists.[8] In the United States, FNA of the kidney is used primarily for the identification or treatment of benign cysts and abscesses.[2] Nonneoplastic mass lesions of the kidney include renal cysts, tuberculosis, abscess,

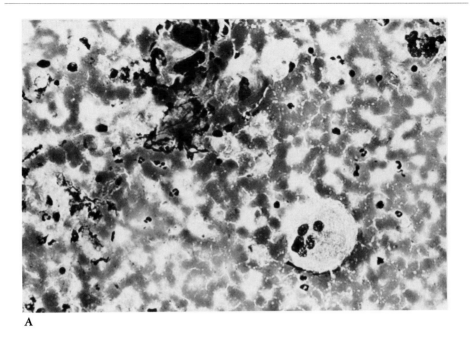

A

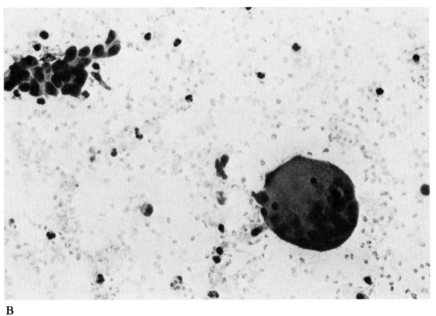

B

Fig. 10.13. A. Multinucleated histiocyte in aspirate of acute pancreatitis (Diff-Quik stain; ×200). B. Scattered multinucleated histiocytes in aspirates of pancreatic carcinoma (Papanicolaou stain; ×200).

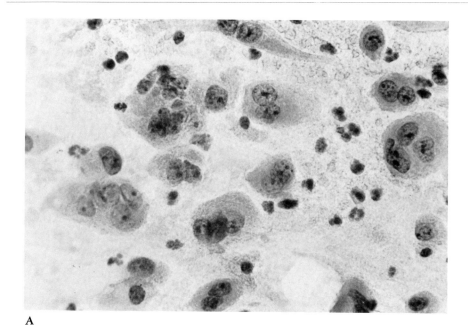

A

B

Fig. 10.14. A. Pleomorphic giant cell carcinoma of the pancreas showing numerous multi-nucleated tumor giant cells arranged in a dissociative fashion (Papanicolaou stain; ×400). **B.** Aspirate of osteoclastic tumor of the pancreas demonstrating numerous multinucleated osteoclastic cells having overlapping nuclei with prominent nucleoli (Diff-Quik stain; ×400). (From Silverman JF, Finley JL, MacDonald KG Jr: Fine-needle aspiration cytology of the pancreas. *Diagn Cytopathol* 6:38–41, 1990. With permission.)

and infarct. The combination of modern imaging techniques such as ultrasonography and computed tomography with percutaneous fine needle biopsy has eliminated the need for surgical exploration of some of these lesions.[1] Renal cysts may be congenital or acquired and single or multiple. Cysts may become infected or hemorrhagic, which can cause acute symptoms of pain and occasionally hematuria.[8] Since renal cell carcinoma may also undergo cystic degeneration with hemorrhage, it is important to aspirate renal cysts for diagnostic purposes.[1,8,41,42]

Cytologic examination of benign renal cysts reveals predominantly scattered macrophages having finely vacuolated cytoplasm with eccentric nuclei. In many cases hemosiderin-laden macrophages are present, indicative of old hemorrhage. Atypical epithelial cells and reactive macrophages can be a potential source for a false-positive diagnosis of malignancy in aspirates of benign cysts.[1,8,38,43] Features in favor of a benign renal cyst include radiologic evidence of a smooth cyst lining, along with cytologic findings of benign cells arranged in small groups or individually scattered and an absence of necrotic cells and debris.[1]

An uncommon cause of renal cyst diagnosed by FNA biopsy is hydatid disease.[44] Frydman and associates reported a case of pulmonary and renal hydatid disease diagnosed by FNA biopsy. The renal hydatid cyst fluid contained scoleces and hooklets of the trematode.

Another unusual finding in renal cysts sampled by FNA biopsy is the presence of Liesegang rings in aspirated hemorrhagic renal cysts.[45] Sneige and associates reported the cytologic findings of Liesegang rings encountered in aspirates of two patients. The periodic ringlike structures ranged in size from 8 microns to 200 microns in diameter and had regularly striated double walls. It is important to recognize Liesegan rings, since they may be readily confused with parasitic organisms such as the giant kidney worm, *Dioctophyma renale*. Although the exact nature of Liesegang rings has yet to be determined, they are believed to represent some form of insoluble precipitate found in hemorrhagic cystic lesions.[45] We have encountered one example of a hemorrhagic cystic lesion of the kidney containing numerous Liesegang rings. The nonpolarizable spherical structures had double walls with equally spaced radial striation. The Liesegang rings were seen both in the smears and in the cell block prepared from the aspirate (Fig. 10.15).

Renal Abscess

Patients with renal abscesses present with chills, fever, severe costovertebral angle pain, tenderness, and pyuria. Renal abscesses are most often seen in patients with acute pyelonephritis or secondary to a systemic inflammatory process. FNA biopsy can be used to both identify and evacuate the abscess.[46] Cytologic examination will demonstrate a purulent exudate consisting of sheets of neutrophils, scattered histiocytes, and necrotic debris in the background. Special stains for organisms including Gram for bacteria, Ziehl–Neelsen for mycobacteria, and GMS for fungi should be performed along with submission of the aspirated material for aerobic, anaerobic, mycobacterial, and fungal cultures.

A potential for a false-positive diagnosis of malignancy exists in aspirates from xanthogranulomatous pyelonephritis and renal infarcts. Misinterpretation of benign foamy histiocytes of xanthogranulomatous pyelonephritis as malignant cells of clear cell carcinoma is possible. In general, an aspirate from well differentiated renal cell

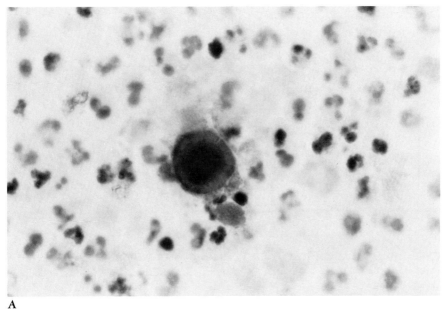

A

B

Fig. 10.15. A. FNA of renal cyst in which numerous Liesegang-like rings were present characterized by periodic ringlike structures having regularly striated double walls (Papanicolaou stain; ×400). **B.** Liesegang ring structures seen in cell block of renal cyst aspirate (H&E stain; ×400).

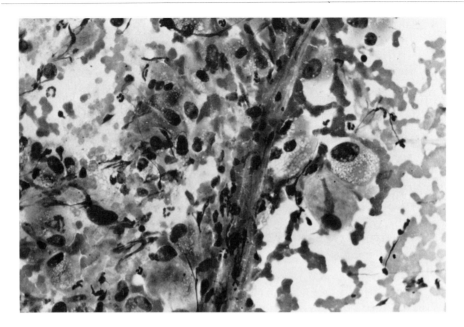

Fig. 10.16. FNA of renal cell carcinoma consisting of clear to vacuolated cells aligned along branching capillaries (Diff-Quik stain; ×200).

carcinoma consists of a cellular specimen in which the cells are arranged in sheets and groups. Many of the clusters will have interspersed thin branching capillaries (Fig. 10.16). The malignant cells, although having abundant clear cytoplasm, will also demonstrate some nuclear enlargement and the presence of nucleoli (Fig. 10.17). The vacuolated appearance of clear cell carcinoma is due to excessive cytoplasmic lipid and glycogen.[1,47,48,49] In contrast, histiocytes from xanthogranulomatous pyelonephritis and fat necrosis are often isolated and associated with other inflammatory cells. Histiocytic nuclei tend to be eccentrically placed within the cell and have a coffee-bean shape. In aspirates from renal infarcts, groups of cells showing atypical changes due to regeneration and repair can be misinterpreted as malignant[50] (Fig. 10.18). Correlation with clinical and radiologic findings is critical.

ADRENAL GLANDS

Although FNA biopsy of the adrenal gland has been used primarily to diagnose primary and metastatic disease, it can be an important tool for the identification of infectious processes.

Granulomatous disease of the adrenal gland is often bilateral.[51] In the past, tuberculosis was an important cause of Addison's disease, accounting for 70% of the cases.[1,52] Today, approximately 30% of Addison's disease is due to tuberculosis. Cytologic findings will demonstrate a granulomatous process with abundant necrotic debris. Ziehl–Neelsen stain should reveal scattered acid-fast bacilli in most cases.

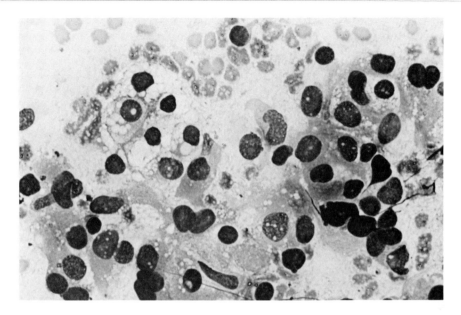

Fig. 10.17. Aspirate of renal cell carcinoma, clear cell type that could be confused with benign histiocytes. Greater degree of nuclear enlargement and nucleoli favor a renal cell carcinoma (Diff-Quik stain; × 400).

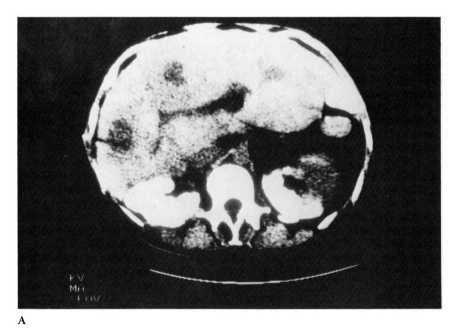

A

Fig. 10.18. A. Renal infarct. CAT scan demonstrating a mass in left kidney along with multiple lesions of the liver. Clinical impression was metastatic renal cell carcinoma to the liver.

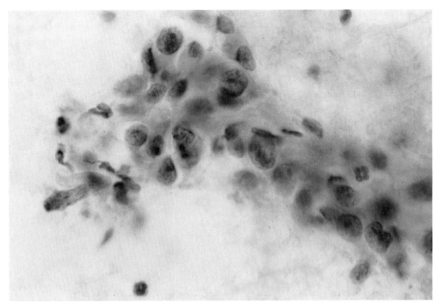

B

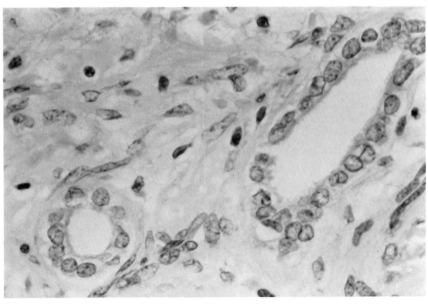

C

Fig. 10.18. B. Aspirate demonstrating scant cellularity consisting of a few clusters of cells arranged in a sheetlike fashion with some variation in nuclear size and shape and small but prominent nucleoli. Aspirate was interpreted as suspicious for malignancy (Papanicolaou stain; ×400). (From Silverman JF, Gurley AM, Harris PT, et al: Fine-needle aspiration cytology of renal infarcts. *Acta Cytol* (in press). With permission.) **C.** Resected renal lesion demonstrating renal infarct with groups of renal tubular cells at the periphery showing features of regeneration and repair.

Tao reported two cases of adrenal tuberculosis diagnosed by FNA biopsy,[1] which is similar to Yee's cytologic report of FNA biopsy of adrenal tuberculosis.[51]

Another cause of granulomatous disease of the adrenal gland is disseminated histoplasmosis. Anderson and associates and Valente and Calafati reported cases of adrenal histoplasmosis diagnosed by FNA biopsy.[53,54] Valente and Calafati commented that with the declining incidence of tuberculosis, *H. capsulatum* may be the most important infectious cause of adrenal failure. In both case reports, diagnostic yeast forms measuring 2 microns to 4 microns in diameter were seen including occasional budding forms and others within macrophages.[53,54] Although disseminated histoplasmosis is rare, when it does occur, it usually involves the adrenal glands.

OTHER RETROPERITONEAL AND ABDOMINAL LESIONS

Nonneoplastic mass lesions of the retroperitoneum are those conditions usually involving retroperitoneal lymph nodes such as chronic lymphadenitis, tuberculosis, lipophagic granulomas following lymphangiography, and Whipple's disease. Other benign lesions that may occur in the retroperitoneum or deep pelvis include abscesses and hematomas. The differential diagnosis should include metastatic tumor undergoing extensive necrosis and inflammation (Fig. 10.19).

Tuberculosis involving the retroperitoneum usually is secondary to periaortic lymph node disease or extension of tuberculosis of the vertebral body (Pott's disease) into the paravertebral soft tissue.[1,55] When it involves the paravertebral soft tissue it may result in little inflammation causing a "cold abscess." The abscess may involve the sheath of the psoas muscle. Cytologic features of granulomatous inflammation will be appreciated, which should suggest the possibility of tuberculosis. Confirmation will be based on special stains for mycobacteria and/or culture.

Most abscesses of the retroperitoneum are bacterial in origin and may be secondary to suppurative abdominal diseases including perforated diverticulitis or pyelonephritis or may appear following trauma or surgery.[1] There have been FNA reports of pelvic actinomycosis in which pyogenic abscesses containing sheets of neutrophils were present, along with colonies of delicately branching, gram-positive organisms ("sulfur granules").[56] Most cases of pelvic actinomycosis have been associated with the use of an IUD. In Lininger and Frable's discussion of pelvic actinomycosis, entities considered in the differential diagnosis include botryomycosis, which consists of dense clusters of rod- or cocci-shaped bacteria and pseudosulfur granules which are noninfectious in origin. Gram stain and culture can assist in making a specific diagnosis.[56]

Kumar and associates recently reported two cases of intestinal malacoplakia diagnosed by aspiration cytology. Malacoplakia is a rare chronic inflammatory disorder that usually involves the urinary tract (especially the bladder), but the disorder has also been reported to involve the gastrointestinal tract, genital structures, skin, lung, bone, brain, soft tissue, and adrenal glands.[57] In two cases reported by Kumar's group, the percutaneous abdominal FNA showed the presence of histiocytes and neutrophils. Within many of the macrophages, target-shape laminated structures

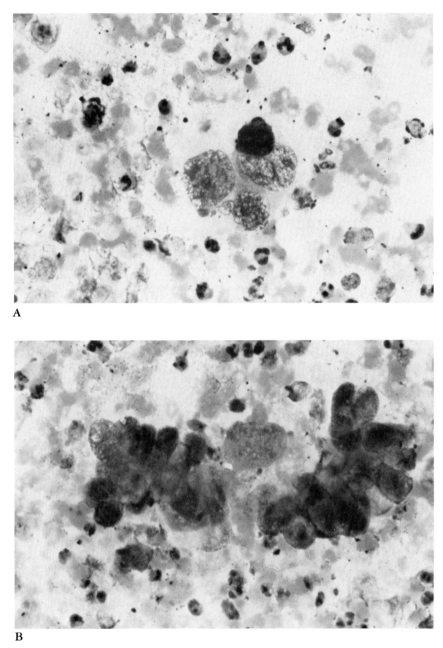

Fig. 10.19. A. Metastatic colonic carcinoma to retroperitoneum undergoing extensive necrosis and acute inflammation. Only rare groups of tumor cells were seen as noted by the small cluster of three malignant cells (Diff-Quik stain; ×400). **B.** Other fields show degenerating and necrotic cells of metastatic colonic carcinoma along with acute inflammation. Note the palisading alignment of the malignant cells (Diff-Quik stain; ×400).

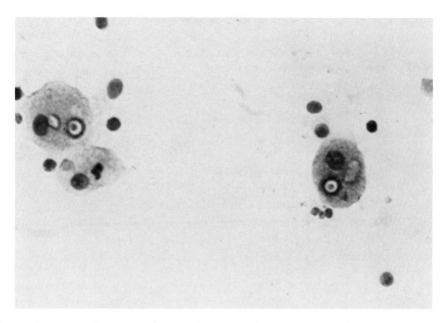

Fig. 10.20. Michaelis-Gutman bodies characterized by target-shaped laminated structures within macrophages (PAS stain; × 100).

termed Michaelis-Gutmann bodies were present, which were periodic acid–Schiff (PAS) positive following diastase digestion (Fig. 10.20). The Michaelis-Gutmann bodies also stained positively with the von Kossa stain for calcium salts. It is important to recognize the target or owl-eyed laminated Michaelis-Gutmann inclusion bodies and not confuse them with fungi.

REFERENCES

1. Tao L-C: Transabdominal Fine-Needle Aspiration Biopsy. New York, Igaku-Shoin, 1990.
2. Kline TS: Handbook of Fine Needle Aspiration Biopsy Cytology, ed. 2, New York, Churchill Livingstone, 1988.
3. Walsh TJ, Berkman W, Brown NL, et al: Cytopathologic diagnosis of extracolonic amebiasis. *Acta Cytol* 27:671–675, 1983.
4. Nosher JL, Plafker J: Fine needle aspiration of the liver with ultrasound guidance. *Radiology* 136:177–180, 1980.
5. Frias-Hidvegi D: Guides to Clinical Aspiration Biopsy. Liver and Pancreas. New York, Igaku-Shoin, 1988.
6. Agarwal PK, Husain N, Singh BN: Cytologic findings in aspirated hydatid fluid. *Acta Cytol* 33:652–654, 1989.
7. Saphir O: A Text on Systemic Pathology. Orlando, FL, Gune & Stratton, 1959.
8. Koss LG, Woyke S, Olszewski W: Aspiration Biopsy. Cytologic Interpretation and Histologic Bases. New York, Igaku-Shoin, 1984.

9. Stormby N, Akerman M: Aspiration cytology in the diagnosis of granulomatous liver lesions. *Acta Cytol* 17:200–204, 1973.

10. Tao LC, Morgan RC, Donat EE: Cytologic diagnosis of intravenous talc granulomatosis by fine needle aspiration biopsy. *Acta Cytol* 28:737–739, 1984.

11. Johansen S, Myren J: Fine-needle aspiration biopsy smears in the diagnosis of liver diseases. *Scand J Gastroenterol* 6:583–588, 1971.

12. Perry MD, Johnston WW: Needle biopsy of the liver for the diagnosis of nonneoplastic liver diseases. *Acta Cytol* 29:385–390, 1985.

13. Brits CJ: Liver aspiration cytology. *S Afr Med J* 48:2207–2214, 1974.

14. Henriques UV, Hasselstrom K: Evaluation of jaundice: fine-needle aspiration liver cytology of a discriminating tool. *Dan Med Bull* 24:104–108, 1977.

15. Lundqvist A: Fine-needle aspiration biopsy of the liver. *Acta Med Scand* 520:1–28, 1971.

16. Nguyen G-K: Fine needle aspiration biopsy cytology of hepatic tumors in adults. *Pathol Annu* 21 (part 1):321–349, 1986.

17. Edmondson HA, Steiner PE: Primary carcinoma of the liver: an autopsy study of 100 cases among 48,900 necropsies. *Cancer* 7:462–502, 1978.

18. Lupovitch A, Chen R, Mishra S: Inflammatory pseudotumor of the liver. Report of the fine needle aspiration cytologic findings in a case initially misdiagnosed as malignant. *Acta Cytol* 33:259–262, 1989.

19. Hales MS, Miller TR: Diagnosis of xanthogranulomatous cholecystitis by fine needle aspiration biopsy. A case report. *Acta Cytol* 31:493–496, 1987.

20. Silverman JF, Finley JL, Berns L, et al: Significance of giant cells in fine-needle aspiration biopsies of benign and malignant lesions of the pancreas. *Diagn Cytopathol* 5:388–391, 1989.

21. Hastrup J, Thommesen P, Frederiksen P: Pancreatitis and pancreatic carcinoma, diagnosed by peroperative fine needle aspiration biopsy. *Acta Cytol* 21:731–734, 1977.

22. Silverman JF, Dabbs DJ, Finley JL: Fine-needle aspiration biopsy of pleomorphic (giant cell) carcinoma of the pancreas. Cytologic, immunocytochemical, and ultrastructural findings. *Am J Clin Pathol* 89:8–14, 1988.

23. Fekete PS, Nunez C, Pitlik DA: Fine-needle aspiration biopsy of the pancreas. *Diagn Cytopathol* 2:301–306, 1986.

24. Hajdu EO, Kumari-Subaiya S, Phillips G: Ultrasonically guided percutaneous aspiration biopsy of the pancreas. *Semin Diagn Pathol* 3:166–175, 1986.

25. Mitchell ML, Carney CN: Cytologic criteria for the diagnosis of pancreatic carcinoma. *Am J Clin Pathol* 83:171–176, 1985.

26. Sneige N, Ordonez NG, Veanattukalathil S, et al: Fine-needle aspiration cytology in pancreatic endocrine tumors. *Diagn Cytopathol* 3:35–40, 1987.

27. Tao LC, Ho CS, McLoughlin MJ, et al: Percutaneous fine needle aspiration biopsy of the pancreas: cytodiagnosis of pancreatic carcinoma. *Acta Cytol* 22:215–220, 1978.

28. Lightwood R, Reber HA, Way LW: The risk and accuracy of pancreatic biopsy. *Am J Surg* 132:189–194, 1976.

29. Schultz NJ, Sanders RJ: Evaluation of pancreatic biopsy. *Ann Surg* 158:1053–1057, 1963.

30. Manci EA, Gardner LL, Pollock WJ, et al: Osteoclastic giant cell tumor of the pancreas. Aspiration cytology, light microscopic, and ultrastructure with review of the literature. *Diagn Cytopathol* 1:105–110, 1985.

31. Silverman JF, Finley JL, MacDonald KG Jr: Fine-needle aspiration cytology of osteoclastic giant cell tumor of the pancreas. *Diagn Cytopathol* 6:38–41, 1990.

32. Walts AE: Osteoclast-type giant cell tumor of the pancreas. *Acta Cytol* 27:500–504, 1983.

33. Rosai J: Carcinoma of pancreas simulating giant cell tumor of bone. Electron-microscopic evidence of its acinar cell origin. *Cancer* 22:333–344, 1968.

34. Baniel J, Konichezky M, Wolloch Y: Osteoclast-like giant cell tumor of the pancreas. *Acta Chir Scand* 153:67–69, 1987.

35. Jeffrey I, Crow J, Willis BL: Osteoclast-type giant cell tumour of the pancreas. *J Clin Pathol* 36:1165–1170, 1983.

36. Cubilla AL, Fitzgerald PJ: Tumors of the Exocrine Pancreas. Atlas of Tumor Pathology. Washington, DC: Armed Forces Institute of Pathology, 1984, Second Series, *fasc* 19, p 60.

37. Pinto MM, Kaye AD, Brogan DA, et al: Diagnosis of cystic lesions of the pancreas. A biochemical and cytologic analysis of material obtained utilizing radiographic or intraoperative technique. *Diagn Cytopathol* 2:40–45, 1986.

38. Helm CW, Burwood RJ, Harrison NW, et al: Aspiration cytology of solid renal tumors. *Br J Urol* 55:249–253, 1983.

39. Juul N, Torp-Pederson S, Grnvall S: Ultrasonically guided fine needle aspiration biopsy of renal masses. *J Urol* 133:579–581, 1985.

40. Linsk JA, Franzen S: Aspiration cytology of metastatic hypernephroma. *Acta Cytol* 28:250–260, 1984.

41. Ambrose SS, Lewis EL, O'Brien DP III, et al: Unsuspected renal tumors associated with renal cysts. *J Urol* 117:704–707, 1977.

42. Deweerd JH: Percutaneous aspiration of selected expanding renal lesions. *J Urol* 87:303–308, 1962.

43. Plowden KM, Erozan YS, Frost JK: Cellular atypia associated with benign lesions of the kidney as seen as fine needle aspirates. *Acta Cytol* 28:648, 1984.

44. Frydman CP, Raissi S, Watson CW: An unusual pulmonary and renal presentation of echinococcosis. Report of a case. *Acta Cytol* 33:655–658, 1989.

45. Sneige N, Dekmezian R, Zaatari GS: Liesegang-like rings in fine needle aspirates of renal/perirenal hemorrhagic cysts. *Acta Cytol* 32:547–551, 1988.

46. Conrad MR, Sanders RC, Mascardo AD: Perinephric abscess aspiration using ultrasound guidance. *AJR* 128:459–464, 1977.

47. Meisels A: Cytology of carcinoma of the kidney. *Acta Cytol* 7:239–244, 1963.

48. Suen KC: Guides to Clinical Aspiration Biopsy: Retroperitoneum and Intestine. New York, Igaku-Shoin, 1988.

49. Zajicek J: Aspiration Biopsy Cytology. Part 2. Cytology of Infradiaphragmatic Organs. Basel, Karger, 1979.

50. Silverman JF, Gurley AM, Harris PJ, et al: Fine-needle aspiration cytology of renal infarcts: cytomorphologic findings and potential diagnostic pitfalls. *Acta Cytol* (in press).

51. Symington T: Functional Pathology of the Human Adrenal Gland. Edinburgh, E & S Livingstone, 1969, pp 78–79.

52. Yee ACN, Gopinath N, Ho C-H, et al: Fine-needle aspiration biopsy of adrenal tuberculosis. *J Can Assoc Radiol* 37:287–289, 1986.

53. Anderson CJ, Pitts WC, Weiss LM: Disseminated histoplasmosis diagnosed by fine needle aspiration biopsy of the adrenal gland. A case report. *Acta Cytol* 33:337–340, 1989.

54. Valente PT, Calafati SA: Diagnosis of disseminated histoplasmosis by fine needle aspiration of the adrenal gland. *Acta Cytol* 33:341–343, 1989.

55. Silverman JF, Larkin EW, Carney M, et al: Fine needle aspiration cytology of tuberculosis of the lumbar vertebrae (Pott's disease). *Acta Cytol* 30:538–542, 1986.

56. Lininger JR, Frable WJ: Diagnosis of pelvic actinomycosis by fine needle aspiration. A case report. *Acta Cytol* 28:601–604, 1984.

57. Kumar PV, Hambarsoomina B, Banani SA, et al: Diagnosis of intestinal malakoplakia by fine needle aspiration cytology. *Acta Cytol* 31:53–56, 1987.

11

Superficial and Deep Lesions of Soft Tissue, Bone, and Prostate

SOFT TISSUE

In aspiration cytology, accurate diagnosis of benign and neoplastic soft tissue lesions can be challenging and difficult. This difficulty is due mainly to the great variety of morphologic patterns seen in both reparative processes and soft tissue neoplasia and the overlapping cytologic features of mesenchymal repair with certain sarcomas.[1] The difficulty in arriving at a correct cytologic diagnosis is compounded by a relatively limited cytologic literature on this topic.[2-5] In addition, tissue repair is a common biologic process closely associated with an inflammatory response. In conventional exfoliative gynecologic and nongynecologic cytology, cells of epithelial repair and regeneration are commonly seen, because these cells are derived from the sampled mucosal surface. It can be anticipated that mesenchymal repair cells will also be encountered in aspirated primary inflammatory soft tissue lesions and followup FNA biopsies from those patients having a prior surgical procedure, irradiation, chemotherapy, or other treatment. It is critical that the cytomorphologic features of mesenchymal repair and other reactive soft tissue lesions be appreciated so that a false-positive diagnosis of malignancy is avoided (Table 11.1).

Mesenchymal Repair

Tissue repair is a common biologic process associated with inflammation as part of the healing process. Although the cytologic features of epithelial regeneration and repair have been well described,[6,7,8] mesenchymal repair has not been adequately studied until recently.[9] James reported the cytologic features of mesenchymal regeneration and repair seen in a series of aspiration biopsies that sampled fibrous connective tissue, skeletal muscle, adipose tissue, and bone.[9] In general, mesenchymal repair is characterized by sparse cellularity set in an inflammatory background and consisting of individual cells and loose cell clusters. There is greater cellular

277

TABLE 11.1. Nonneoplastic Soft Tissue Legions

Mesenchymal repair
Fat necrosis
Endometriosis
Granular cell tumor
Nodular fasciitis
Fibromatosis
Proliferative fasciitis
Proliferative myositis
Rheumatoid and pseudorheumatoid nodule
Myospherulosis
Ganglion cysts
Granulomatous inflammation
Myositis ossificans

variability in mesenchymal repair than epithelial repair, whereas cells usually occur in greater numbers in epithelial repair (Table 11.2).[6-9] Depending on the site, there may be evidence of cellular maturation and differentiation in some examples of mesenchymal repair.[9]

Fibrous Tissue Repair

In fibrous connective tissue repair, cells derived from granulation tissue or active fibrosis can be seen (Figs. 11.1 and 11.2). In general, the cellularity of granulation tissue is sparse but is associated with a background of hemorrhage, inflammation, and granular debris. Active fibrosis shows greater cellularity and tends to have a cleaner background.[9] The predominant cell type in granulation tissue are the reactive fibroblasts and/or myofibroblasts, which usually are arranged singly and in widely spaced, loosely cohesive clusters (Fig. 11.3). In early granulation tissue, the fibroblasts are somewhat enlarged with poorly delineated cytoplasm having a fibrillar quality. The fibroblast nucleus is centrally located and has a kidney-bean shape that expands the midportion of the cell. The nuclei tend to taper at both ends, although an occasional twisted nucleus can be present. The nuclear chromatin may be mildly hyperchromatic with a small nucleolus. In organizing granulation-type tissue, the fibroblasts tend to have a more bland appearance with a delicate chroma-

TABLE 11.2. Differences Between Epithelial and Mesenchymal Repair

	Epithelial Repair	Mesenchymal Repair
Cellularity	Variable	Usually sparse
Background	Inflammatory	Inflammatory
Cellular arrangement	Cohesive sheets	Loose aggregates; single cells
Cell uniformity	Uniform	Variable
Evidence of cell maturation	Variable	Common (dependent on site)

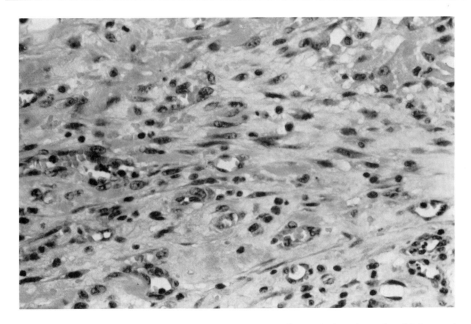

Fig. 11.1. Example of mesenchymal repair consisting of granulation tissue in which reactive fibroblasts and myofibroblasts are present associated with blood vessels and a sprinkling of a few chronic inflammatory cells (H&E stain; ×400).

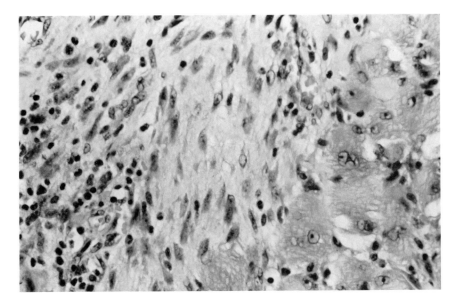

Fig. 11.2. Active fibrosis in which fibroblastic cells are arranged in a more cohesive fashion. Also present are foci of skeletal muscle repair and some chronic inflammation (H&E stain; ×400).

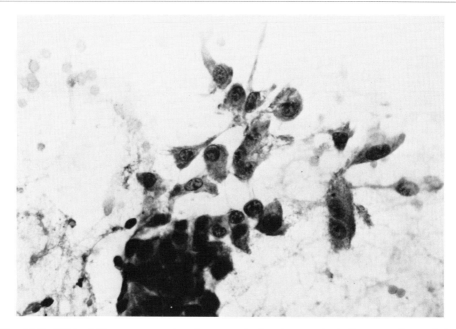

Fig. 11.3. FNA of fibrous connective tissue repair showing cytologic features of granulation tissue, characterized by scattered fibroblasts having tapering cytoplasm and centrally located nuclei that expand the midportion of the cell (Papanicolaou stain; ×400).

tin pattern. In active fibrosis, fibroblasts show features similar to those of granulation tissue, although there is a greater tendency of the cells to be arranged in loose clusters and small tissue fragments (Fig. 11.4). In James' experience, aspirates from fibromatosis show similar features to active fibrosis including sparse cellularity, clean background, and no significant pleomorphism.[9] This is similar to other reports of fibromatosis, in which the aspirates had limited cellularity and consisted of occasional clusters of uniform spindle-shaped cells.[10,11]

Aspirates of fibromatoses should generate cytologic diagnoses that include mesenchymal reactive lesions, benign connective tissue tumors, and some low grade sarcomas.[10,11,12] Tani and associates reported a case of bilateral fibromatosis of the breast in a 22-year-old woman which demonstrated cellular smears consisting of numerous fibroblastic-type stromal cells and small fragments of collagen.[12] In our experience, fibromatosis tends to be more cellular than fibroblastic-type mesenchymal repair although there are overlapping morphologic features that can be cytologically challenging in some cases (Fig. 11.5).

Nodular fasciitis is another benign proliferation of connective tissue that shares cytologic features with fibroblastic mesenchymal repair and fibromatosis.[13,14] Nodular fasciitis most often occurs in the upper extremities, especially the forearm, but can be present in any location as demonstrated in Fritsches' FNA report of nodular fasciitis of the breast.[13] In Dahl and Akerman's series, besides fibroblastic type cells, ganglion-like cells were also appreciated, raising the possibility of proliferative fasciitis. The ganglion-like cells were plump and had polyhedral or triangular shapes with one to two nuclei and prominent nucleoli. In some of the cases, increased numbers of neutrophils, eosinophils, and macrophages were seen, whereas other

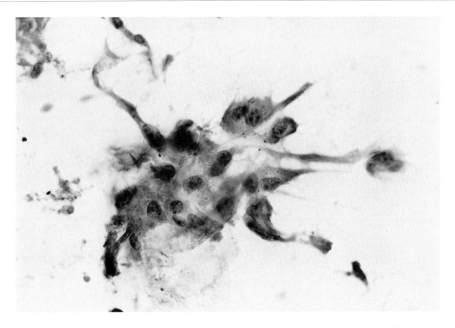

Fig. 11.4. FNA of fibrous connective tissue repair showing features of active fibrosis characterized by greater tendency of the cells to be arranged in loose clusters and small tissue fragments (Papanicolaou stain; ×400).

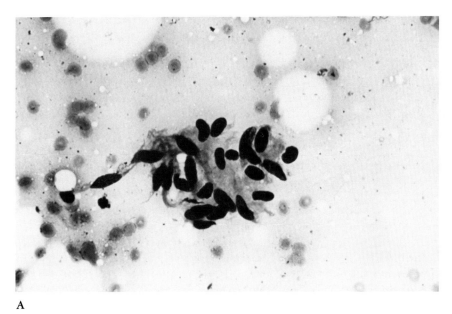

A

Fig. 11.5. A. FNA of fibromatosis of arm in 18-year-old woman showing cytologic features overlapping with mesenchymal repair and fasciitis. The cohesive nature of the fragment is more in keeping with fibromatosis (Diff-Quik stain; ×200).

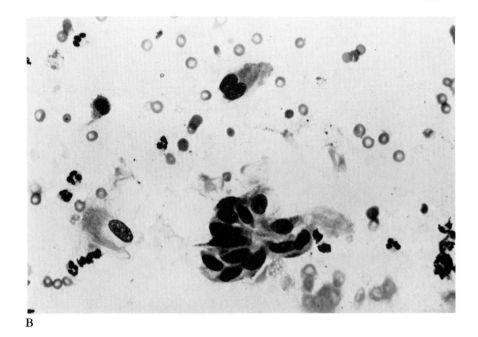

B

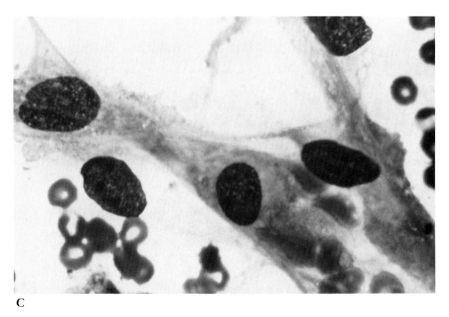

C

Fig. 11.5. B. Overall scanty cellularity in aspirate of fibromatosis. Note cohesive group of fibroblastic type cells along with a few individually scattered cells (Diff-Quik stain; ×400). C. High-power view of fibromatosis demonstrating spindle-shaped cells arranged in a loosely cohesive fashion and having oval to slightly elongated nuclei and surrounding fibrillary cytoplasm (Diff-Quik stain; ×630).

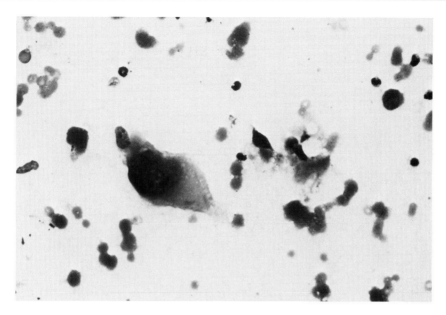

Fig. 11.6. Aspirate showing cells demonstrating skeletal muscle repair. The myoblasts are fusiform in shape and possess large irregular hyperchromatic nuclei (Diff-Quik stain; ×400).

cases had a myxoid fibrillary background stroma. In our experience, nodular fasciitis shares similar features with fibromatosis and some cases of mesenchymal repair. Also considered in the differential diagnosis are sarcomas, especially when the aspirate is cellular and shows increased numbers of mitotic figures.[14] Dahl and Akerman believe that low grade fibrosarcomas have a more uniform population of cells in contrast to the varied cellular composition of nodular fasciitis.[14]

Skeletal Muscle Repair

Fine-needle aspiration biopsies of masses demonstrating skeletal muscle repair will generally contain sparse cellularity with an inflammatory and/or hemorrhagic background consisting of granular debris, occasional neutrophils, and histiocytes. Owing to the biologic ontogeny of skeletal muscle, skeletal muscle repair demonstrates greater morphologic variation and cellular heterogeneity than other types of mesenchymal regeneration and repair.[9] Some of the myoblasts are spindled to fusiform in shape and are arranged singly or in small groups. At this stage of development, cross-striations are not usually identified. Instead, a small to moderate amount of ill-defined pale fibrillar cytoplasm is seen with eccentrically placed irregular to oval nuclei that tend to be large and hyperchromatic (Fig. 11.6). Occasional myoblasts will align and fuse to form early myotubes.[9] These cells are round, contain more abundant cytoplasm, and are multinucleated (Fig. 11.7). Again, the cytoplasm is granular to fibrillar with no evidence of cross-striations. Although many of the nuclei in the myotube stage show similar features to the myoblasts, other cells have a peripheral arrangement of the nuclei with prominent nucleoli. Multinucleated myofibers will have cross-striations in the cytoplasm (Fig. 11.8). All of the foregoing

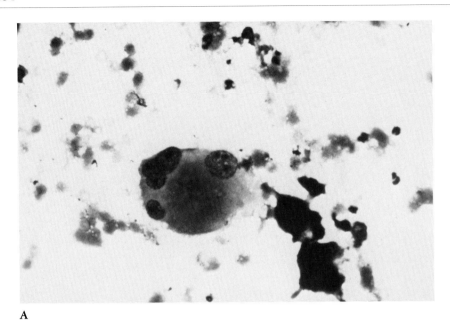

A

B

Fig. 11.7. A. Polygonal shape myoblast demonstrating multinucleation and abundant cyto-plasm (Diff-Quik stain; ×400). **B.** Aspirate of mesenchymal repair demonstrating myoblastic and fibroblastic cells. The myoblasts are polygonal to irregular in shape, including some demonstrating multinucleation. The fibroblasts have a more spindled configuration (Diff-Quik stain; ×400).

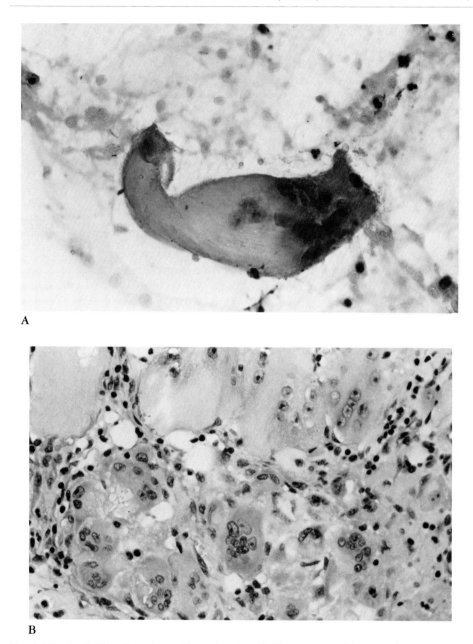

A

B

Fig. 11.8. A. Multinucleated myofibers showing fibrillary nature of the cytoplasm (Papanico-laou stain; ×630). **B.** Histologic section demonstrating skeletal muscle repair characterized by proliferation of myoblastic cells, the majority of which are multinucleated and vary from oval to elongated in shape (H&E; ×400).

cytologic features demonstrate the great variability and pleomorphism of regenerating skeletal muscle fibers. Considered in the differential diagnosis of skeletal muscle repair and regeneration are benign entities such as proliferative fasciitis and myositis ossificans, and malignancies such as pleomorphic sarcomas.

Proliferative fasciitis usually presents as an ill-defined mass involving subcutaneous tissue and/or underlying skeletal muscle in adults with a peak age incidence between 40 to 70 years.[15] Anglo-Henry reported a case of proliferative fasciitis examined by FNA biopsy in a 35-year-old woman presenting with a rapidly growing nodule of the right forearm.[15] Cytologic findings demonstrated variably sized spindle-shaped cells arranged predominantly in a dissociative fashion along with numerous larger polygonal ganglion-type cells having one or two eccentric nuclei with prominent nucleoli. In the air-dried Wright–Giemsa stain, the cytoplasm had a finely vacuolated appearance. Considered in the differential diagnosis was proliferative myositis, which is the intramuscular counterpart of proliferative fasciitis. Therefore, these two entities cannot be cytologically distinguished.[15] An FNA report of myositis ossificans demonstrated immature fibroblasts and scattered skeletal muscle cells in various stages of degeneration.[16] The authors noted that the reactive proliferating nature of the cells could potentially lead to a false-positive diagnosis of sarcoma. This is especially true in the early phase of skeletal muscle repair when nuclear enlargement, hyperchromasia, and nucleolar prominence may simulate the cytomorphologic features of pleomorphic sarcomas. Therefore, to avoid a false-positive diagnosis of malignancy, a conservative approach is needed in interpreting aspirates of soft tissue lesions. In general, pleomorphic sarcomas are more cellular and consist of atypical-appearing cells arranged singly and in syncytial clusters. Often, necrosis will be noted in the background. A definite diagnosis of sarcoma should not be rendered in sparsely cellular FNA specimens of soft tissue lesions.

Repair of Adipose Tissue and Fat Necrosis

Aspirates of repair and regeneration of adipose tissue will generally be moderately cellular and set in an inflamed, necrotic, and hemorrhagic background in which some granular type debris will be present. Most often, the inflammatory exudate will consist of macrophages and lymphocytes. Fibroblastic cells will also be identified. Diagnostic cells are lipoblasts, lipocytes, and macrophages (Fig. 11.9). Macrophages generally have abundant cytoplasm containing small lipid vacuoles (Fig. 11.10). Lipocytes may have enlarged nuclei and multivacuolated cytoplasm with sharp cytoplasmic borders giving the cells a globoid shape.[9] Individual lipid vacuoles tend to be sharply outlined and can give the nucleus a scalloped border. This feature may simulate cytologic findings of myxoid liposarcoma.[17] Diagnostic cytomorphologic features favoring the diagnosis of myxoid liposarcoma in FNA biopsy include cellular smears containing lipoblasts set in a myxoid background and having an associated branching capillary network (Fig. 11.11).

Fat necrosis has a greater degree of inflammation and necrotic debris, along with numerous macrophages and lipoblast-like cells smaller than the lipoblasts of myxoid liposarcoma.[18] Akerman and Rydholm reported the cytologic findings of 20 liposarcomas in an FNA series of 72 lipomatous tumors. The authors discussed the cytologic similarities and differences that can occur in aspirates of soft tissue tumors that

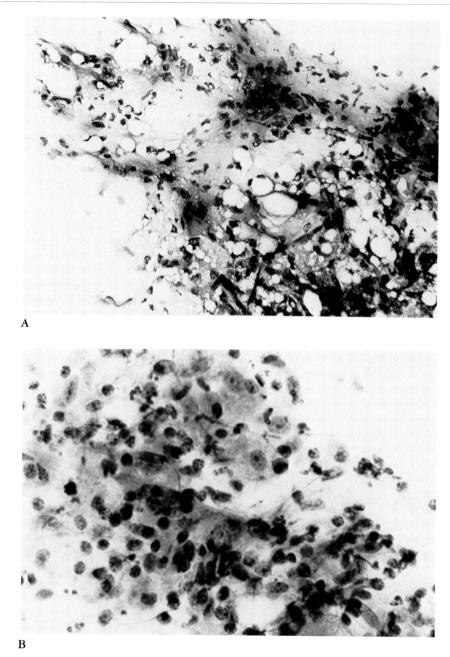

A

B

Fig. 11.9. A. Aspirate of fat necrosis consisting of lobules of fat undergoing necrosis with associated granulation type tissue and some inflammation (Diff-Quik stain; ×100). **B.** High-power view showing loose sheets of histiocytes along with granulation-type tissue and acute inflammation in aspirate of fat necrosis (Diff-Quik stain; ×200).

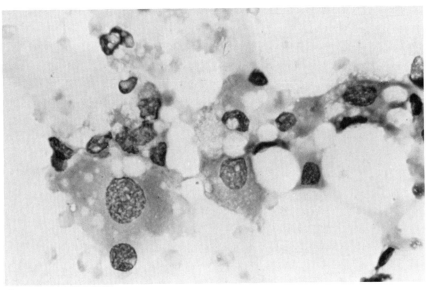

A

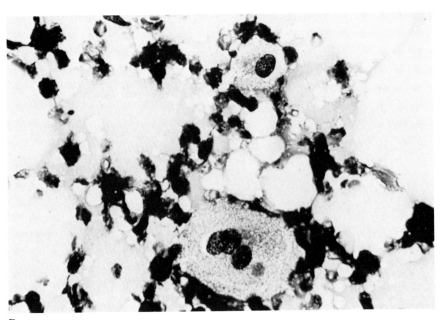

B

Fig. 11.10. **A.** Scattered macrophages having abundant cytoplasm and intracytoplasmic small vacuoles in an aspirate of fat necrosis (Diff-Quik stain; ×400). **B.** Coarsely vacuolated histiocytes including one showing multinucleation in aspirate of fat necrosis (Diff-Quik stain; ×400).

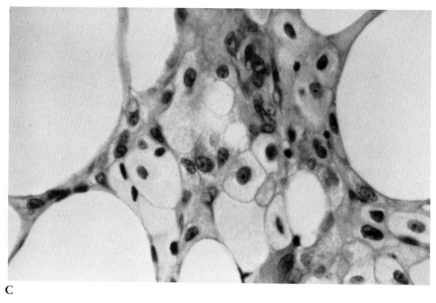

C

Fig. 11.10. C. Histologic section of fat necrosis showing lobules of fat in which interspersed collections of vacuolated histiocytes are present (H&E stain; ×400).

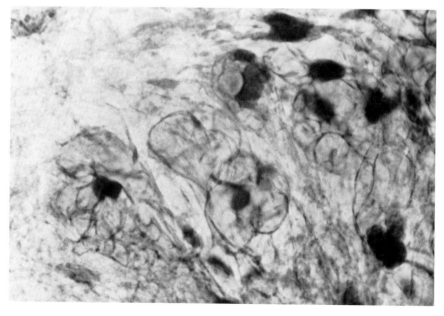

Fig. 11.11. Aspirate of liposarcoma in which lipoblasts are present having coarsely vacuolated cytoplasm and scalloping of the nuclei (Papanicolaou stain; ×600).

could potentially be misdiagnosed as liposarcoma.[17] These include intramuscular myxoma, myxofibrosarcoma, and malignant fibrous histiocytoma. Mucin-producing adenocarcinomas metastatic to subcutaneous tissue and metastatic clear cell carcinoma to soft tissue can potentially be misdiagnosed as fat necrosis.[18] Metastatic adenocarcinoma will show evidence of glandular differentiation and cytologic features of malignancy. Mucin-containing signet cells may also be present. In clear cell carcinoma of the kidney, the cells have a greater degree of nuclear atypicality with the presence of more prominent nucleoli, in contrast to the usually bland vacuolated macrophages of fat necrosis (Fig. 11.12).

Soft Tissue Neoplasms

In general, FNAs of sarcomas are more cellular and atypical than reparative processes. Benign and malignant soft tissue tumors make up a large heterogeneous group of neoplasms because of their different cells of origin. This factor along with the differentiation or grade of the tumors accounts for the great morphologic variability encountered in aspirates of sarcomas.[19-42] Clinical information such as the patient's age and the site of the lesion is often quite helpful in arriving at a correct diagnosis. Although the cytologic features will occasionally suggest the correct diagnosis, often a specific classification cannot be rendered from the cytologic material.[42,43] A useful simple cytologic classification of sarcoma consists of categorizing the malignancy into spindle cell, pleomorphic, round cell, epithelioid, or poorly differentiated neoplasms. Spindle cell sarcomas include fibrosarcoma, synovial sarcoma, some malignant fibrous histiocytomas, leiomyosarcoma, malignant schwannoma, and hemangiopericytoma.

Malignant schwannomas have cells with an elongated spindle shape and a characteristic thin nucleus. The nuclei are uniformly long with a pyknotic structure and the cytoplasm is finely fibrillar and variable in length. The cells are often arranged in small clusters or twisted conglomerates (Fig. 11.13).

Cytologically, fibrosarcomas consist of medium-sized, round, or oval cells and/or short, uniform, spindle-shaped cells. The nuclei are well defined and pale and are surrounded by well preserved cytoplasm with no vacuoles or granularity. Mononucleated or multinucleated giant cells are uncommon.

Synovial sarcomas consist of spindle to round epithelioid cells with a high nuclear to cytoplasmic ratio. In smears, the cells are characteristically arranged in small clusters or cords and have definite cohesion. Solitary cells are rarely seen and mononucleated or multinucleated giant cells are not a feature.

Leiomyosarcomas demonstrate long spindle-shaped to oval cells showing only slight variation in size and shape, although a rare giant tumor cell or bizarre single or multinucleated cell may be present. The nuclei are cigar-shaped and elongated and therefore blunter than those of fibroblasts and shorter than those of malignant schwannoma (Fig. 11.14). A prominent longitudinal and transverse "fishbone" alignment of the nuclear chromatin is said to be a diagnostic feature.[42] The tumor cells have little cytoplasmic cohesion but are arranged in clusters or side by side.

Malignant fibrous histiocytoma demonstrates a variety of cell types, with spindle-shaped cells, pleomorphic giant cells, undifferentiated mesenchymal-type cells, and rare signet-ring lipoblastic-like cells present (Fig. 11.15).

Pleomorphic sarcomas include malignant fibrous histiocytoma, some liposarco-

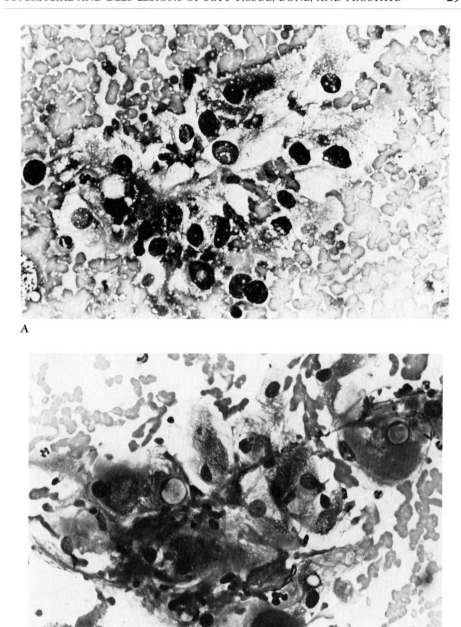

Fig. 11.12. A. Aspirate of clear cell carcinoma of the kidney metastatic to soft tissue consisting of loose sheets of clear to vacuolated cells demonstrating a greater degree of nuclear enlargement and hyperchromasia than would be seen in histiocytes from fat necrosis. Also note prominent nucleoli (Diff-Quik stain; ×200). **B.** High-power view of metastatic clear cell carcinoma of kidney to soft tissue. Loose cluster of atypical cells is seen, including some possessing intranuclear cytoplasmic inclusions (Diff-Quik stain; ×400).

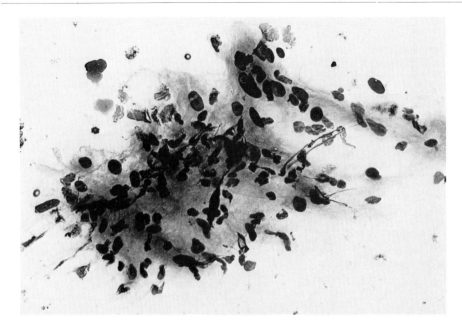

Fig. 11.13. FNA of low grade malignant schwannoma demonstrating cells arranged in small clusters set in a fibrous type matrix. Neoplastic cells have spindled nuclei that have a twisted configuration (Diff-Quik stain; ×200).

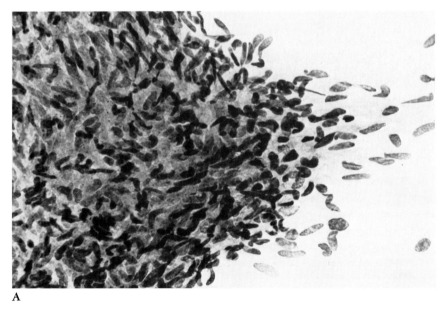

A

Fig. 11.14. A. FNA of retroperitoneal leiomyosarcoma consisting of microtissue fragment of spindle-shaped cells (Diff-Quik stain; ×200).

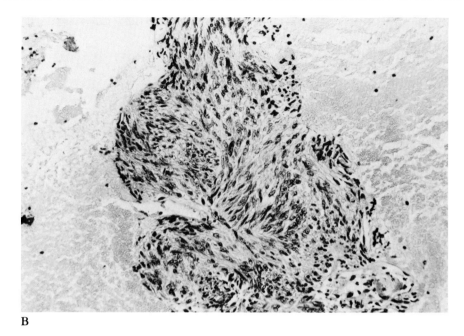

B

C

Fig. 11.14. B. Cell block from aspirate of leiomyosarcoma demonstrating interlacing fascicles of malignant smooth muscle cells (H&E; ×200). **C.** High power view of immunoperoxidase stain for desmin demonstrating positive cytoplasmic staining of the neoplastic muscle cells (×630).

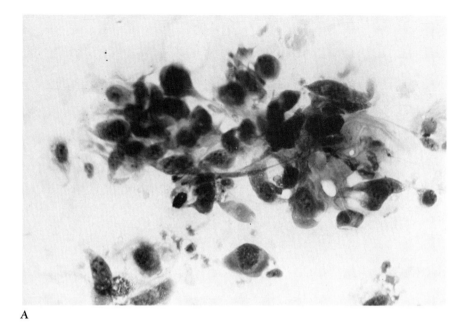

A

B

Fig. 11.15. A. Loose cluster of spindle-shaped cells in aspirate of malignant fibrous histiocytoma (Papanicolaou stain; ×400). **B.** Loose aggregate of neoplastic spindle-shaped cells
including demonstrating atypical mitotic figures in aspirate of malignant fibrous histiocytoma
(Papanicolaou stain; ×200).

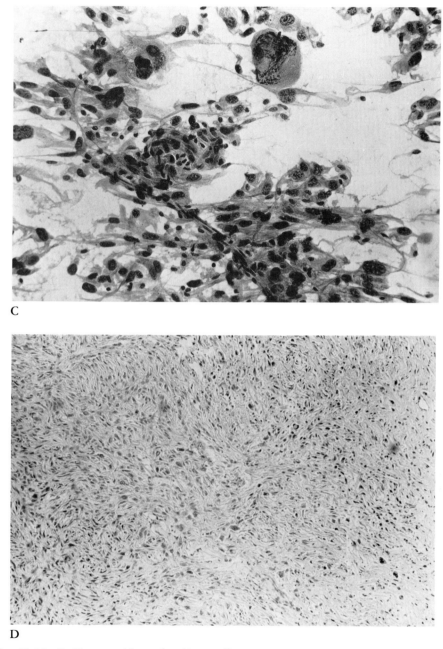

Fig. 11.15. C. Pleomorphism of malignant fibrous histiocytoma in aspirate of malignant fibrous histiocytoma. Note the presence of both atypical spindled and multinucleated tumor giant cells (Papanicolaou stain; × 200). D. Resected lesion showing characteristic storiform pattern of malignant fibrous histiocytoma (H&E; × 100).

mas, and rhabdomyosarcoma. Poorly differentiated or undifferentiated round cell sarcomas include some liposarcomas, rhabdomyosarcoma, Ewing's sarcoma, and some epithelioid sarcomas. Epithelioid patterns can be seen in high grade leiomyoblastoma, chordoma, chondroid sarcoma, clear cell sarcoma of tenosynovium, and epithelioid sarcoma, along with a number of benign neoplasms.[42] Aspirates from many sarcomas of skeletal muscle or adipose derivation may show differentiated cytologic features such as cross-striations of rhabdomyoblasts that can suggest the cell of origin. In some cases of malignant fibrous histiocytoma, a storiform pattern will be seen, and aspirates of angiosarcoma may demonstrate the vascular nature of the neoplasm[41] (Fig. 11.16). In many aspirates of soft tissue sarcoma, however, correct classification will require immunocytochemical studies or ultrastructural examination of the aspirated material for a more definitive diagnosis. Often, examination of the resected specimen with ancillary studies is needed for a specific diagnosis.[22,25,31,36,39,41,42] The presence or absence of background matrix, such as myxoid stroma, cartilage, or osteoid or fibroconnective tissue may also aid in better classifying the sarcoma.

In general, although most aspirates from sarcomas will show cells arranged either individually or in a loosely cohesive fashion, microtissue fragments can be present. Useful parameters to evaluate the grade of the sarcoma include differentiation, cellularity, necrosis, amount of stroma, vascularity, and number of mitoses. Some of these features can be estimated from the cytologic examination.[42]

Uncommon Soft Tissue Lesions

A number of other uncommon soft tissue lesions have been encountered in FNA biopsy. A case of *subcutaneous endometriosis* has been reported in which the diagnosis was suggested when three-dimensional clusters of epithelial cells were appreciated in an aspirate of the soft tissue.[44] The uniform cytologic appearance of these epithelial cells should not suggest a malignant diagnosis (Fig. 11.17).

With the Romanovsky stain, aspirates from *granular cell tumors* will generally reveal a cellular specimen consisting of scattered groups of cells with abundant granular cytoplasm and indistinct cell borders.[45] With the Papanicolaou stain, the cytoplasm has a reddish hue (Fig. 11.18). Granular cells have oval to round, uniform nuclei having an evenly dispersed chromatin pattern and occasional nucleoli. Granular cells are positive with the PAS stain. Immunocytochemical studies performed on the cytologic material will demonstrate S-100 and CEA positivity, although the S-100 staining may be decreased in alcohol-fixed smears.[46] Ultrastructural examination shows the presence of autophagosome and angulate body granules[47] (Fig. 11.19).

Zamora and associates reported the FNA cytologic findings of solitary *pseudorheumatoid nodules* in two pediatric patients.[48] Both children presented with subcutaneous nodular masses involving the left elbow and forearm, respectively. Neither patient had clinical or laboratory evidence of rheumatoid arthritis. Grossly, the aspirate had a creamy consistency. Cytologically it was found to consist of necrotic granular and filamentous background material accompanied by a granulomatous inflammatory infiltrate. The differential diagnosis of other necrotizing granulomatous, inflammatory-type lesions of the soft tissue should be considered, including tuberculosis, leprosy, sarcoid, and fungal infections. The authors point out the

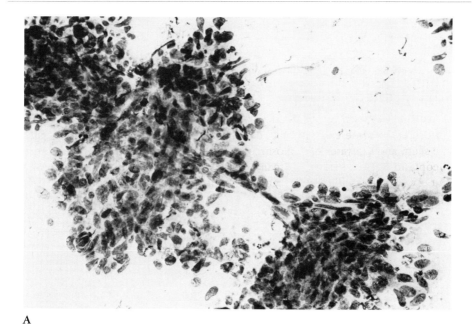

A

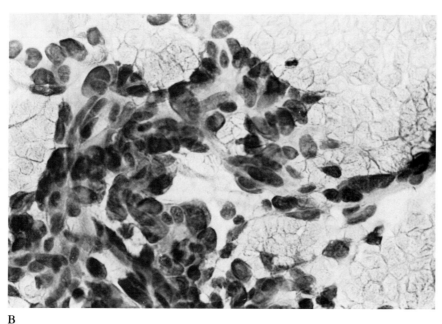

B

Fig. 11.16. A. Aspirate of retroperitoneal angiosarcoma demonstrating neoplastic cells arranged in clusters, including areas showing atypical cells lining vascular spaces (Diff-Quik stain; ×100). **B.** High-power view demonstrating vascular nature of the neoplasm in an aspirate of angiosarcoma of the retroperitoneum (Diff-Quik stain; ×400).

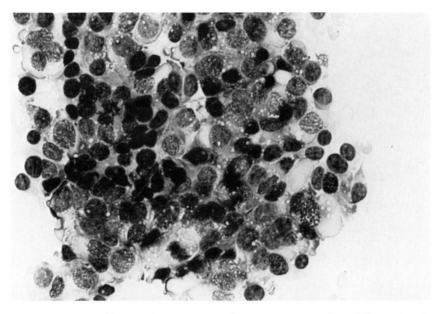

Fig. 11.17. Aspirate of benign follicular cyst of the ovary attached to abdominal wall and thereby causing a mass lesion thought to represent a soft tissue neoplasm. Uniform cuboidal nature of the cells suggests the possibility of a benign epithelial lesion (Diff-Quik stain; ×400).

helpful role of special stains for organisms in arriving at a correct diagnosis. Cytologically, aspirates from leprosy will show multinucleated histiocytes with numerous vacuoles (globus cells) and positive staining for mycobacteria. In sarcoidosis, besides granulomatous inflammation, Schaumann and asteroid bodies may be present.

Vuong reported a case of FNA cytologic diagnosis of *myospherulosis of the soft tissue* secondary to intramuscular injections of petrolatum-based hormones.[49] Myospherulosis is a disease process characterized by subcutaneous and intramuscular inflammatory pseudocystic masses containing saccular structures resembling a bag of marbles.[49,50] This iatrogenic lesion is believed to be secondary to erythrocytes sequestered by petrolatum-based material arranging themselves into characteristic saccular structures. Cytologic findings from an aspirate of the gluteal region demonstrated numerous saccular formations of variable sizes and shapes including structures containing spherules or endobodies the size of red blood cells (Fig. 11.20). These structures can be confused with fungi such as *Coccidioides immitis*.

Another type of soft tissue lesion examined by FNA biopsy is *ganglion cyst*.[51,52] The aspirate grossly has a colorless to pale yellow gelatinous appearance and consists of monotonous smears containing abundant metachromatically staining mucoid material along with individually scattered histiocytes, small clusters of vacuolated macrophages, and some collagen fibers (Fig. 11.21).

FNA biopsy has also been used to diagnose *soft tissue infections*.[53] Conditions that have been sampled include decubitus, diabetic, ischemic, venous, and traumatic ulcers, cellulitis, and infected surgical wounds. Often the entire specimen is submit-

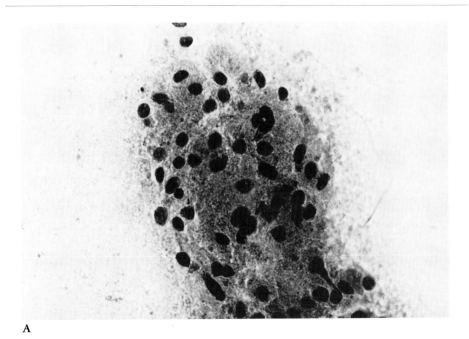

A

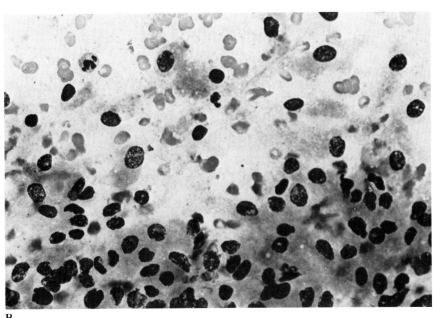

B

Fig. 11.18. A. FNA biopsy of soft tissue mass involving shoulder. Features of granular cell tumor are appreciated including oval to spindled cells having prominent reddish cytoplasmic granularity (Papanicolaou stain; ×200). **B.** Aspirate of granular cell tumor consisting of loose sheets of oval to spindle cells with granular cytoplasm (Diff-Quik stain; ×200).

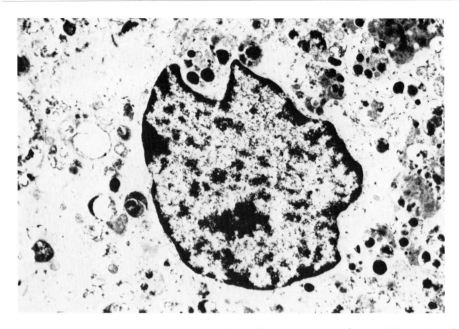

Fig. 11.19. Ultrastructural examination performed on the aspirated material showing the presence of autophagosomes and angulate body granules.

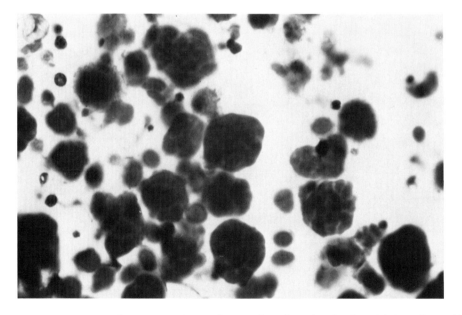

Fig. 11.20. Aspirate of myospherulosis of cervical neck region in the vicinity of parotid gland showing the presence of saccular-like structures containing endobodies. Note that these structures could easily be confused with fungi such as the spherules of coccidioidomycosis (Papanicolaou stain; ×400).

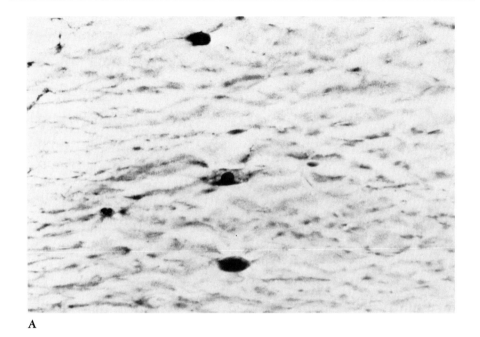

A

B

Fig. 11.21. **A.** Aspirate of ganglion cyst consisting of a few scattered histiocytic cells set in a metachromatically staining mucoid stroma (Diff-Quik stain; × 200). **B.** High-power view of vacuolated histiocytes and background mucoid material in aspirate of ganglion cyst (Diff-Quik stain; × 400).

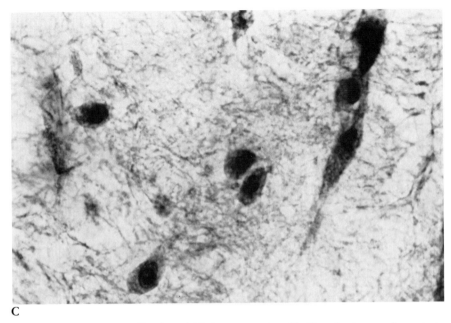

C

Fig. 11.21. C. Oval to spindle-shaped histiocytes set in a fibrillary background matrix in an aspirate of ganglion cyst (Papanicolaou stain; ×400).

ted for culture. We recommend that cytologic smears also be prepared so that the cellular reaction can be ascertained and organisms, if present, can be rapidly identified. It is suggested that FNA biopsy of deep tissue infection is a reliable and clinically useful technique that helps provide guidelines for further antimicrobial therapy.

BONE

In general, a combined clinical, radiologic, and pathologic examination is necessary for an accurate diagnosis of bone lesions.[1,54-57] Traditionally, open bone biopsy has been required to obtain adequate tissue for examination. FNA biopsy has been shown to be of value in the diagnosis of both primary and metastatic malignant tumors of the bone, since many of these lesions are lytic or have soft tissue extension.[55,56] Aspiration cytology is also beneficial for the evaluation of nonneoplastic bone lesions (Table 11.3).

TABLE 11.3. Nonneoplastic Bone Lesions

Bone repair and fracture
Granulomatous inflammation
Acute or chronic osteomyelitis
Eosinophilic granuloma

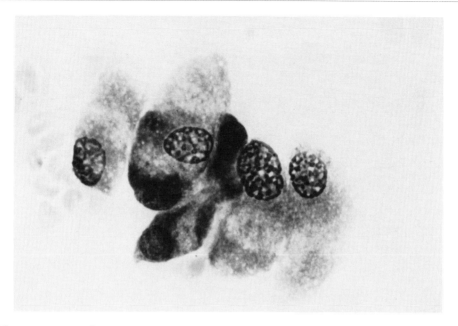

Fig. 11.22. Osteoblast having columnar to flame shape with indistinct cell borders and eccentrically placed nuclei. Note midzonal area of cytoplasmic clearing which is different from paranuclear clearing of plasma cells (Diff-Quik stain; × 1000).

Bone Regeneration and Repair

Bone regeneration and repair is usually synonymous with healing fractures or changes secondary to osteomyelitis or tumor.[9] In bone aspirates demonstrating repair, the cellularity is generally sparse and consists of osteoblasts arranged singly and in loose clusters. Osteoid may be identified as metachromatically staining dense acellular material in the Wright–Giemsa stains. Reactive osteoblasts tend to be columnar to flame-shaped with indistinct cell borders and an eccentrically placed nucleus (Fig. 11.22). A midzonal band of cytoplasmic clearing is present, in contrast to paranuclear clearing of plasma cells. Osteoclasts may be present in more destructive bone lesions and are characterized by large multinucleated cells with indistinct to ruffled cytoplasmic borders[9] (Fig. 11.23). The cells can have up to several dozen nuclei possessing delicate chromatin with small nucleoli. In osteomyelitis, an inflammatory background is present. In contrast, aspirates from osteosarcoma tend to be cellular with necrosis and contain a variable amount of osteoid in the background. Besides atypical osteoblasts, undifferentiated spindled and giant cells are present, arranged singly and in loose clusters. The greater cellularity and pleomorphism help differentiate osteosarcoma from osteoblastic repair.

Specific Nonneoplastic Bone Lesions

There have been only a few reports describing the FNA cytologic findings of specific nonneoplastic bone lesions.[53,56-60] We have previously reported the cytomorphologic features of tuberculosis of the lumbar vertebrae.[54] FNA biopsy was

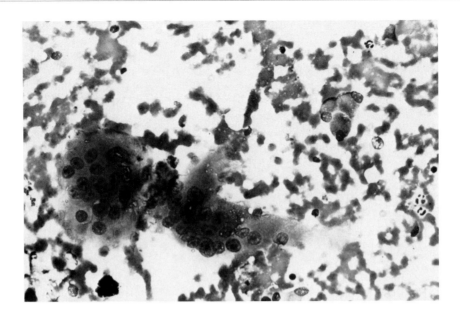

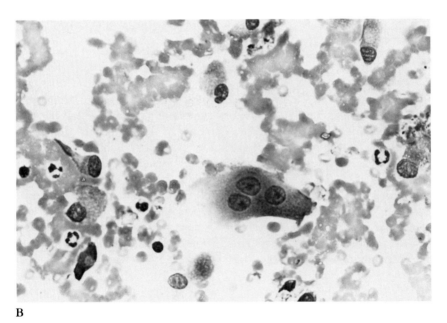

B

Fig. 11.23. A. Scattered osteoclasts having abundant cytoplasm with multiple nuclei possessing delicate chromatin with small nucleoli (Diff-Quik stain; × 200). **B.** High-power view of osteoclast demonstrating multinucleation with prominent nucleoli. A few scattered osteoblasts are also present (Diff-Quik stain; × 400).

performed in a 72-year-old woman with a prior history of malignant lymphoma treated by chemotherapy. Cytologic examination revealed microtissue fragments of cohesive cells including epithelioid histiocytes and scattered multinucleated Langhans'-type giant cells (Fig. 11.24). The diagnosis was confirmed by culture of the aspirated material. FNA biopsy has also been of value in diagnosing nonneoplastic bony lesions, such as histiocytosis X,[59,62,63] eosinophilic granuloma,[1,60] cryptococcosis,[58] actinomycosis,[65] and osteomyelitis.[61,66]

Thommesen and associates reported a series of 16 patients in whom the diagnosis of histiocytosis X was confirmed in five of nine patients by FNA cytology.[63] We have examined FNA biopsies of three cases of *Langerhans' cell histiocytosis* (eosinophilic granuloma) of bone in children (mean age 8.3 years; range 5–11 years). Two patients presented with vertebral lesions and the third had a femoral mass. Cytomorphologic features of eosinophilic granuloma were seen in all cases, including the presence of Langerhans' cell histiocytes having oval to reniform nuclei with nuclear grooving and abundant pale cytoplasm (Fig. 11.25). The background showed a polymorphic population of cells including neutrophils, lymphocytes, foamy histiocytes, and osteoclasts (Fig. 11.26). A moderate number of eosinophils were seen in two cases, but eosinophils were sparse in the third case. Ancillary immunocytochemical studies performed on the aspirated material demonstrated positive staining for S-100 protein (all three cases) and T-6 antigen (one case). Ultrastructural examination performed in one case demonstrated characteristic Birbeck granules in the histiocytes (Fig. 11.27). A specific cytologic diagnosis was made in all cases, enabling proper chemotherapy in one case, surgical excision in another, and spontaneous resolution in the third case. Our experience demonstrates that FNA cytology can make a definitive diagnosis of eosinophilic granuloma, especially when coupled with ancillary studies such as immunocytochemistry and ultrastructural examination on the aspirated material.

Lupovitch and associates reported a case of *osteomyelitis of the pubis* diagnosed by FNA biopsy.[61] As expected, an acute inflammatory cell exudate of neutrophils, necrotic bone, and intracytoplasmic bacteria was present, both in the FNA smears and cell block (Fig. 11.28). The presence of bacteria was confirmed by Gram staining of the FNA smears and positive culture of the aspirate. Frable[65] emphasized the efficacy of culturing the FNA material from bone lesions when diagnosing inflammatory lesions, since the inflammatory findings can be limited or nonspecific. Lee and associates also support the submission of aspirates from osteomyelitis for culture confirmation.[53]

PROSTATE

Aspiration biopsy cytology of the prostate is a common diagnostic procedure.[67] The procedure is used mainly to differentiate benign prostatic hyperplasia from prostatic carcinoma, although occasionally, inflammatory conditions will be encountered[67-70] (Table 11.4). Aspiration biopsy of the prostate is containdicated when active prostatitis is present.[69,70,71] However, even experienced urologists may find it difficult to distinguish prostatitis from prostatic carcinoma on the basis of physical examination. This is reflected by a number of reports documenting cases of prostatitis

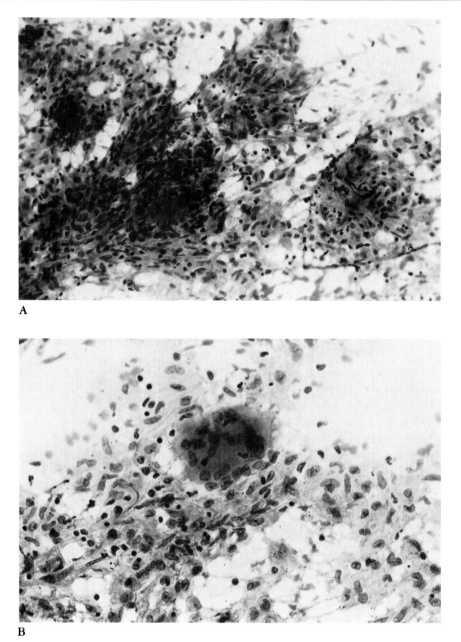

A

B

Fig. 11.24. A. FNA biopsy of Pott's disease (tuberculosis of vertebrae). Note microtissue fragments of granulomatous inflammation (Papanicolaou stain; × 200). **B.** High-power view of aspirate of tuberculosis of lumbar vertebra demonstrating multinucleated Langhans'-type giant cells, along with loose clusters of epithelioid histiocytes (Papanicolaou stain; × 400).

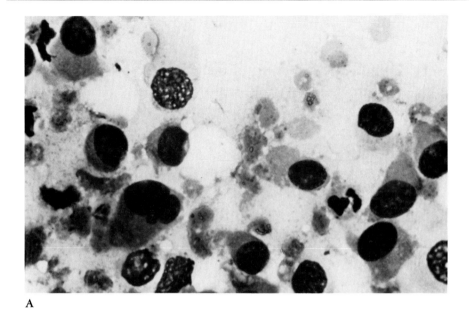

A

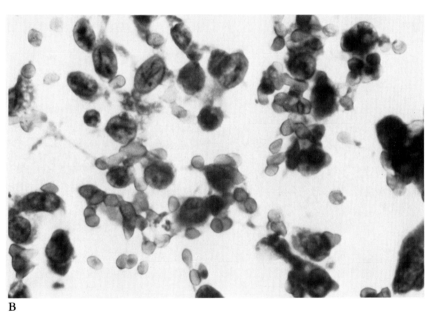

B

Fig. 11.25. **A.** Aspirate of eosinophilic granuloma of bone demonstrating numerous Langerhans'-type histiocytes having oval nuclei with surrounding pale cytoplasm. A few multinucleated cells are present (Diff-Quik stain; × 400). **B.** Langerhans' cells from aspirate of eosinophilic granuloma of bone. Note delicate chromatin pattern and nuclear grooving (Papanicolaou stain; × 400).

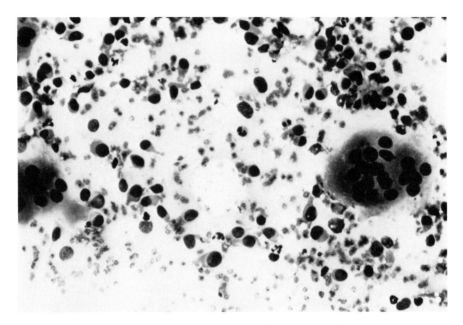

Fig. 11.26. Low-power view of Langerhans' cell histiocytosis of bone showing numerous individually scattered Langerhans' cells, along with some neutrophils and occasional osteo-clast (Diff-Quik stain; ×100).

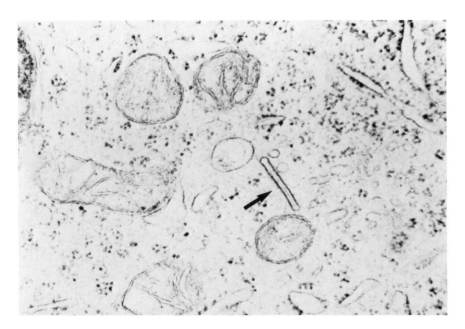

Fig. 11.27. Ultrastructural examination of aspirated material showing trilaminar Birbeck granules in the histiocytes consistent with Langerhans' cell histiocytosis (*arrow*).

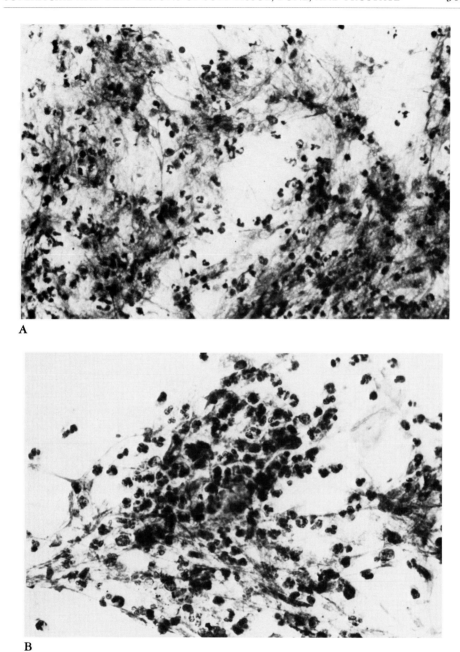

Fig. 11.28. A. Aspirate of acute osteomyelitis of clavicle in 27-month-old child. Note sheets of neutrophils and debris in the background (Diff-Quik stain; × 100). **B.** Aspirate of staphylococcal abscess of lumbar vertebra showing sheets of neutrophils (Papanicolaou stain; × 400).

TABLE 11.4. Nonneoplastic Prostate Lesions

Acute prostatitis
Chronic prostatitis
Infectious granulomatous inflammation
Noninfectious granuloma
Spermatic granuloma
Malakoplakia
Prostatic infarct
Radiation and/or chemotherapy–induced atypia

diagnosed by FNA biopsy.[68,69,72,73] When prostatitis is sampled, there is a potential for a false-positive diagnosis of malignancy owing to the accompanying epithelial changes.[67,69,70,72] This is compounded by prostatitis coexisting with carcinoma in a number of cases.[69] In a recent report detailing the results of 250 consecutive aspiration biopsy specimens of the prostate, prostatitis was found in over 45% of the patients.[69] However, in 14.1% of the patients with prostatitis, concomitant adenocarcinoma was present. Therefore, an accurate diagnosis depends on adhering to strict cytologic criteria for malignancy and awareness of the cellular patterns of inflammatory atypias encountered in aspirates from patients with prostatitis.

Acute Prostatitis

Acute prostatitis results in a tender swollen prostate gland which, owing to its firmness, may clinically simulate carcinoma.[67] The infection is most often due to bacteria with gonococci, staphylococci, streptococci, or *E. coli* the most common agents. Rarely, fungi such as cryptococci or *Blastomyces* may cause acute prostatitis. Aspiration biopsy cytology of acute prostatitis produces cellular smears consisting predominantly of neutrophils with a few histiocytes, lymphocytes, and some debris. The acinar cells may be arranged in loosely cohesive groups in which there may be loss of polarity of the cells. The individual cells may also have indistinct cell borders. Some nuclear enlargement with anisonucleosis, clumped chromatin, and prominent nucleoli may be present, leading to a possible false-positive diagnosis of malignancy (Fig. 11.29). However, adenocarcinoma of the prostate will usually demonstrate increased cellularity and discohesion of the cells along with greater anisonucleosis, nuclear membrane irregularity, and more prominent macronucleoli.[74] Other features of malignancy including loss of nuclear polarity, nuclear crowding, cell enlargement and acinar formation may also be present in aspirates of prostatic adenocarcinoma (Figs. 11.30, 11.31). Since prostatitis (especially acute prostatitis), can also demonstrate some of these features, a conservative diagnostic approach is recommended whenever significant inflammation is present in the smears. Usually, however, acute prostatitis will also contain some epithelial sheets maintaining a honeycomb configuration along with other benign features.

Chronic Prostatitis

Chronic prostatitis can clinically simulate carcinoma on palpation. The prostate gland is characteristically firm, enlarged, and focally nodular.[67] In Faul and Schmidt's

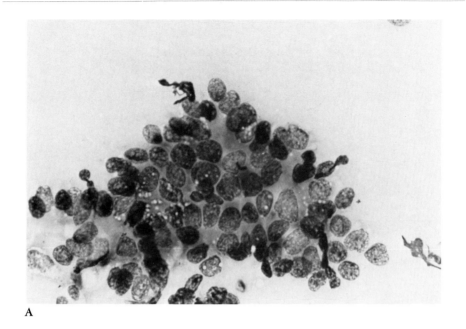

A

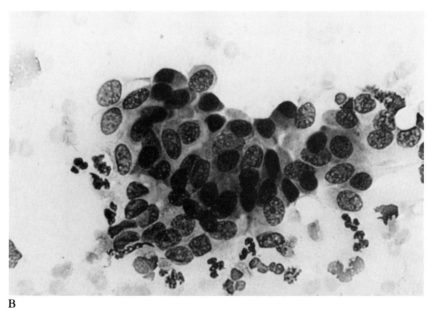

B

Fig. 11.29. **A.** Aspirate of acute prostatitis demonstrating atypical prostatic acinar cells. Note the presence of nuclear enlargement with anisonucleosis and overlapping of nuclei (Diff-Quik stain; ×400). **B.** Atypical acinar cells in aspirate of acute prostatitis. Note nuclear enlargement with some overlapping. The presence of neutrophils should elicit a conservative approach (Diff-Quik stain; ×400).

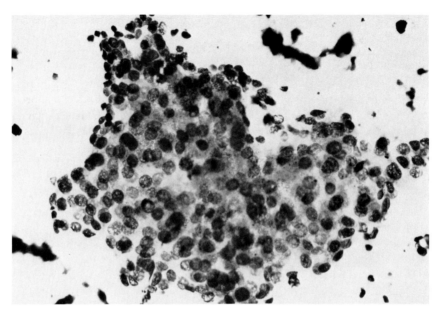

Fig. 11.30. Aspirate of well differentiated prostatic carcinoma showing features that overlap with inflammatory atypia seen in acute prostatitis. Note the presence of nuclear overlapping with loss of honeycomb pattern (Diff-Quik stain; × 200).

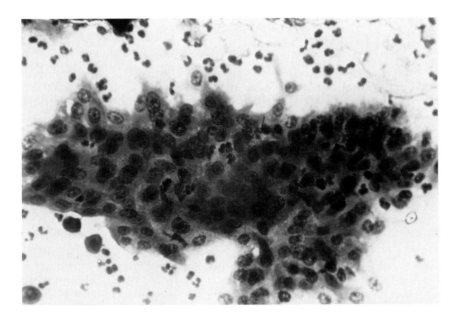

Fig. 11.31. Syncytial sheet of atypical acinar cells in aspirate of acute prostatitis. Note nuclear overlapping with presence of small nucleoli in many of the cells. A conservative diagnostic approach is recommended whenever significant acute inflammation, as noted in this specimen, is appreciated (Diff-Quik stain; × 200).

study of 350 patients with lesions clinically suspicious for prostatic carcinoma on palpation, nearly half the patients had chronic prostatitis. ABC of chronic prostatitis will demonstrate cellular smears with a polymorphic population of inflammatory cells including histiocytes, lymphocytes, and some neutrophils. In comparison with acute prostatitis, neutrophils are decreased in numbers, but increased numbers of histiocytes will be present. Epithelial atypia is generally less than what is appreciated in acute prostatitis. However, as reported by Kline, epithelial changes such as dyshesion of the cells with anisonucleosis, nuclear enlargement, hyperchromasia, and prominence of nucleoli including eosinophilic macronucleoli may be present in chronic prostatitis, creating a potential for a false-positive diagnosis of malignancy.[67] Kline notes that prostatitis can be mistaken for well differentiated carcinoma.[67,70,75,76,77] This potential for a misdiagnosis of carcinoma has been noted by others such as Epstein, who reported that the first eight cases of prostatitis she encountered in a series of 118 prostatic biopsies were interpreted as malignant.[77] Kline recommends that when prostatitis is present along with epithelial atypia, aspiration biopsy should be repeated 4 to 8 weeks after antibiotic therapy, unless there is a concomitant core biopsy that can either exclude or confirm the presence of carcinoma.[67] Another potential source for a false-positive diagnosis of malignancy is the presence of immature metaplastic cells in chronic prostatitis.[69]

Granulomatous Prostatitis

Granulomatous prostatitis is an uncommon inflammatory process which may have a number of different causes.[72,78-81] It may clinically present as a diffuse or nodular enlargement of the prostate with increased induration of the gland that can also simulate carcinoma. Granulomatous prostatitis has been subclassified into noninfectious and infectious types.[72] The noninfectious type may have an allergic or nonallergic origin. The noninfectious, nonallergic type of prostatitis is most common, with an incidence in biopsy material of approximately 3%.[80] It has been proposed that this form of granulomatous prostatitis represents an autoimmune reaction to prostatic secretions released following obstruction of the prostatic ducts. A variant of granulomatous prostatitis having increased numbers of eosinophils has been associated with asthma, vasculitis, and allergies.[82] Infectious granulomatous prostatitis may be due to fungi, tuberculosis, syphilis, or protozoan infections. Other causes of granulomatous prostatitis include prior prostatic surgery, herpes zoster infection, bacillus Calmette-Guerin (BCG) immunotherapy for bladder carcinoma, and vasculitis.[83] Cytologic findings of granulomatous prostatitis include the presence of epithelioid histiocytes and multinucleated giant cells associated with predominantly chronic inflammatory cells (Fig. 11.32). The epithelioid cells can be found singly or in small to large clusters. The multinucleated giant cells may also demonstrate some phagocytosis including digestion of degenerating granulocytes, corpora amylacea, and amorphous prostatic secretions. In tuberculous prostatitis, granular eosinophilic material and cellular debris consistent with caseation necrosis may be present.[72] The diagnosis can be confirmed with special stains for AFB on the smears and/or culture of the aspirate. In eosinophilic prostatitis the aspirate will contain numerous eosinophils associated with small clusters of epithelioid histiocytes but no multinucleated giant cells.[72] Special stains for fungi and/or culture will be helpful in diagnosing specific infectious agents such as *Blastomyces,* cryptococci, or other

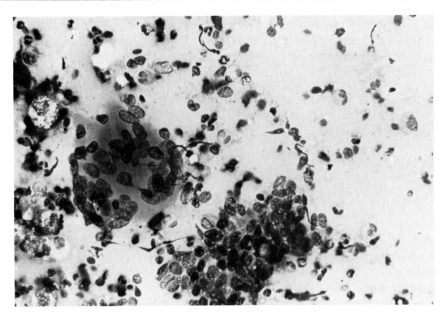

Fig. 11.32. Aspirate of granulomatous prostatitis showing the presence of clusters of atypical prostatic acinar cells along with multinucleated histiocytes. Note the extensive inflammation in the background (Diff-Quik stain; × 200).

fungi (Fig. 11.33). In Miralles' series of 868 prostatic aspirates, 18 examples (2%) of granulomatous prostatitis were encountered.[72] Stilmant and associates reported four patients having cytologic evidence of granulomatous prostatitis induced by BCG immunotherapy for bladder cancer.[83] Almost all the authors have noted that granulomatous prostatitis can also be misdiagnosed as carcinoma if the cytologic features of the inflammatory process are not recognized.[67,68,70,72,83]

Other Urologic Granulomatous Lesions

Other unusual urologic granulomatous processes diagnosed by FNA cytology include spermatic granuloma.[84] *Spermatic granulomas* are tumorlike lesions that occur adjacent to the testis or seminal vesicles and are usually associated with infection, trauma, or prior surgery. Perez-Guillermo and associates described the cytologic findings of three cases characterized by granulomatous inflammation, intrahistiocytic and extracellular spermatozoids, lymphoid cells, and rare plasma cells and eosinophils.[84] Epididymal epithelium may also be present. The spermatozoids could easily be overlooked since they often lack tails. Diagnostic features of sperm heads include well defined edges and pointed ends best seen in the Papanicolaou-stained smears as well as a two-toned basophilic staining with the May–Grunwald–Giemsa stain.

Another unusual type of granulomatous process that can involve the urologic system is *malakoplakia*. The etiology of malakoplakia is not certain, although it is believed to be secondary to abnormal intraphagosomal digestion of bacteria by histiocytes.[85-89] Cazzaniga and associates reported three cases of prostatic mala-

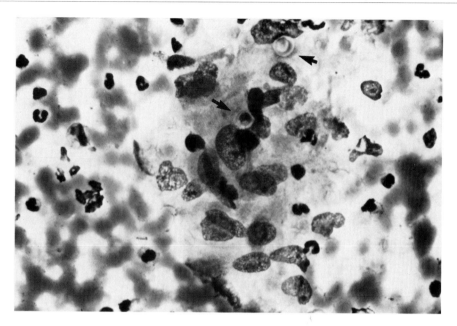

Fig. 11.33. Aspirate of granulomatous prostatitis due to blastomycosis. Note the cluster of epithelioid histiocytes in which a rare intracytoplasmic organism is present (*arrow*) (Diff-Quik stain; ×400).

koplakia diagnosed by FNA biopsy and compared the aspirated specimens with simultaneously obtained histologic material obtained by transrectal punch biopsies.[85] Diagnostic cytologic findings include the presence of large scattered histiocytes having abundant foamy cytoplasm and containing the diagnostic concentrically laminated Michaelis–Gutmann (M–G) bodies (Fig. 11.34). Extracellular M–G bodies were also present in the background. The cytologic findings were similar to another FNA report of malakoplakia.[90]

Other Nonneoplastic Potential Sources for a False-Positive Diagnosis of Malignancy

Besides acute and chronic granulomatous prostatitis, false-positive interpretation of malignancy can result from misinterpretation of normal benign elements and induced atypias. Cells from the seminal vesicles are present in up to 2% of prostatic aspirates and are especially likely to be seen if the biopsy is from a laterally located nodule.[67] Seminal vesicle cells may be arranged singly or in sheets and have atypical features such as individually scattered large cells having pleomorphic, hyperchromatic nuclei (Fig. 11.35). Cytologic features to suggest the correct diagnosis include the triangular to columnar shape of the seminal vesicle cells, along with the presence of cytoplasmic yellowish lipochrome granules. Generally, few seminal vesicle cells are seen, whereas in aspirates of prostatic carcinoma, malignant cells are numerous.

Another potential source for a false-positive diagnosis of malignancy includes contamination of the specimen by rectal cells. Some of these cells may be arranged

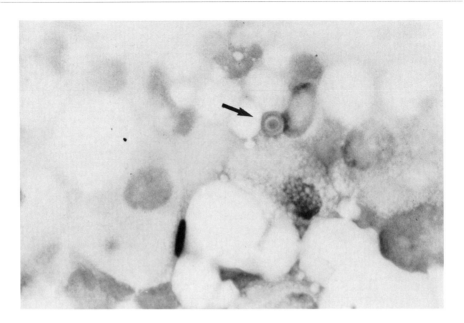

Fig. 11.34. Aspirate of prostatic malakoplakia demonstrating a few foamy macrophages ("von Hansemann cells") containing intracytoplasmic Michaelis–Gutman bodies (*arrow*) (PAS stain; ×400). (Courtesy of Dr. Marco Cazzaniga, Department of Pathology, General Hospital, Milano, Italy.) (From Cazzaniga MG, Tommasini-Degma A, Negri R, et al: Cytologic diagnosis of prostatic malakoplakia. Report of three cases. *Acta Cytol* 31:41–52, 1987. With permission.)

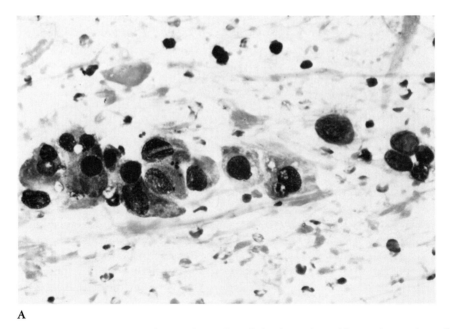

A

Fig. 11.35. A. Loose cluster of seminal vesicle cells having enlarged hyperchromatic nuclei. (Diff-Quik stain; ×400).

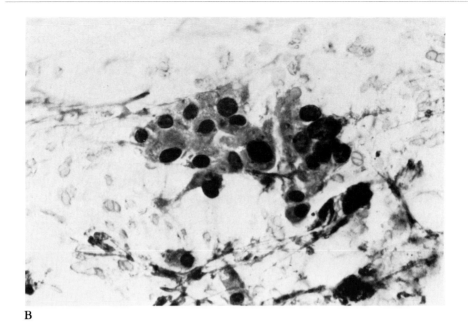

B

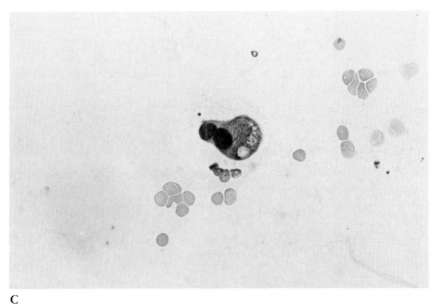

C

Fig. 11.35. B. Loose sheet of seminal vesicle cells having cuboidal to columnar shape and demonstrating anisonucleosis and hyperchromasia of the nuclei (Diff-Quik stain; ×200). **C.** Single atypical seminal vesicle cell having triangular shape with the presence of cytoplasmic yellowish lipochrome granules (Papanicolaou stain; ×400).

in loose cellular groupings resembling microacini and showing nucleolar prominence, which may falsely suggest the possibility of well differentiated prostatic carcinoma. Helpful diagnostic features for the identification of rectal cells include the arrangement of the tall columnar cells in small monolayer sheets with evidence of peripheral palisading or a picket-fence alignment. Cytoplasmic vacuolization may also be noted.[70]

Radiation- and chemotherapy-induced atypia can produce a variety of cytologic changes that could be potential sources for false-positive diagnoses of malignancy. These include squamous metaplasia, epithelial atypia, and the presence of atypical fibroblasts.[91,92] Kline noted that radiation- and chemotherapy-induced atypia of the prostate will result in only a few poorly preserved atypical cells which "must be interpreted cautiously." Kline recommends that unless abundant cells are present, the aspiration should be repeated after 3 to 4 months. Prostatic infarcts can also cause epithelial atypia which may potentially be confused with carcinoma.[91]

REFERENCES

1. Koss LG, Woyke S, Olszewski W: Aspiration Biopsy. Cytologic Interpretation and Histologic Bases, ed. 1. New York, Igaku-Shoin, 1984.

2. Nguyen G-K: What is the value of fine-needle aspiration biopsy in the cytodiagnosis of soft-tissue tumors? *Diagn Cytopathol* 4:352–355, 1988.

3. Miralles TG, Gosalbez F, Menendez P, et al: Fine needle aspiration cytology of soft-tissue lesions. *Acta Cytol* 30:671–678, 1986.

4. Layfield LJ, Anders KH, Glasgow BJ, et al: Fine-needle aspiration of primary soft-tissue lesions. *Arch Pathol Lab Med* 110:420–424, 1986.

5. Golouh R, Us-Krasovec M: Differential diagnosis of the pleomorphic aspiration biopsy sample of nonepithelial lesions. *Diagn Cytopathol* 1:308–316, 1985.

6. Bibbo M, Keebler CM, Wied GL: The cytologic diagnosis of tissue repair in the female genital tract. *Acta Cytol* 15:133–137, 1971.

7. Geirsson G, Woodworth FE, Patten SF, et al: Epithelial repair and regeneration in the uterine cervix. I. An analysis of the cells. *Acta Cytol* 21:371–378, 1977.

8. Sugimori H, Kashimura Y, Kashimura M, et al: Analytical study of repair cells. *Acta Cytol* 26:434–444, 1982.

9. James LP: Cytopathology of mesenchymal repair. *Diagn Cytopathol* 1:91–104, 1985.

10. El-Naggar A, Abdul-Karim FW, Marshalleck JJ, et al: Fine-needle aspiration of fibromatosis of the breast. *Diagn Cytopathol* 3:320–322, 1987.

11. Lin BPC, Scott GS, Loughman NT, et al: Mesenteric fibromatosis: cytologic, histologic, and ultrastructural findings in a case. *Diagn Cytopathol* 5:69–74, 1989.

12. Tani EM, Stanley MW, Skoog L: Fine needle aspiration cytology presentation of bilateral mammary fibromatosis. Report of a case. *Acta Cytol* 32:555–558, 1988.

13. Fritsches HG, Muller EA: Pseudosarcomatous fasciitis of the breast. Cytologic and histologic features. *Acta Cytol* 27:73–75, 1983.

14. Dahl I, Akerman M: Nodular fasciitis. A correlative cytologic and histologic study of 13 cases. *Acta Cytol* 25:215–223, 1981.

15. Anglo-Henry MR, Seaquist MB, Marsh WL Jr: Fine needle aspiration of proliferative fasciitis. A case report. *Acta Cytol* 29:882–886, 1985.

16. Popok SM, Naib ZM: Fine needle aspiration cytology of myositis ossificans. *Diagn Cytopathol* 1:236–240, 1985.

17. Akerman M, Rydholm A: Aspiration cytology of lipomatous tumors: a 10-year experience at an orthopedic oncology center. *Diagn Cytopathol* 3:295–302, 1987.

18. James LP: Myxoid liposarcoma: diagnosis by fine-needle aspiration biopsy. *ASCP* Check Sample 2:1–6, 1983.

19. Akerman M, Idvall I, Rydholm A: Cytodiagnosis of soft tissue tumors and tumor-like conditions by means of fine needle aspiration biopsy. *Arch Orthop Trauma Surg* 96: 61–67, 1980.

20. Akerman M, Rydholm A, Persson BM: Aspiration cytology of soft-tissue tumors. The 10-year experience at an orthopedic oncology center. *Acta Orthop Scand* 56:407–412, 1985.

21. Rydholm A, Akerman M, Idvall I, et al: Aspiration cytology of soft tissue tumours. A prospective study of its influence on choice of surgical procedure. *Int Orthop* 6:209–214, 1982.

22. Kindblow L-G: Light and electron microscopic examination of embedded fine-needle aspiration biopsy specimens in the preoperative diagnosis of soft tissue and bone tumors. *Cancer* 51:2264–2277, 1983.

23. Kanter MH, Duane GB: Angiomatoid malignant fibrous histiocytoma. Cytology of fine-needle aspiration and its differential diagnosis. *Arch Pathol Lab Med* 109:564–566, 1985.

24. Massoni EA, Hajdu SI: Cytology of primary and metastatic uterine sarcomas. *Acta Cytol* 28:93–100, 1984.

25. Navas-Palacios JJ, de Agustin de Agustin PP, de los Heros FA, et al: Ultrastructural diagnosis of facial nerve schwannoma using fine needle aspiration. *Acta Cytol* 27:441–445, 1983.

26. Kapila K, Chopra P, Verma K: Fine needle aspiration cytology of alveolar soft-part sarcoma. A case report. *Acta Cytol* 29:559–561, 1985.

27. Ryd W, Mugal S, Ayyash K: Ancient neurilemoma: a pitfall in the cytologic diagnosis of soft-tissue tumors. *Diagn Cytopathol* 2:244–247, 1986.

28. Seidal T, Mark J, Hagmar B, et al: Alveolar rhabdomyosarcoma: a cytogenetic and correlated cytological and histological study. *Acta Path Microbiol Immunol Scand* 90:345–354, 1982.

29. Bondeson L, Andreasson L: Aspiration cytology of adult rhabdomyoma. *Acta Cytol* 30:679–682, 1986.

30. Brehaut LE, Anderson LH, Taylor DA: Extraskeletal Ewing's sarcoma. Diagnosis of a case by fine needle aspiration cytology. *Acta Cytol* 30:683–687, 1986.

31. Geisinger KR, Silverman JF, Cappellari JO, et al: Fine needle aspiration cytology of malignant hemangiopericytomas with ultrastructural and flow cytometric analyses. *Am J Clin Pathol* 91:361, 1989.

32. Kim K, Naylor B, Han IH: Fine needle aspiration cytology of sarcomas metastatic to the lung. *Acta Cytol* 30:688–694, 1986.

33. Perry MD, Furlong JW, Johnston WW: Fine needle aspiration cytology of metastatic dermatofibrosarcoma protuberans. A case report. *Acta Cytol* 30:507–512, 1986.

34. Wakely PE Jr, Giacomantonio M: Fine needle aspiration cytology of metastatic malignant rhabdoid tumor. *Acta Cytol* 30:533–537, 1986.

35. Hales M, Bottles K, Miller T, et al: Diagnosis of Kaposi's sarcoma by fine-needle aspiration biopsy. *Am J Clin Pathol* 88:20–25, 1987.

36. Finley JL, Silverman JF, Dabbs DJ, et al: Chordoma: Diagnosis by fine-needle aspiration biopsy with histologic, immunocytochemical, and ultrastructural confirmation. *Diagn Cytopathol* 2:330–337, 1986.

37. Merck C, Hagmar B: Myxofibrosarcoma. A correlative cytologic and histologic study of 13 cases examined by fine needle aspiration cytology. *Acta Cytol* 24:137–144, 1980.

38. Walaas L, Angervall L, Hagmar B, et al: A correlative cytologic and histologic study of malignant fibrous histiocytoma: an analysis of 40 cases examined by fine-needle aspiration cytology. *Diagn Cytopathol* 2:46–54, 1986.

39. Kim K, Goldblatt PJ: Malignant fibrous histiocytoma. Cytologic, light microscopic and ultrastructural studies. *Acta Cytol* 26:507–511, 1982.

40. Akerman M, Rydholm A: Aspiration of cytology of intramuscular myxoma. A comparative clinical, cytologic and histologic study of ten cases. *Acta Cytol* 27:505–510, 1983.

41. Silverman JF, Lannin DL, Larkin EW, et al: Fine-needle aspiration cytology of postirradiation sarcomas, including angiosarcoma, with immunocytochemical confirmation. *Diagn Cytopathol* 5:275–281, 1989.

42. Hajdu SI, Hajdu EO: Cytopathology of Soft Tissue and Bone Tumors. *In:* Weid GL, Ed. Monographs in Clinical Cytology, Vol. 12. Karger, Switzerland, 1989.

43. Orell SR, Sterrett GF, Walters MN-I, et al: Manual and Atlas of Fine Needle Aspiration Cytology, ed. 1. New York, Churchill Livingstone, 1986.

44. Griffin JB, Betsill WL Jr: Subcutaneous endometriosis diagnosed by fine needle aspiration cytology. *Acta Cytol* 29:584–588, 1985.

45. Lowhagen T, Rubio C: The cytology of the granular cell myoblastoma of the breast. *Acta Cytol* 21:314–345, 1977.

46. Feldman PS, Covell JL: Breast and lung. *In:* Fine Needle Aspiration Cytology and Its Clinical Application. Chicago, American Society of Clinical Pathologists Press, 1985, pp 27–43.

47. DeMay RM, Kay S: Granular cell tumor of the breast. *Pathol Annu* 19:121–148, 1984.

48. Zamora T, Vargas J, de Agustin P, et al: Fine needle aspiration cytologic findings and differential diagnosis of solitary pseudorheumatoid nodule. *Acta Cytol* 33:393–396, 1989.

49. Vuong PN: Acquired gluteal myospherulosis secondary to intramuscular injections of petrolatum-based hormones: a case report diagnosed by fine-needle aspiration cytology. *Diagn Cytopathol* 4:137–139, 1988.

50. McClatchie S, Warambo MW, Brenner AD: Myospherulosis: a previously unreported disease? *Am J Clin Pathol* 51:699–704, 1969.

51. Oertel YC, Beckner ME, Engler WF: Cytologic diagnosis and ultrastructure of fine-needle aspirates of ganglion cysts. *Arch Pathol Lab Med* 110:938–942, 1986.

52. Esteban JM, Oertel YC, Mendoza M, et al: Fine needle aspiration in the treatment of ganglion cysts. *South Med J* 79:691–693, 1986.

53. Lee P-C, Turnidge J, McDonald PJ: Fine-needle aspiration biopsy in the diagnosis of soft tissue infections. *J Clin Microbiol* 22:80–83, 1985.

54. Silverman JF, Larkin EW, Carney M, et al: Fine needle aspiration cytology of tuberculosis of the lumbar vertebrae (Pott's disease). *Acta Cytol* 30:538–542, 1986.

55. Nathanson L, Cohen W: A statistical and roentgen analysis of two hundred cases of bone and joint tuberculosis. *Radiology* 36:550–567, 1941.

56. Palombini L, Marino D, Vetrani A, et al: Fine needle aspiration biopsy in primary malignant and metastatic bone tumors. *Appl Pathol* 1:76–81, 1983.

57. Stormby N, Akerman M: Cytodiagnosis of bone lesions by means of fine needle aspiration biopsy. *Acta Cytol* 17:166–172, 1973.

58. Ganjei P, Evans DA, Fischer ML: Diagnosis of cryptococcal osteomyelitis by fine needle aspiration cytology: a case report. *Acta Cytol* 26:224–226, 1982.

59. Katz RL, Silva EG, De Santos LA, et al: Diagnosis of eosinophilic granuloma of bone by cytology, histology, and electron microscopy of transcutaneous bone aspiration biopsy. *J Bone Joint Surg* 62:1284–1290, 1980.

60. Elsheikh T, Silverman JF, Wakely PE, et al: Fine-needle aspiration cytology (FNA) of Langerhans' cell histiocytosis (eosinophilic granuloma) of bone in children. *Am J Clin Pathol* 93:444, 1990.

61. Lupovitch A, Elie JC, Wysocki R: Diagnosis of acute bacterial osteomyelitis of the pubis by means of fine needle aspiration. *Acta Cytol* 33:649–651, 1989.

62. Sloth M, Bartholdy N, Andersen MJF, et al: Fine-needle aspiration biopsy of bone lesions in the spine: diagnostic value. *Rontgenblatter* 37:388–390, 1984.

63. Thommesen P, Bartholdy N, Bunger E: Histiocytosis X. VIII: Histiocytosis X stimulating tuberculosis. *Acta Radiol Oncol* 22:295–297, 1983.

64. Elsheikh T, Silverman JF, Wakely PE, et al: Fine-needle aspiration cytology of Langerhans' cell histiocytosis (eosinophilic granuloma) of bone in children. *Diagn Cytopathol* (in press).

65. Frable WJ: Thin Needle Aspiration Biopsy. *In:* Major Problems in Pathology, ed. 14. Philadelphia, WB Saunders, 1983, pp 298–304.

66. Linsk JA, Franzen S: Clinical Aspiration Cytology. Philadelphia, JB Lippincott, 1983, pp 357–358.

67. Kline TS: Guides to Clinical Aspiration Biopsy: Prostate. New York, Igaku-Shoin, 1985.

68. Stilmant MM, Freedlund MC, de las Morenas A, et al: Expanded role for fine needle aspiration of the prostate. *Cancer* 63:583–592, 1989.

69. Maksem JA, Johenning PW, Galang CF: Prostatitis and aspiration biopsy cytology of prostate. *Urology* 32:263–268, 1988.

70. Kline TS: Handbook of Fine Needle Aspiration Biopsy Cytology, ed 2. New York, Churchill Livingstone, 1988, pp 365–392.

71. Frable WJ: Thin-Needle Aspiration Biopsy. Vol 14 in the series Major Problems in Pathology. Philadelphia, WB Saunders Company, 1983, pp 275–285.

72. Miralles T, Gosalbez F, Menendez P: Fine needle aspiration cytology of granulomatous prostatitis. *Acta Cytol* 34:57–62, 1990.

73. Taylor EW, Wheeler RF, Correa RJ Jr, et al: Granulomatous prostatitis: Confusion clinically with carcinoma of the prostate. *J Urol* 117:316–318, 1977.

74. Kline TS, Kohler FP, Kelsey DM: Aspiration biopsy cytology (ABC). Its use in diagnosis of lesions of the prostate gland. *Arch Pathol Lab Med* 106:136–139, 1982.

75. Faul P, Schmiedt E: Cytologic aspects of diseases of the prostate. *Int Urol Nephrol* 5:297–310, 1974.

76. Ekman H, Hedberg K, Persson PS: Cytological versus histological examination of needle biopsy specimens in the diagnosis of prostatic cancer. *Br J Urol* 39:544–548, 1967.

77. Epstein NA: Prostatic biopsy: A morphologic correlation of aspiration cytology with needle biopsy histology: *Cancer* 38:2078–2087, 1976.

78. Epstein JI, Hutchins GM: Granulomatous prostatitis: distinction among allergic, nonspecific and post-transurethral resection lesions. *Hum Pathol* 15:818–825, 1984.

79. Ney CH, Miller H, Levy J: Granulomatous prostatitis (classification): special reference to radiologic finding. *Urology* 21:320–323, 1983.

80. Tanner FJ, McDonald JR: Granulomatous prostatitis: a histologic study of a group of granulomatous lesions collected from prostate glands. *Arch Pathol* 36:358–370, 1943.

81. Tuero J, Alonso de la Campa JM, Lacort J, et al: Granulomatous prostatitis. *Urol Int* 43:97–101, 1988.

82. Towfighi J, Deghees SA, Wheeler JE, et al: Granulomatous prostatitis with emphasis on the eosinophilic variety. *Am J Clin Pathol* 58:630–641, 1972.

83. Stilmant M, Siroky MB, Johnson KB: Fine needle aspiration cytology of granulomatous prostatitis induced by BCG immunotherapy of bladder cancer. *Acta Cytol* 29:961–966, 1985.

84. Perez-Guillermo M, Thor A, Lowhagen T: Spermatic granuloma. Diagnosis by fine needle aspiration cytology. *Acta Cytol* 33:1–5, 1989.

85. Cazzaniga MG, Tommasini-Degna A, Negri R, et al: Cytologic diagnosis of prostatic malakoplakia. Report of three cases. *Acta Cytol* 31:48–52, 1987.

86. Stanton MJ, Maxted W: Malakoplakia: a study of the literature and current concepts of pathogenesis, diagnosis and treatment. *J Urol* 125:139–146, 1981.

87. Lou TY, Teplitz CL: Malacoplakia, pathogenesis and ultrastructural morphogenesis: a problem of altered macrophage (phagolysosomal) response. *Hum Pathol* 5:191–707, 1974.

88. Lewin KJ, Harell GS, Lee AS, et al: Malacoplakia: An electron microscopic study: demonstration of bacilliform organisms in malacoplakic macrophages. *Gastroenterology* 66:28–45, 1974.

89. Lewin KJ, Fair WR, Steigbigel RT, et al: Clinical and laboratory studies into the pathogenesis of malacoplakia. *J Clin Pathol* 29:354–363, 1976.

90. Akhtar M, Ali MA, Robinson C, et al: Role of fine needle aspiration biopsy in the diagnosis and management of malacoplakia. *Acta Cytol* 29:457–460, 1985.

91. Bostwick DG: Premalignant lesions of the prostate. *Semin Diagn Pathol* 5:240–253, 1986.

92. Bostwick DG, Egbert BM, Fajardo LF: Radiation injury of the normal and neoplastic prostate. *Am J Surg Pathol* 6:541–551, 1982.

12

Central Nervous System

There have been only a limited number of series reporting the results of FNA biopsy of the central nervous system (CNS).[1-4] However, the crush-smear cytologic preparation as first described by Cushing has been used for more than 50 years in the rapid intraoperative diagnosis of CNS lesions.[5-8] Although the crush-smear technique has not gained wide acceptance in the United States, it has been shown to be extremely reliable in the past with an accuracy rate of up to 95%.[2,5,6,9] In addition, the nuclear and cytoplasmic detail in cytologic preparations is often superior to that found in the histologic sections.[6,10,11] Recently, FNA cytology has been used for the diagnosis of brain lesions.[1,2,8,10-14] In our review of the four largest FNA biopsy series of the CNS in the literature, we found a sensitivity of the procedure of 92%, a specificity of 100%, and a positive predictive value of 96%; the efficiency of the test of 89%. Most of the series have emphasized the use of FNA biopsy for the diagnosis of primary and metastatic neoplasms of the brain and spinal cord. However, we can expect a greater reliance on cytologic diagnosis of infectious diseases with the introduction of stereotactic brain biopsy[15-18] and the concomitant increase in neurologic complications seen in the acquired immune deficiency syndrome (AIDS) (Table 12.1).

OBTAINING THE SPECIMEN BY STEREOTACTIC BIOPSY

As noted by Neal and Apuzzo, "Rational treatment of intracranial lesions must be based on accurate diagnosis. Inflammatory and infectious lesions must be differentiated from neoplastic lesions."[15] The evaluation of brain masses has undergone a dramatic change in recent years with the use of stereotactic biopsy. Previously, major surgery through a craniotomy was the only means of obtaining tissue for pathologic diagnosis. However, stereotactic biopsy can be performed through a small burr hole in the skull under local anesthesia. A number of different stereotactic instruments are currently available. In our institution, we use the

TABLE 12.1. Infectious CNS Complications in AIDS

HIV
Meningitis
Encephalopathy
Other
OTHER VIRUSES
Cytomegalovirus
Herpes zoster virus
Herpes simplex
Papovavirus (JC virus, progressive multifocal leukoencephalopathy)
PROTOZOA
Toxoplasma gondii
Acanthamoeba
FUNGI
Cryptococcus neoformans (meningitis, cryptococcoma)
Other fungi: *Candida, Aspergillus, Coccidioides, Histoplasma* (rarely)
BACTERIA (rarely)
Listeria (meningitis, abscess)
Nocardia (abscess)
Escherichia coli (meningitis)
Treponema pallidum (neurosyphilis)
MYCOBACTERIA
Mycobacterium tuberculosis (abscess, meningitis)
Mycobacterium avium-intracellulare (encephalitis, meningitis)

Brown–Roberts–Wells (BRW) stereotactic frame, which interfaces with a three-dimensional database derived by computed tomography (CT). The BRW system (Figs. 12.1 through 12.4) consists of

1. A nickel-plated aluminum base head ring that is fixed to the skull of the patient at four points.
2. A localizing unit attaches to the head ring (Fig. 12.1). This unit is composed of vertical and diagonal carbon fiber rods arranged in three groups, each one shaped like the letter **N**. Axial scanning through the localizing unit results in nine points or fiducials which establish the target coordinates for the lesion.
3. An arc guidance system that allows for an infinite number of approaches to the target lesion (Fig. 12.2).
4. A phantom base that allows for verification of entry point, trajectory, and target (Fig. 12.3).
5. An Epson HX-20 microcomputer with software that provides calculation of target coordinates and arc angle settings (Fig. 12.4).

Although initially quite expensive, the unit has declined in cost to approximately $60,000. The reader is referred to other sources for a more complete description on the workings of the instrument.[19,20,21]

The principal advantage of stereotactic biopsy is that it is extremely accurate, obtaining tissue within 1 to 3 millimeters from the CT scan–selected target. With this great accuracy, deep-seated regions such as the basal ganglia, third ventricle,

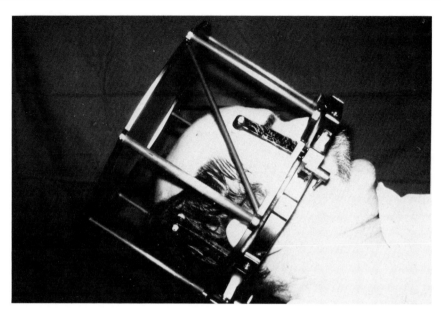

Fig. 12.1. Brown–Roberts–Wells stereotactic frame. Nickel-plated, aluminum-based head ring is fixed to the skull of the patient at four points and a localizing unit attached to the head ring.

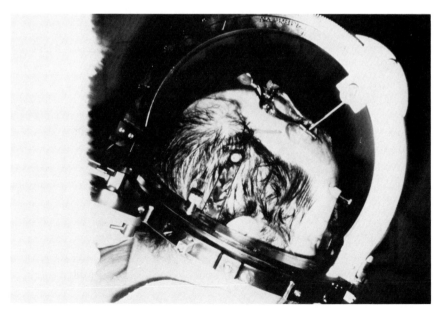

Fig. 12.2. Arc guidance system for BRW stereotactic frame allows for an infinite number of approaches to the target lesion.

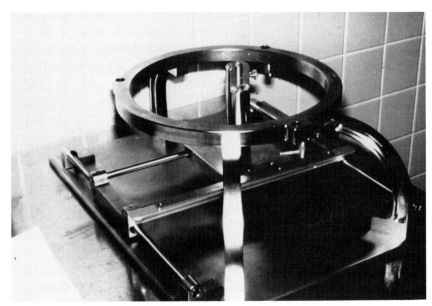

Fig. 12.3. A phantom base for the BRW unit allows for verification of entry point, trajectory, and target.

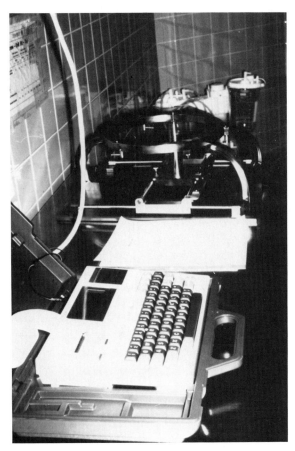

Fig. 12.4. Microcomputer in the operating room calculates target coordinates and arc angle settings.

326

and pineal gland can be sampled with relatively few complications. The main disadvantage of stereotactic biopsy is the relatively small size of the sample, consisting of tissue cores measuring approximately 2 mm in greatest dimension. However, we concur with Chandrasoma and Apuzzo that the specimen can be maximized for diagnosis by first relying on cytologic smear preparations to make a preliminary diagnosis.[15]

The usual specimen consists of one to three small fragments of tissue from the target point. A small portion of each fragment is cut with a scalpel blade and placed on a glass slide. A second glass slide is then used to make crush preparations. We generally fix some of the smears in 95% alcohol and stain with a rapid hematoxylin and eosin (H&E) procedure in the frozen section room adjacent to the neurosurgery suite. We also perform Diff-Quik staining of air-dried smears, although this is not preferred by Chandrasoma and Apuzzo. Romanowsky stains, thought by some to be less than optimal for the evaluation of CNS neoplasms, have proved to be superior when a lymphomatous or an infectious/inflammatory lesion is encountered. If the initial material is not diagnostic, the remaining small tissue cores are submitted for frozen section. If the initial crush preparations are diagnostic, the tissue cores can be submitted for permanent section and/or ancillary techniques, such as electron microscopy, immunocytochemistry, or culture. It is also not unusual to ask a neurosurgeon to obtain additional tissue for permanent sections from the target lesion if the initial specimen appears to be diagnostic but is used in its entirety for the immediate interpretation, or to select a different target point if nondiagnostic tissue is encountered. The maximum utilization of stereotactic biopsy requires a team approach consisting of radiologist, neurosurgeons, and pathologists.

BRAIN ABSCESS

Pyogenic brain abscess is most often of bacterial origin, with *Staphylococcus aureus*, hemolytic streptococci, *Streptococcus viridans,* and aerobic gram-negative rods the most common agents.[22] Anaerobic organisms probably account for many of the so-called sterile abscesses. Brain abscesses produce considerable morbidity and a 5 to 20% mortality. There is a striking male:female ratio (3:1) and increased involvement in the 30 to 40 age group, although no age is spared. Brain abscess is usually related to an initial infection in a contiguous site such as the middle ear, mastoid, sinus, teeth, nose, or scalp. Some brain abscesses are secondary to penetrating cranial trauma or postsurgical infection. Often the location of the brain abscess is closely linked to the contiguous infection. Hematogenous spread from an extracranial site is another source of brain abscess, especially in a patient with a lung infection (bronchiectasis, lung abscess, empyema), congenital heart defect with bacterial endocarditis, or immunocompromised state. In 10 to 20% of cases, the source of the abscess is unknown.

Aspiration biopsy cytologic findings of brain abscess consist of numerous neutrophils. Often the specific organism can be identified cytologically, for example, bacteria in Diff-Quik stained smears or fungi in the H&E, Papanicolaou, or the Wright–Giemsa stained preparation (Fig. 12.5). Besides a diagnostic procedure, FNA or stereotactic biopsy can also be used for drainage of the purulent material

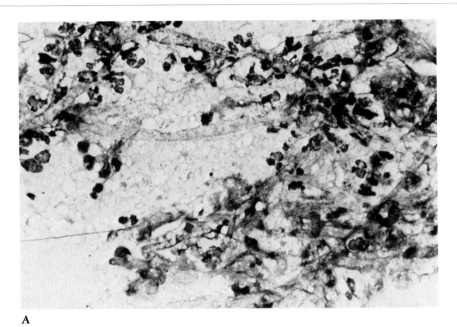

A

B

Fig. 12.5. A. FNA of brain abscess in which sheets of neutrophils and faintly staining hyphae of *Aspergillus* are present (Diff-Quik stain; × 200). **B.** GMS stain demonstrating branching hyphae of *Aspergillus*. Note acute-angle branching and septation (GMS stain; × 200). (From Silverman JF: Cytologic Diagnosis In Acquired Immunodeficiency Syndrome. In: *Pathology Of Aids And Other Manifestations Of HIV Infection,* Ed. Joshi VV. New York, Igaku-Shoin, 1990.)

or instillation of specific antibiotics.[15] When an abscess is encountered, material should be especially submitted for fungal and anaerobic and aerobic bacterial culture.

Nocardia asteroides, a gram-positive bacterium, can cause a localized brain abscess and/or meningitis in usually debilitated patients, although occasional cases appear in individuals having no predisposing factors.[22] Nocardiosis of the brain is often hematogenously spread from the lung. The inflammatory response is usually suppurative, although rare granulomatous reactions can occur. GMS and Gram stains will demonstrate the delicate branching filaments of *Nocardia* (Fig. 12.6). The organism is also weakly acid-fast when an acid in aqueous solution is employed in the decolorizing process.[22] Chandrasoma and Apuzzo reported one case of *Nocardia* encephalitis diagnosed by stereotactic brain biopsy.[15]

FUNGAL INFECTIONS

Aspergillosis of the CNS is usually an opportunistic infection but can occur in immune-competent individuals as a result of hematogenous spread or extension from an adjacent infection of the paranasal sinus. Clinical settings in which hematogenous spread occurs include pulmonary aspergillosis, mycotic endocarditis, cranial surgery, trauma, or narcotic addition.[22] The fungus can invade blood vessel walls and produce vascular thombosis with secondary cerebral infarction. We have encountered a case of aspergillosis of the brain diagnosed by FNA biopsy in a 13-year-old female undergoing treatment for Burkitt's lymphoma. A scattering of neutrophils and necrotic brain tissue was seen along with septated acute angle–branching hyphae. When examining the H&E and Diff-Quik stained smears at the time of immediate interpretation in the frozen section room, we have found that the visualization of the organisms can be enhanced by lowering the condenser of the microscope (see Fig. 12.5[b]).

Bigner and associates reported a case of cerebral mucormycosis diagnosed by FNA biopsy in a 59-year-old woman receiving corticosteroid therapy. The patient presented with a sudden onset of left hemiparesis and a mass lesion of the right caudate nucleus.[23] Besides large, branching, nonseptated fungal hyphae consistent with Zygomycetes (Phycomycetes), fragments of infarcted brain tissue containing pyknotic neurons, glial cells, and capillaries were present. The cerebral infarction was due to thrombosis of blood vessels occluded with fungal hyphae. The most common pattern of infection by members of the Phycomycetes class of fungi is the rhinocerebral form in which the organisms originate in the nasal cavity or paranasal sinuses in individuals with diabetic ketoacidosis or who are immunocompromised.[22,23] Occasionally cerebral involvement with Phycomycetes is by vascular dissemination from a pulmonary, gastrointestinal, or cutaneous site.[24]

Central nervous system cryptococcosis can occur in immune-competent patients, although it is a frequently encountered infection in individuals with AIDS. We have encountered one case of cryptococcal abscess in an individual with a cryptococcal infection of the lung (Fig. 12.7). Both a fine-needle and a stereotactic biopsy were performed (Fig. 12.8). The diagnostic material was seen only in the aspirated material (Fig. 12.9). Other central nervous system fungal infections include blastomycosis and histoplasmosis.

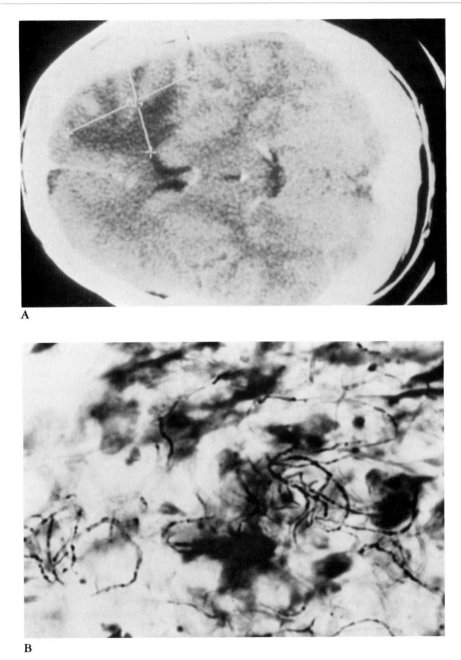

A

B

Fig. 12.6. **A.** CT scan in which coordinates note the location of the lesion undergoing aspiration. **B.** Delicate, branching filaments of *Nocardia* having a beaded appearance (Acid-fast stain; × 1000).

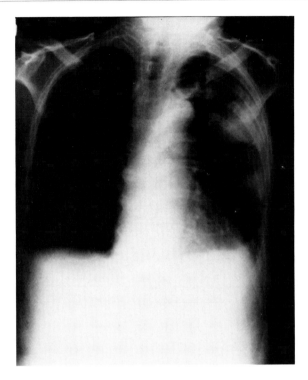

Fig. 12.7. Chest X-ray demonstrating cavitary lesion of left lung in patient with pulmonary and central nervous system cryptococcosis.

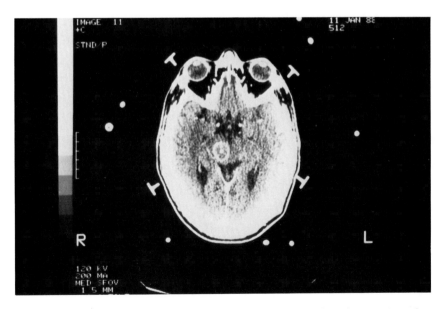

Fig. 12.8. Stereotactic biopsy under CT scan guidance sampling deep brain lesion of cryptococcosis (Same patient as in Fig. 12.7).

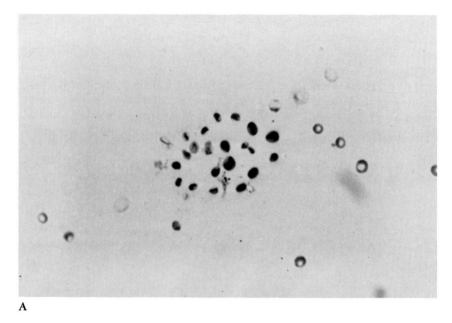

A

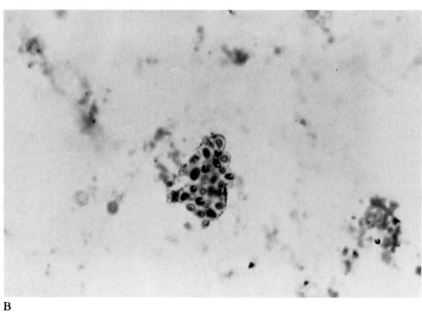

B

Fig. 12.9. A. Aspirate obtained under stereotactic guidance revealed fungal yeast forms including some budding consistent with cryptococcosis (Diff-Quik stain; ×200). **B.** Cluster of cryptococci including some having refractile quality characteristic of the organism (Papanicolaou stain; ×200) (Same patient as in Figs. 12.7 and 12.8).

STEREOTACTIC BIOPSY IN AIDS

Many patients with AIDS have several neurologic complications during their course. Progressive dementia is seen in approximately two thirds of adult patients.[25] Individuals with AIDS also develop opportunistic infections of the central nervous system and primary CNS lymphomas, both of which can be diagnosed by fine-needle or stereotactic biopsy. The most frequently encountered central nervous system infections in AIDs patients are cytomegalovirus encephalitis, cryptococcosis, toxoplasmosis, and progressive multifocal leukoencephalopathy.[25]

Mass lesions of the central nervous system can occur in a small percentage of AIDS patients having neurologic symptoms. The most common causes of mass lesions in this patient population are primary CNS lymphoma and cerebral toxoplasmosis, although CT scan abnormalities due to other infectious conditions such as progressive multifocal leukoencephalopathy and cytomegalovirus encephalitis can occur.[15]

CEREBRAL TOXOPLASMOSIS

Toxoplasma gondii is the etiologic agent of an infection in adults worldwide; it usually has a benign self-limiting course.[25] In immunosuppressed patients, however, latent toxoplasmosis can become symptomatic. Central nervous system toxoplasmosis is found in 3 to 40% of adult AIDS patients at autopsy. The clinical manifestations of toxoplasmosis are variable, ranging from headache and fever to coma. The clinical and radiologic appearance can be very similar to malignant lymphoma.[28] CT scans commonly demonstrate multiple ring-enhancing lesions.[29] Initially, all AIDS patients with mass lesions suspected to be toxoplasmosis underwent stereotactic biopsy. Currently, in many centers, only those patients failing anti-*Toxoplasma* therapy undergo biopsy.[15]

Cytologic and tissue diagnosis depends on identifying the *Toxoplasma gondii* pseudocyst, which has a well defined wall surrounding numerous organisms. The pseudocyst can resemble enlarged nuclei in air-dried smears, making the identification of *Toxoplasma* trophozoites in routine preparations difficult. Immunoperoxidase stains using anti-*Toxoplasma* antibodies can be useful in confirming the diagnosis.[15,25] The cytologic and histologic findings will depend on the stage of the disease. During the acute phase of the infection, a cellular infiltrate consisting of lymphocytes, plasma cells, and occasional neutrophils may be seen along with vascular proliferation and necrosis (Fig. 12.10). Typically, numerous organisms will be present. In more chronic lesions undergoing organization, central coagulative necrosis surrounded by a rim of lipid-laden macrophages will be present along with evidence of cavity formation.[25] In contrast to the acute phase, organisms are not as abundant and may be difficult to identify. The resolved *Toxoplasma* lesions are cystic, containing a small number of macrophages and evidence of old hemorrhage.

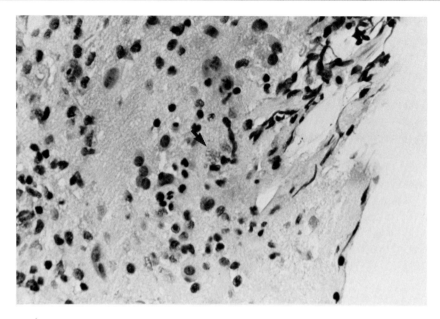

Fig. 12.10. Stereotactic biopsy of brain in AIDs patient demonstrating lymphocytes, reactive astrocytes, and a single pseudocyst of toxoplasmosis (*arrow*) (H&E stain; × 200).

PROGRESSIVE MULTIFOCAL LEUKOENCEPHALOPATHY

Progressive multifocal leukoencephalopathy (PML) is a rapidly progressive neurologic disease characterized by multiple foci of demyelination. The central nervous system involvement is believed to be due to infection of oligodendrocytes by JC polyoma virus (Papovavirus).[30] PML typically occurs in immunosuppressed patients including those with lymphoproliferative disorders, sarcoidosis, or tuberculosis; renal transplant recipients on immunosuppressive therapy; and more recently AIDS patients.[31,32,33] Once considered to be a very rare CNS infection, it has been a frequent complication in AIDS patients (seen in 2–4% of these individuals at autopsy).

Although the CT scans reveal nonenhancing lesions in the white matter, usually there is no evidence of a clinical mass effect.[30] Recently, Suhrland and associates reported two cases of PML diagnosed by stereotactic biopsy.[34] Cytologic findings demonstrated increased cellularity consisting of numerous individually scattered atypical cells, many of which were stripped of cytoplasm. The nuclei were enlarged, ranging from 14 to 21 microns, and the chromatin had a smudged appearance with focal areas of coarsely clumped chromatin often marginated along the nuclear membrane.[34] These cells correspond to the pathognomonic oligodendrocyte nuclei containing ground glass or basophilic viral inclusion bodies.[25] In addition, a second population of atypical cells were seen which appeared to be astrocytic in nature and had either normal or enlarged nuclei having a smudged chromatin pattern (Fig.

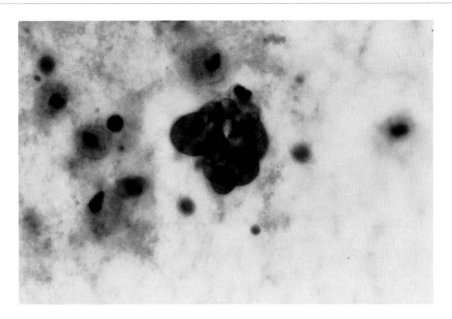

Fig. 12.11. Scattered atypical cells, most likely astrocytic in nature, having enlarged lobulated nuclei with smudged chromatin pattern in aspirate of patient with progressive multifocal leukoencephalopathy (H&E stain; × 1000). Courtesy of M. J. Suhrland, New York University, New York City. (From Suhrland MJ, Koslow M, Perchick A, et al: Cytologic findings in progressive multifocal leukoencephalopathy. Report of two cases. *Acta Cytol* 31:505–511, 1987.)

12.11). These cells were multilobulated and had abundant dense eosinophilic cytoplasm forming multiple cytoplasmic stellate processes.

Confirmation of PML can be facilitated by immunocytochemical studies or recognizing polyoma virions in electron microscopy examination. The differential diagnosis of the large atypical cells in the biopsies include malignant cells of astrocytic or metastatic origin.[34] However, in PML the large atypical cells are few in number, and identification of the smudged inclusion bodies should suggest the correct diagnosis. Other viral infections that may enter into the differential diagnosis include herpes simplex, cytomegalovirus, and subacute sclerosing panencephalitis (SSPE). Changes similar to the basophilic smudging of nuclear chromatin noted in PML can also be present in herpes encephalitis and SSPE. However, specimens in both of the latter two entities will have cells possessing large eosinophilic intranuclear viral inclusion bodies separated by a halo from the nuclear membrane.[34]

In conclusion, Chandrasoma and Apuzzo state that the likelihood that a specific infectious agent will be cytologically identified when a smear pattern shows inflammation and gliosis is increased in AIDS when compared with findings in individuals not at an increased risk for AIDS. In their series, 15 specific infectious agents were encountered in stereotactic brain biopsies of 58 patients.[15] Eleven of these cases were in 25 patients at risk for AIDS. Infections encountered in the AIDS risk group include six examples of toxoplasmosis, one cytomegalic encephalitis, one cryptococcosis, and three PML.

GRANULOMATOUS INFLAMMATION

A rare cause of CNS parenchymal lesions is granulomatous inflammation, usually due to tuberculosis or fungal infections.[15,22] Sarcoidosis is a very unusual cause of parenchymal granulomas, whereas meningeal lesions are more common.[22] Granulomatous inflammation is also a potential source for a false-negative diagnosis in biopsies of pineal germinoma (seminoma). Kraichoke and associates reported four patients with pineal germinomas initially evaluated by stereotactic biopsy.[35] All of the biopsies showed granulomatous inflammation with epithelioid cells and lymphocytes. In two of the cases, the entire specimen consisted of granulomatous inflammation with no malignant cells. The authors caution that finding granulomatous inflammation in the stereotactic biopsy specimen of a pineal mass should suggest a diagnosis of germinoma and encourage additional sampling of the lesion. Acute and chronic inflammation are other potential sources for a false-negative diagnosis of a central nervous system neoplasm. Chandrasoma and Apuzzo reported that they have encountered stereotactic biopsies of glioblastoma multiforme having a predominant neutrophilic infiltrate and craniopharyngiomas and astrocytomas with increased numbers of lymphocytes. The authors caution that the presence of necrosis, foamy macrophages, or neutrophils may represent degenerative areas of a high grade malignant neoplasms, especially when the CT appearance of the lesion and clinical course are not typical for an inflammatory process.

CYSTIC LESIONS

Aspirations from cystic lesions of the brain should generate a differential diagnosis that includes primary epidermoid cyst, arachnoid or leptomeningeal cyst, Rathke's cleft cyst, dermoid cyst, necrotic metastatic tumor, necrotic glioblastoma, cystic astrocytoma, craniopharyngioma, colloid cyst, cystic pituitary adenoma, and abscess.[36] Some leptomeningeal cysts are postinflammatory in nature and therefore not true cysts. They are believed to form from distended subarachnoid spaces lined by pia–arachnoid adhesions. In contrast, true arachnoid cysts are usually lined by delicate fibrovascular membranes covered by attenuated meningothelial cells, although some are lined by choroidal or ependymal epithelium. Necrotic glioblastoma and metastatic carcinoma should contain a few degenerating pleomorphic tumor cells in addition to the necrotic debris. Cystic astrocytomas may be paucicellular with only a few histiocytes and white blood cells present. Colloid cysts will contain a viscous fluid and a few cells whereas cystic pituitary adenomas should cytologically demonstrate a monomorphic population of uniform pituitary cells and occasional psammoma bodies. Epidermoid and dermoid cysts and craniopharyngiomas contain squamous cells and/or cholesterol crystals. In contrast, an abscess will demonstrate neutrophils and necrotic debris. Often the offending organism can be identified.[36,37]

REFERENCES

1. Silverman JF, Timmons RL, Leonard JR III, et al: Cytologic results of fine-needle aspiration biopsies of the central nervous system. *Cancer* 58:1117–1121, 1986.

2. Willems J, Alva-Willems JM: Accuracy of cytologic diagnosis of central nervous system neoplasms in stereotactic biopsies. *Acta Cytol* 28:243–249, 1984.

3. Liwnicz BH, Henderson KS, Masakawa T, et al: Needle aspiration cytology of intracranial lesions: a review of 84 cases. *Acta Cytol* 26:779–786, 1982.

4. Zaharopoulos P, Wong JY: Cytology of common primary midline brain tumors. *Acta Cytol* 24:384–390, 1980.

5. Cahill EM, Hidvegi DF: Crush preparations of lesions of the central nervous system. a useful adjunct to the frozen section. *Acta Cytol* 29:279–285, 1985.

6. Adams JH, Graham DI, Doyle D: The smear technique for neurosurgical biopsies. In Brain Biopsy. Philadelphia, JB Lippincott, 1981.

7. Eisenhardt L, Cushing H: Diagnosis of intercranial tumors by supravital technique. *Am J Pathol* 6:541–542, 1930.

8. Liwnicz GH, Rodriguez CA: The central nervous system. In: *Aspiration Biopsy: Cytologic Interpretation and Histologic Bases,* eds Koss LG, Woyke S, Olszewski W. New York, Igaku-Shoin 457–490, 1984.

9. Marshall LF, Adams H, Doyle D, et al: The histological accuracy of the smear technique for neurosurgical biopsies. *J Neurosurg* 39:82–88, 1973.

10. Silverman JF: Cytopathology of fine-needle aspiration biopsy of the brain and spinal cord. *Diagn Cytopathol* 2:312–319, 1986.

11. Silverman JF, Timmons RL, Leonard JR, et al: Fine-needle aspiration cytology of the central nervous system. *Cancer* 58:1117–1121, 1986.

12. Silverman JF, Timmons R, Harris LS: Fine needle aspiration cytology of primary epidermoid cyst of the brain. *Acta Cytol* 29:989–993, 1985.

13. Silverman JF, Dabbs DJ, Leonard JR, et al: Fine needle aspiration cytology of hemangioblastoma of the spinal cord with immunocytochemistry and ultrastructural studies. *Acta Cytol* 30:303–308, 1986.

14. Zaharopoulos P, Wong JY: Cytology of common primary midline brain tumors. *Acta Cytol* 24:384–390, 1980.

15. Chandrasoma PT, Apuzzo MLJ: *Stereotactic Brain Biopsy.* New York, Igaku-Shoin, 1989.

16. Apuzzo MLJ, Chandrasoma PT, Cohen D, et al: Computed imaging stereotaxy: experience and perspective related to 500 procedures applied to brain masses. *Neurosurgery* 20:930–937, 1987.

17. Ostertag CB, Mennel HD, Kiessling M: Stereotactic biopsy of brain tumors. *Surg Neurol* 14:275–283, 1980.

18. Apuzzo MLJ, Chandrasoma PT, Zelman V, et al: Applications of computerized tomographic guidance stereotaxis. In: *Surgery of the Third Ventricle,* ed Apuzzo MLJ. Baltimore, Williams & Wilkins, 751–792, 1987.

19. Brown RA: A computerized tomography–computer graphics approach to stereotaxic localization. *J Neurosurg* 50:715–720, 1979.

20. Brown RA: A stereotactic head frame for use with CT body scanners. *Invest Radiol* 14:300–304, 1979.

21. Brown RA, Roberts TS, Osborn AG: Stereotaxic frame and computer software for CT-directed neurosurgical localization. *Invest Radiol* 15:308–312, 1980.

22. Burger PC, Vogel FS: *Surgical Pathology of the Nervous System and Its Coverings.* New York, John Wiley & Sons, 1982.

23. Bigner SH, Burger PC, Dubois PJ, et al: Diagnosis of cerebral mucormycosis by needle aspiration biopsy: a case report. *Acta Cytol* 26:699–704, 1982.

24. Meyer RD, Rosen P, Armstrong D: Phycomycosis complicating leukemia and lymphoma. *Ann Intern Med* 77:871–879, 1972.

25. Cho E-S, Sharer LR: Central nervous system in HIV infection. In: Pathology of AIDS and Other Manifestations of HIV Infection, ed. Joshi VV. New York, Igaku-Shoin, 1990, pp 43–63.

26. Brynes RK, Joshi VV: Precautions for safe handling of biopsy and autopsy specimens. In: *Pathology of AIDS and Other Manifestations of HIV Infection,* ed. Joshi VV. New York, Igaku-Shoin, 1990, pp 367–369.

27. Spire B, Barre-Sinoussi F, Montagnier L, et al: Inactivation of lymphadenopathy associated virus by chemical disinfectants. *Lancet* 2:899–901, 1984.

28. Levy RM, Bredesen DE, Rosenblum ML: Neurological manifestations of the acquired immunodeficiency syndrome (AIDS): experience at UCSF and review of the literature. *J Neurosurg* 62:475–495, 1985.

29. Navia BA, Petito CK, Gold JWM, et al: Cerebral toxoplasmosis complicating the acquired immune deficiency syndrome: clinical and neuropathological findings in 27 patients. *Ann Neurol* 19:224–238, 1986.

30. Walker DL: Progressive multifocal leukoencephalopathy. In: *Handbook of Clinical Neurology: Demyelinating Diseases,* vol 3, ed Koitsier JC. Amsterdam, Elsevier, 1985, pp 503–524.

31. Lyon LW, McCormick WF, Schochet SS: Progressive multifocal leukoencephalopathy. *Arch Intern Med* 128:420–426, 1971.

32. Walker DL: Progressive multifocal leukoencephalopathy: an opportunistic viral infection of the central nervous system. In: *Handbook of Clinical Neurology,* vol 34, eds PJ Vinken, GW Bruyn. Amsterdam, North-Holland Publishing, 1978, pp 307–329.

33. Moskowitz LB, Hensky GT, Chan JC, et al: The neuropathology of the acquired immunodeficiency syndrome. *Arch Pathol Lab Med* 108:867–872, 1984.

34. Suhrland MJ, Koslow M, Perchick A, et al: Cytologic findings in progressive multifocal leukoencephalopathy. Report of two cases. *Acta Cytol* 31:505–511, 1987.

35. Kraichoke S, Cosgrove M, Chandrasoma PT: Granulomatous inflammation in pineal germinoma. A cause of diagnostic failure at stereotaxic brain biopsy. *Am J Surg Pathol* 12:655–660, 1988.

36. Silverman JF, Timmons R, Harris LS: Fine needle aspiration cytology of primary epidermoid cyst of the brain. *Acta Cytol* 29:989–993, 1983.

37. Fratkin JD, Ward MW, Roberts DW, et al: CT-guided stereotactic biopsy of intracranial lesions: correlation between core biopsy and aspiration smear. *Diagn Cytopathol* 2:126–132, 1986.

13

Opportunistic Infections and Neoplasia in Acquired Immunodeficiency Syndrome (AIDS)

Although acquired immunodeficiency syndrome is partially discussed elsewhere in this monograph, a brief review of this disease and the role of cytology in its diagnosis and management is warranted since an increasing number of cytologic specimens are obtained from this patient population. Many of the organisms encountered in AIDS are either not culturable or are difficult to culture. A rapid morphologic diagnosis of the etiology of the infection is critical since results of cultures can take several days to weeks depending on the organism. FNA cytology is virtually the only way to make the cytologic diagnosis of the infection in some patients with AIDS.

The Centers for Disease Control (CDC) estimates that approximately one million persons in the United States are infected with human immunodeficiency virus (HIV) and that the number of cases of acquired immunodeficiency syndrome (AIDS) will continue to increase.[1,2,3] A projection that between 52,000 and 57,000 cases of AIDS will be diagnosed in 1990 is based on AIDS case surveillance data, HIV seroprevalence totals and information provided by epidemiologists, statisticians, and mathematical models. The current case definition of AIDS is presented in Table 13.1. The essential features of the definition are (1) a disease that is at least moderately indicative of underlying cellular immunodeficiency, (2) absence of adequate explanation for the immunodeficiency, other than infection by human immunodeficiency virus, and (3) positive test for antibody to HIV and/or a positive culture for HIV.[4]

TABLE 13.1. 1987 Revision of CDC Surveillance Case Definition of AIDS (Abridged)

Any patient with one or more of the following reliably diagnosed diseases in the absence of known cause of immunodeficiency; laboratory evidence regarding HIV infection either positive or not available:
→ Candidiasis of esophagus, trachea, bronchi, or lungs
→ Cryptococcosis, extrapulmonary
→ Cryptosporidiosis with diarrhea persisting >1 month
→ Cytomegalovirus disease, extranodal, in patient >1 month of age
→ Herpes simplex virus infection with ulceration persisting >1 month
→ Kaposi's sarcoma in patient <60 years of age
→ Lymphoma, brain (primary), in patient <60 years of age
→ Lymphoid interstitial pneumonia and/or pulmonary lymphoid hyperplasia in child <13 years of age
→ *Mycobacterium avium-intracellulare* or *M. Kansasii* disease, disseminated
→ Pneumocystosis
→ Progressive multifocal leukoencephalopathy
→ Toxoplasmosis, brain, in patient >1 month of age
Any patient with one or more of the following reliably diagnosed diseases plus laboratory evidence of HIV infection:
→ Bacterial infections, multiple or recurrent, in child <13 years of age
→ Coccidioidomycosis, disseminated
   HIV encephalopathy
→ Histoplasmosis, disseminated
   Isosporiasis with diarrhea persisting >1 month
→ Kaposi's sarcoma at any age
→ Lymphoma, brain (primary), at any age
→ Other non-Hodgkin's lymphoma of certain types
→ Mycobacteriosis caused by mycobacteria other than *M. tuberculosis,* disseminated
→ Tuberculosis, extrapulmonary
   Salmonella (nontyphoid) septicemia, recurrent
   HIV wasting syndrome

Modified from Ewing EP Jr. In: *Pathology of AIDS and Other Manifestations of HIV Infection,* ed. Vijay V. Joshi. Igaku-Shoin, New York.
→ Cytologic diagnosis possible.

PATHOGENESIS AND ASSOCIATED DISORDERS

The human immunodeficiency virus (HIV-1) is a retrovirus discovered by French and American investigators in 1983 and 1984, respectively. HIV has a major lipoprotein envelope (gp120) that has an epitope which recognizes and binds to CD4 receptor molecules normally found on the surface of helper T lymphocytes (CD4), follicular dendritic cells, Langerhans' cells, pulmonary macrophages, brain macrophages and neurons, and glial cells.[5,6] The virus-specific DNA copies can enter the host cell nucleus and become integrated into the host chromosomal DNA. The viral cytopathic effect of HIV includes multinucleation of the infected cell secondary to cell fusion and cell death.

HIV-1 shows a particular tropism for T4 (CD4) lymphocytes resulting in retroviral infection and destruction of helper T cells. Absolute lymphocyte counts are frequently below 1,000 cells per μl, with the T-4:T-8 ratio usually less than 1:1 (normal ratio is approximately 2:1. A number of sensitive and specific tests for the antibody to HIV-1 have been developed, including the enzyme-linked immunosorbant assay (ELISA), Western blot immunophoresis, radioimmunoprecipitation (RIP), and cytoplasmic membrane immunophoresence assay (IFA). Viral culture of peripheral blood and HIV antigen detection assays can also be used.

Persons at risk for HIV infection include homosexual and bisexual men (approximately 70% of estimated infected individuals in the United States in 1987), intravenous (IV) drug users, recipients of infected blood or blood products, female prostitutes, and heterosexual partners of infected individuals. Modes of transmission include sexual contact with an HIV-positive individual and nonsexual transmission, including transmission of HIV-infected blood or blood products through transfusion, IV drug use, or needle-stick accidents. Very rarely, HIV infection has been transmitted by blood or other body fluid contamination of health care workers via breaks in the skin or mucous membranes. In the pediatric AIDS patient, transplacental or perinatal transmission is the most common route of infection.

By definition, patients with AIDS have opportunistic infections and/or certain neoplastic disorders, and they develop additional complications throughout the clinical course of the disease. The diagnosis and clinical management of persons with AIDS requires a definitive means of rapid morphologic diagnosis of these lesions. A number of studies based on autopsy and surgical specimens have documented many of the complications and sequelae of this syndrome, but there have been few reviews of the role of cytology in the diagnosis and management of patients with AIDS.[7] This is ironic, since cytologic examination represents one of the most frequently used methods of making a rapid diagnosis of especially opportunistic infections in this patient population. Although exfoliative cytologic specimens are frequently used, occasionally FNA biopsy will be performed. The most common sites to undergo aspirations include lymph node, lung, soft tissue, and brain. Most often the presence of an opportunistic infection is documented in the aspirated material, although occasionally a neoplasm will be encountered.

The FNA biopsy has been used to diagnose a number of infectious and neoplastic conditions in AIDS patients. An increased incidence of neoplasia, particularly Kaposi's sarcoma and non-Hodgkin's lymphoma has been found in patients with AIDS.[8] Kaposi's sarcoma is the most common neoplasm in AIDS patients; seen in approximately 40 to 45% of homosexual males and 10% or fewer of IV drug users and hemophiliacs with AIDS[8] (Fig. 13.1). The incidence of Kaposi's sarcoma in AIDS patients has declined in the last few years, possibly owing to falling incidence of AIDS in homosexual men. Bottles and associates reported one of the largest series of FNA biopsy of AIDS patients, in which 125 FNA biopsies of lymph node were performed on 113 men who were observed in an outpatient clinic of San Francisco General Hospital.[9] Twelve patients (10%) demonstrated Kaposi's sarcoma of the lymph nodes with 60 (50%) aspirates showing lymphoid hyperplasia, 24 (20%) non-Hodgkin's lymphoma, 21 (17%) mycobacterial infection, and one each Hodgkin's disease, giant cell carcinoma, nasopharyngeal carcinoma, and squamous cell carcinoma. Other neoplasms that have been reported in AIDS, which may be encountered with FNA biopsy include plasmacytoma, head and neck squa-

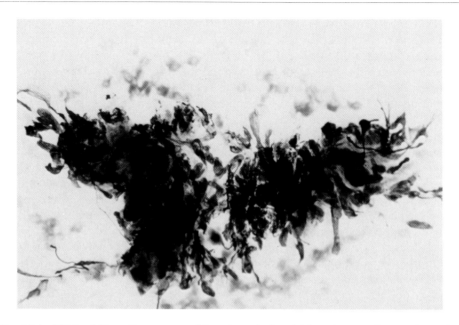

Fig. 13.1. FNA of Kaposi's sarcoma of lymph node in which a cluster of atypical spindle cells is present (May–Grunwald–Giemsa stain; ×200) (Courtesy of R. Michael Cohen, University of Iowa, Iowa City, IA).

mous cell carcinoma, anorectal carcinoma, germ cell tumors, adenocarcinoma of the pancreas and colon, malignant melanoma, basal cell carcinoma, thymoma, squamous cell carcinoma of the skin, liposarcoma, and angiolipomas.[10-20] Anorectal carcinoma and squamous cell carcinoma of the oral cavity are the most frequently reported malignancies with the exception of Kaposi's sarcoma and hematopoietic neoplasms. Kaposi's sarcoma of the lung, although suspected when increased numbers of hemosiderin-laden macrophages are found in the bronchoalveolar lavage specimen, can seldom be diagnosed definitely by FNA biopsy.[21] Open lung biopsy is the procedure of choice to diagnose pulmonary Kaposi's sarcoma.

A previously unusual parotid lesion, cystic benign lymphoepithelial lesion, has been recently described in patients with AIDS or HIV infection.[22] The FNA cytologic features include lymphoid cells and foamy macrophages along with superficial and/or anucleated squamous cells (Fig. 13.2), corresponding to the histologic finding of an intraparotid squamous-lined cyst surrounded by a reactive lymphoid population.[23,24] The differential diagnosis includes other cervical neck lesions that may contain benign squamous cells and lymphocytes, including Warthin's tumor and branchial cleft cyst.[24] The diagnosis of cystic benign lymphoepithelial lesion should be suspected when a cystic parotid lesion is aspirated in a patient at risk for or having AIDS.

Percutaneous FNA biopsy of the lung has been used to diagnose pneumonitis in patients with AIDS.[25-30] The procedure is most commonly employed to diagnose *Pneumocystis carinii,* but other organisms including bacteria, *Legionella,* viruses, my-

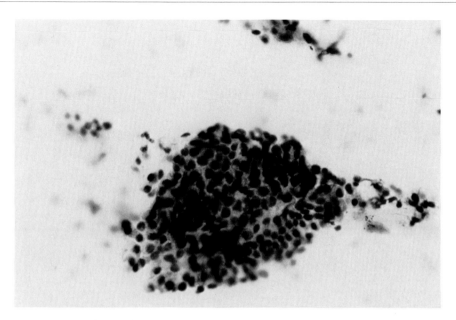

Fig. 13.2. FNA of cystic benign lymphoepithelial lesion in a patient with AIDS, consisting of a clump of benign squamous cells and scattered lymphocytes in the background (Papanicolaou stain; × 100) (Courtesy of R. Michael Cohen, University of Iowa, Iowa City, IA).

cobacteria and fungi have been identified by cytomorphologic or culture examination. Although bronchoalveolar lavage is the cytologic procedure of choice for the diagnosis of *Pneumocystis* pneumonia, FNA biopsy may be performed occasionally, particularly in patients with atypical radiologic presentations, including cavitary or nodular lesions.[31]

A number of infectious and neoplastic processes can involve the gastrointestinal tract of HIV-infected persons. Strigle and associates reported cytopathologic findings based on their personal experience at a large county hospital.[32] Their report included FNA biopsy findings of abdominal masses not accessible to endoscopic sampling and thereby to exfoliative cytology. FNA biopsy of the liver, pancreas, and abdomen accounted for over 6% of all HIV-related aspirations at their institution. The main pathologic processes encountered were B-cell lymphoma and mycobacterial infection.

Mycobacterium avium-intracellulare can be readily visualized in the Diff-Quik stained smears of FNA biopsies of suspected lesions.[25,33] The organisms appear as "negative images" characterized by unstained, rod-shaped structures against a deep blue background of the stain (Fig. 13.3). Whenever negative images are appreciated in cytologic smears, additional material should be submitted for mycobacterial culture. A number of the infectious complications seen in AIDS are discussed throughout this monograph in the specific organ-related chapters. FNA of CNS lesions in AIDS is discussed in detail in Chapter 12 and pulmonary lesions in Chapter 9. The organisms that can involve the lung and gastrointestinal tract are listed in Tables 13.2 and 13.3.

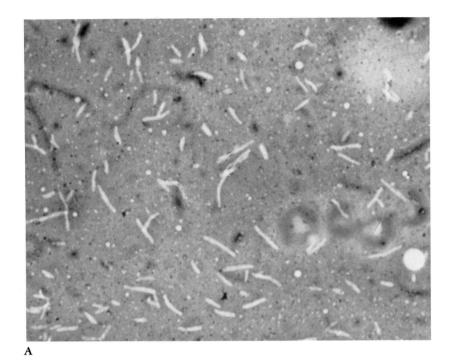

A

B

Fig. 13.3. **A.** FNA of retroperitoneal lymph node demonstrating numerous individual rod-shaped negative images (Diff-Quik stain; × 1000) (Courtesy of Dr. Susan Maygarden, Medical College of Virginia, Richmond, VA). (From Maygarden SJ, Flanders EL: Mycobacteria can be seen as "negative images" in cytology smears from patients with acquired immunodeficiency syndrome. *Mod Pathol* 2:239–243, 1989.) **B.** Ziehl–Neelsen stain reveals scattered beaded acid-fast bacilli (× 1000). Courtesy of Dr. Maygarden. (From Maygarden SJ, Flanders EL: Mycobacteria can be seen as "negative images" in cytology smears from patients with acquired immunodeficiency syndrome. *Mod Pathol* 2:239–243, 1989.)

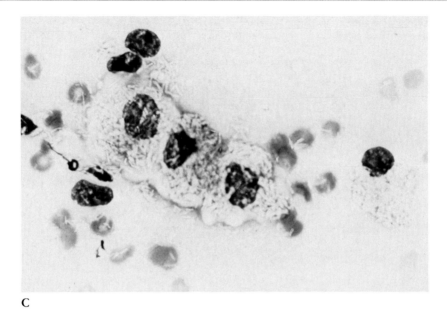

C

Fig. 13.3. C. Touch imprint of lymph node demonstrating histiocytes containing numerous linear striations in the cytoplasm corresponding to the presence of bacilli of *Mycobacterium avium-intracellulare* (Diff-Quik stain; ×1000). Courtesy of Dr. Mary K. Sidawy, George Washington University Medical Center, Washington, DC. (From Jannotta FS, Sidawy MK: The recognition of mycobacterial infections by intraoperative cytology in patients with acquired immunodeficiency syndrome. *Arch Pathol Lab Med* 113:1120–1123, 1989.)

TABLE 13.2. Pulmonary Infections in AIDS

→ *Pneumocystis carinii* pneumonia
Bacterial pneumonia
Streptococcus pneumoniae
Haemophilus influenzae
Staphylococcus aureus
→ Cryptococcosis
→ Disseminated *Mycobacterium avium* complex or *Mycobacterium kansasii*
→ Tuberculosis
→ Cytomegalovirus pneumonia
Toxoplasmosis
→ Strongyloidiasis
→ Bronchopulmonary candidiasis
→ Disseminated histoplasmosis
→ Disseminated coccidioidomycosis
→ Herpes simplex pneumonia
Cryptosporidiosis

→Cytologic diagnosis possible.

TABLE 13.3. Agents Causing Diarrhea in AIDS

> BACTERIA
>   *Salmonella* species
>   *Shigella* species
> → *Campylobacter (Helicobacter)* species
>   *Neisseria gonorrhoeae*
> → *Mycobacterium avium-intracellulare*
>   *Chlamydia trachomatis*
>   *Treponema pallidum*
> PROTOZOA
> → *Entamoeba histolytica*
> → *Giardia lamblia*
> → *Cryptosporidium*
> → *Isopora belli*
>   Microsporidium (diagnosis by
>   electron microscopy)
> VIRUSES
> → Cytomegalovirus
> → Herpes simplex
>   AIDS-associated enteropathy
> FUNGI
> → *Candida albicans*

→Cytologic diagnosis possible.

PRECAUTIONS IN FNA BIOPSY

When performing an FNA biopsy or handling the smears, clinicians should regard all patients as potentially infectious with the HIV-1 virus. Therefore, universal precautions should apply to both the handling of FNA specimens and performance of the procedure, since unfixed tissue and/or blood products are involved.[34-37] It has been estimated that the risk of HIV transmission from a single percutaneous exposure to HIV-infected blood is 0.4%,[38,39] while the risk following a parenteral exposure to blood from a patient who is antigen positive for hepatitis B virus ranges from 23% to 43% per exposure.[40,41,42] General precautions include double gloving when performing the FNA biopsy. Usually there is no need to wear gowns, masks, or protective eyewear. Most needle sticks occur when drawing blood and especially when one is recapping the needle. There are devices available that allow positioning the needle and attached syringe into rigid holders or containers that provide a mechanism to minimize exposure of the hand to the needle when recapping (Fig. 13.4). Following the aspiration, the needle must be handled with extreme care and promptly placed in a rigid puncture-proof container that should contain a disinfectant solution. HIV can survive storage in various liquid media, dry state, and freezing. However, the usual pathology fixatives inactivate HIV.[34] It has been reported that ethanol used as a fixative for cytologic preparation inactivates HIV at a concentration as low as 20%, and neutral buffered formalin inactivates HIV at a concentration as low as 1%. After the biopsy specimen has been processed, the working preparatory area needs to be decontaminated using commercial and simple chemical

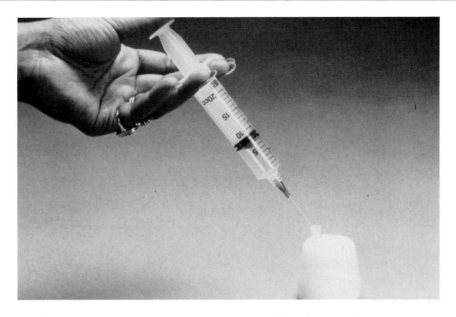

Fig. 13.4. Simple device that allows inserting the needle and attached syringe into the cap and thereby minimizing exposure of the hand to the needle when recapping.

disinfectants, such as 0.5% sodium hypochloride (1:10 dilution of household bleach).

REFERENCES

1. Morgan M, Curran JW, Berkelman RL: The future course of AIDS in the United States. Editorial comment. *JAMA* 263:1539–1540, 1990.

2. Gail MH: Projecting the incidence of AIDS. Editorial comment. *JAMA* 263:1538–1539, 1990.

3. Lemp GF, Payne SF, Rutherford GW, et al: Projections of AIDS morbidity and mortality in San Francisco. *JAMA* 263:1497–1501, 1990.

4. Brynes RK, Ewing EP Jr, Joshi VV: Pathology of the acquired immune deficiency syndrome (AIDS). American Society of Clinical Pathologists National Meeting, 1987.

5. McDougal JS, Kennedy MS, Sligh JM, et al: Binding of HTLV-III/LAV to T4 + T cells by a complex of the 110K viral protein and the T4 molecule. *Science* 231:382–385, 1986.

6. Funke I, Hahn A, Rieber EP, et al: The cellular receptor (CD4) of the human immunodeficiency virus is expressed on neurons and glial cells in human brain. *J Exp Med* 165:1230–1235, 1987.

7. Silverman JF: Cytologic diagnosis in acquired immunodeficiency syndrome. In: *Pathology of AIDS and Other Manifestations of HIV Infection,* ed Joshi VV. New York, Igaku-Shoin, 1990, pp 347–365.

8. Knowles DM, Chadburn A: The neoplasms associated with AIDS. In: *Pathology of AIDS and Other Manifestations of HIV Infection,* ed Joshi VV. New York, Igaku-Shoin, 1990, pp 83–120.

9. Bottles K, McPhaul L, Volberding P: Fine-needle aspiration biopsy of patients with the acquired immunodeficiency syndrome (AIDS): experience in an outpatient clinic. *Ann Intern Med* 108:42–45, 1988.

10. Kaplan MH, Susin M, Pahwa SG, et al: Neoplastic complications of HTLV-III infection: lymphomas and solid tumors. *Am J Med* 82:389–396, 1987.

11. Longo DL, Steis RG, Lane HC, et al: Malignancies in the AIDS patient: natural history, treatment strategies and preliminary results. In: Acquired immune deficiency syndrome, eds Selikoff IJ, Teirstein AS, Hirschman SZ. *Ann NY Acad Sci* 437:421–429, 1984.

12. Steis RG, Longo DL: Clinical, biologic, and therapeutic aspects of malignancies associated with the acquired immunodeficiency syndrome. Part I. *Ann Allergy* 60:310–314, 1988.

13. Cappell MS, Yao F, Cho KC: Colonic adenocarcinoma associated with the acquired immunodeficiency syndrome. *Cancer* 62:616–619, 1988.

14. Tessler AN, Catanese A: AIDS and germ cell tumors of testis. *Urology* 30:203–204, 1987.

15. Grieger TA, Carl M, Liebert HP, et al: Mediastinal liposarcoma in a patient infected with the human immunodeficiency virus. *Am J Med* 84:366, 1988.

16. Bluff DD, Greenberg SD, Leong P, et al: Thymoma, *Pneumocystis carinii* pneumonia, and AIDS. *NY State J Med* 88:276–277, 1988.

17. Overly WL, Jakubek DJ: Multiple squamous cell carcinomas and human immunodeficiency virus infection. *Ann Intern Med* 106:334, 1987.

18. Sitz KV, Keppen M, Johnson DF: Metastatic basal cell carcinoma in acquired immunodeficiency syndrome–related complex. *JAMA* 257:340–343, 1987.

19. Gupta S, Imam A: Malignant melanoma in a homosexual man with HTLV-III/LAV exposure. *Am J Med* 82:1027–1030, 1987.

20. Alhashimi MM, Krasnow SH, Johnston-Early A, et al: Squamous cell carcinoma of the epiglottis in a homosexual man at risk for AIDS. *JAMA* 253:2366, 1985.

21. Strigle SM, Gal AA: A review of pulmonary cytopathology in the acquired immunodeficiency syndrome. *Diagn Cytopathol* 5:44–54, 1989.

22. Finfer MD, Schinella RA, Rothstein SG, et al: Cystic parotid lesions in patients at risk for acquired immune deficiency syndrome. *Arch Otolaryngol Head Neck Surg* 114:1290–1294, 1988.

23. Weidner N, Geisinger KR, Sterling RT, et al: Benign lymphoepithelial cysts of the parotid gland: a histologic, cytologic, and ultrastructural study. *Am J Clin Pathol* 85:395–401, 1986.

24. Finfer MD, Gallo L, Perchick A, et al: Fine needle aspiration biopsy of cystic benign lymphoepithelial lesion of the parotid gland in patients at risk for the acquired immune deficiency syndrome. *Acta Cytol* 34:821–826, 1990.

25. Jannotta FS, Sidawy MK: The recognition of mycobacterial infections by intraoperative cytology in patients with acquired immunodeficiency syndrome. *Arch Pathol Lab Med* 113:1120–1123, 1989.

26. Wallace JM, Batra P, Gong Jr H, et al: Percutaneous needle lung aspiration for diagnosing pneumonitis in the patient with acquired immunodeficiency syndrome (AIDS). *Am Rev Respir Dis* 131:389–391, 1985.

27. Batra P, Wallace JM, Ovenfors C-O: Efficacy and complications of transthoracic needle biopsy of lung in patients with *Pneumocystis carinii* pneumonia and AIDS. *J Thorac Imag* 2:79–80, 1987.

28. Bandt PD, Blank N, Castellino RA: Needle diagnosis of pneumonitis. *JAMA* 110:1578–1580, 1972.

29. Jacobs JB, Vogel C, Powell RD, et al: Needle biopsy in *Pseudocystis carinii* pneumonia. *Radiology* 93:525–530, 1969.

30. Castellino RA: Percutaneous pulmonary needle diagnosis of *Pneumocystis carinii* pneumonitis. *Natl Cancer Inst Monogr* 43:137–140, 1976.

31. Saldana MJ, Mones JM: Cavitation and other atypical manifestations of *Pneumocystis carinii* pneumonia. *Semin Diagn Pathol* 6:273–286, 1989.

32. Strigle SM, Gal AA, Martin SE: Alimentary tract cytopathology in human immunodeficiency virus infection: a review of experience in Los Angeles. *Diagn Cytopathol* 6:409–420, 1990.

33. Maygarden SJ, Flanders EL: Mycobacteria can be seen as "negative images" in cytology smears from patients with acquired immunodeficiency syndrome. *Mod Pathol* 2:239–243, 1989.

34. Brynes RK, Joshi VV: Precautions for safe handling of biopsy and autopsy specimens. In: *Pathology of AIDS and Other Manifestations of HIV Infection,* ed VV Joshi. New York, Igaku-Shoin, 1990, pp 367–369.

35. Wenk RE, Dutta D, Mellema S, et al: Needle accidents and disease transmission. ASCP Check Sample 26:1988.

36. Thurn J, Willenbring K, Crossley K: Needlestick injuries and needle disposal in Minnesota physicians' offices. *Am J Med* 86:575–579, 1989.

37. Bonnett KA: How to prevent needle sticks. *J Pract Nurs* 38:32–35, 1988.

38. Ciesielski CA, Bell DM, Chamberland ME, et al: Correspondence. *N Engl J Med* 322:1156, 1990.

39. Henderson DK: HIV-1 in the health care setting. In: *Principles and Practice of Infectious Diseases,* 3rd ed, eds., Mandell GL, Douglas RG, Bennett JE. New York, Churchill Livingstone, 1990:2221–2236.

40. Grady GF, Lee VA, Prince AM, et al: Hepatitis B immune globulin for accidental exposures among medical personnel: final report of a multicenter controlled trial. *J Infect Dis* 138:625–638, 1978.

41. Werner BJ, Grady GF: Accidental hepatitis-B-surface-antigen-positive inoculations: use of e-antigen to estimate infectivity. *Ann Intern Med* 97:367–369, 1982.

42. Seefe LB, Wright EC, Zimmerman HJ, et al: Type B hepatitis after needle stick exposure: prevention with hepatitis B immune globulin: final report of the Veterans' Administration Cooperative Study. *Ann Intern Med* 88:285–293, 1978.

Index

Page numbers in italics refer to illustrations

DATE DUE

DEMCO 38-296